STRATEGIES IN DENTAL DIAGNOSIS AND TREATMENT PLANNING

To my patients: some were friends first, many have become friends since. I have been privileged to serve them, and I am grateful for the confidence they have placed in me.

STRATEGIES IN DENTAL DIAGNOSIS AND TREATMENT PLANNING

Robert B Morris DDS FICD FACD
Adjunct Professor (Clinical)
Marquette University School of Dentistry
Milwaukee, Wisconsin, USA

MARTIN DUNITZ

© **Martin Dunitz Ltd 1999**

First published in the United Kingdom in 1999
by Martin Dunitz Ltd, The Livery House,
7–9 Pratt Street, London NW1 0AE

Telephone (44) (171) 482 2202
Facsimile   (44) (171) 267 0159
Website   http://www.dunitz.co.uk

A CIP catalogue record for this book is available from the British Library.

ISBN 1–85317–568–4

Distributed in the United States and Canada by:
Thieme New York
333 Seventh Avenue
New York, NY 10001
USA
Tel. 212 760 0888

Composition by Scribe Design, Gillingham, Kent
Printed and bound in Singapore

CONTENTS

PREFACE

I'll keep this short. This book is not intended as an exhaustive treatise covering diagnosis and treatment planning in and of every conceivable dental discipline (look at the many excellent references cited for that). What I have tried to do is provide the dental student or general practitioner dentist with a framework for effective and rational diagnosis and treatment planning. I have offered a number of strategies to approach problems, both simple and complex, that the dentist is likely to face from time to time.

The process is illustrated with case examples, and they are just that – examples. I have not tried to cover every possible condition or situation. The text approximates the chronological sequence of the examination, diagnosis, and treatment planning process, and the chapters titles are self-explanatory.

This book is intended to be practical, realistic, and clinically oriented. It takes a common sense approach to general dentistry and to the art and science of diagnosis and treatment planning. I hope you find it useful.

ACKNOWLEDGEMENTS

For giving me life, and a solid framework in which to live it, I thank my beloved parents, Bernard and Maysel. For making my life complete, I thank my dear wife, Dianne; for making it interesting, my daughters, Allison and Amie, of whom I could not be more proud.

I have had so many fine teachers that singling out any is tremendously difficult. Nevertheless, I must mention Drs Ben Karr and Bill Nequette, my mentors, friends, and role models, who shared with me so generously their time and experience. So much of what I think of as 'my' knowledge came from others. To all my teachers, undergraduate and CE, who were patient and kind and willing to stay behind to answer my questions, this book is but another payment on the debt I owe.

My daughter Allison was my dispassionate and effective editor. My associates and office staff were all understanding and supportive. My patients have provided me with both material for the text and my primary livelihood. I thank them all.

Jim Brozek made digital the hundreds of color images in this book. Supplementing those images were Drs Drew Dentino, Sara Jean Donegan, Donald Ferguson, and Cesar Gonzalez. All the clinical cases illustrated are my own, with the following exceptions: Dr Bill Nequette permitted me to show some of his masterful reconstructions of lost vertical dimension; and Dr Ken Waliszewski allowed me to document his heroic effort involving implants to regain form and function in a patient following a hemimandibulectomy. My thanks also go to the fine surgeons involved in that case, Dr Phil Hawkins (oral surgeon) and Drs Ben VanRaalte and David Larson (plastic surgeons). Drs John Cheek (orthodontist), Donald Pricco (oral surgeon), Brian Blocher (oral surgeon), and John Newman (endodontist) provided excellent specialty treatment and documentation in three other cases shown in this text.

Drs Jim Hove and Robin Ferguson acted as doctor and patient for the comprehensive examination series.

Finally, my thanks are due to Dr Vincent Williams for his kind thoughts regarding my previous text, *Principles of dental treatment planning*, and to Robert Peden, commissioning editor at Martin Dunitz, for his help and patience. I think that's everybody.

INTRODUCTION

WHERE I'M COMING FROM . . .

My dear reader, in this age of instant world-wide electronic communication, the fact that you are actually holding a book in your hand suggests that you are more literate than most, and that you appreciate some of the qualities that are unique to words and images on a printed page, bound together with a hard cover, no less.

As you have shown such discrimination in your search for knowledge I must promise you a reward. I will not waste your time or your energy. I will be succinct, always; brief, when possible. I will also attempt to avoid the stiff, ponderous, formal style which is the curse of so many textbooks.

I am just a dentist. I can offer you the benefit of over a quarter of a century of clinical experience, during which a great many trusting people have allowed me to do rather unpleasant things to them, for which they actually paid me money, in the firm belief that they would be healthier, happier, better-looking, or achieve whatever goal motivated them to submit to my ministrations. To those patients I owe a great debt. They have allowed me to live well, to educate my children, to call myself 'doctor.' They have taught me much of what I know about diagnosis and planning, occasionally by proving me wrong. They have been variously appreciative and loyal, critical and difficult, a pleasure to serve and a penance to endure. It has been my pleasure to see and care for the children, and now the grandchildren, of patients who knew me when I had hair, and it has been my painful privilege to offer condolences to families of patients whose dental work did indeed last them a 'lifetime,' and who went to their graves with my dentistry in their mouths.

I have also been a continuing education 'junkie,' seeking knowledge across a wide range of topic areas, some only distantly related to dentistry. I have also used my friends and colleagues in dentistry to enhance my own knowledge and experience, and have shamelessly stolen every good idea I could find to benefit my patients. I always try to give credit, and will in this text, if I can but remember the source.

I have had the good fortune to be called 'teacher' for the past 25 years, and to be challenged by some students who obviously knew as much or more than I, and by other students who seemed to know less after my lectures than before. On the whole, however, teaching undergraduate dental students and graduate dentists who are seeking continuing education is an excellent reality check for a clinician. You find out what you really know, and what you really don't know, and I have tried very hard to include mostly the former in this book.

If you are uncomfortable with this approach, this informal and slightly irreverent style, this intensely personal voice, then I can recommend several large, exhaustively researched, and heavily footnoted texts which have accompanied me to bed (and too often to sleep) over the years. Otherwise I invite you to read further, or just look at the pictures and read the text where it looks interesting. If I can offer you just a few good 'nuggets,' an insight or two, a strategy you haven't thought of, I'll be content. Perhaps I can cause you to rethink your approach to some clinical situations, or I may simply reinforce your existing biases. In any event I thank you for the effort in reading this book, and I wish you all the best in caring for your patients.

WHERE WE'RE GOING . . .

We probably ought to get straight on to what this book is about. Diagnosis and treatment planning books are notoriously bad about finding a focus and staying with it. The subject matter is simply too broad; it encompasses potentially the entire field of dentistry and some of medicine as well. The whole subject of dentistry, both normal and pathologic, is impossible to capture. The results have always been a compromise. Too much emphasis on this, too little on that, too detailed, too cursory.

This is my second attempt to offer a treatise on treatment planning. The first, now out of print, had a small but enthusiastic following, which provided the impetus for this new effort. Changes in both the market and printing technology have made it possible to focus on what really interests me about diagnosis and treatment planning, without having to do lip service to the entire field of diagnosis, oral pathology, and all the disciplines of dentistry along the way.

I will concentrate, then, on the rudiments of diagnosis and treatment planning – the basic tools – without going into great detail on the pathology and pathogenesis of oral diseases. The first part of the book offers an outline of the process of examination and diagnosis for the typical adult patient, with a few modifications suggested for pediatric and geriatric* patients. In doing so, I hope to establish a minimum baseline for data gathering which is necessary to derive an effective diagnosis and treatment plan.

Given these basics, I will proceed to discuss and illustrate the process of treatment planning, offering a number of strategies aimed at getting it 'right,' that is, to select for any given patient that plan of dental treatment that is most appropriate and effective for him or her at this time.

As we learn best with our minds turned 'on,' many of the topics in this book will be introduced and developed as clinical case histories, which I hope will both interest and challenge you. Please analyze them as if they were yours and, if you see issues in some of the cases that are not addressed in the text, good for you. If you see more or better treatment options than I may have suggested, even better.

The goal is not to demonstrate the 'best' treatment plan, but to offer some creative ways of thinking about dental planning and some strategies to employ in that process, which you may choose to add to your own repertoire. In the process, I hope to share some of the enjoyment of doing comprehensive dentistry in a general practice, and the

Gather data	History: Personal, dental, medical Radiographic examination Clinical examination Other diagnostic aids	General appraisal Soft tissue examination Periodontal examination Oral hygiene status Dental examination Functional examination Other considerations

Arrive at diagnosis
      Differential and/or problem list

Develop treatment plan
      which is in a rational **sequence** based on **urgency** first,
                      then on   **efficiency**

     and which Addresses all known problems
                  Deals with etiologic factors (preventive)
                  Relates effectively to the patient

* Defined as someone much older than me.

deep satisfaction which can come from being a help to someone in one small but important aspect of their lives.

To complete this introduction, let's look at the process schematically, and establish some common terminology which will be used through the text.

DIAGNOSIS AND TREATMENT PLANNING IN A NUTSHELL

The simple schematic outline summarizes the process. The succeeding chapters will address the individual steps in order, and explore strategies for treatment planning.

DEFINITION OF KEY TERMS

This definition of key terms will be useful in following the text.

ROUTINE SYSTEMATIC APPROACH

Doing examination and diagnosis the same way every time (routine) and in a logical order (systematic) saves a great deal of time while avoiding serious omissions and mistakes in the process.

DATA GATHERING

Refers to the comprehensive collection of bits of information about the patient through interview, history, examination, and other aids.

PATIENT HISTORY

Usually the first means of data gathering, the history consists of all information given to us by the patient. It includes basic demographic information, chief complaint (and history of same), medical history, and dental history. Although written forms are often used to obtain the history, these must always be supplemented with the interview, through which the dentist can communicate directly with the patient, reviewing any written information, and eliciting additional information specific to that patient.

EXAMINATION

The examination includes all additional methods used by the dentist beyond the interview and history, such as radiographs, clinical examination, and other diagnostic aids and modalities.

TYPES OF EXAMINATION

Every patient visit does not demand the totality of the diagnostic process. This would be too exhaustive and time-consuming. There are several types of examinations which may be performed for various purposes.

Emergency examination

When an emergency arises it is often necessary to proceed quickly, and this examination should include basic patient information, a good health history, and only the dental history necessary to assess the chief complaint being addressed as an emergency. Radiographs, clinical examination, and other tests are limited to the specific problem at hand. Patients should be reminded that this is not a complete examination.

Screening examination

When large numbers of people are to be treated in, for example, an institutional setting, screening examinations are often employed as a means of **triage** to allocate time and resources most efficiently. Screening examinations may be employed also in research, to gather specific bits of information about a population. Once again, the limitations of this procedure should be discussed with the patient.

Triage

This is a concept developed by the military for dealing with multiple casualties most effectively. Patients are quickly assessed and divided into three (hence the term 'triage') groups: those who can safely wait for treatment; those who need immediate treatment for survival but have a reasonable prognosis if treated; and those who are likely to expire despite treatment, or whose treatment would use so much of the available resources as to preclude treating those in the second group. Most dental screening examinations do not have implications quite this grave, but the term has come into more general use to include screenings intended to classify patient groups.

Comprehensive examination

Given the appropriate setting and adequate time, the comprehensive examination is employed in order to gather ALL the relevant data about a dental patient. It includes a number of critical items, which will be the focus of the next few chapters.

TECHNIQUES OF EXAMINATION

The dentist may use a number of techniques in the examination process.

Inspection

This is the gathering of visual evidence: observing the patient, reading radiographs, analyzing diagnostic casts, and so forth.

Palpation

This involves touching the patient, pressing and rolling the fingers over tissues to determine their texture, consistency, and degree of pain or tenderness experienced by the patient as a result. In dentistry, the use of an explorer to detect caries, cracked teeth, open margins, and subgingival calculus might also be included, because it is most certainly a tactile method.

Percussion

In medicine this refers to a tapping of various body cavities to elicit sounds and sensations of diagnostic value. In dentistry, it more commonly refers to tapping of teeth to elicit information from the patient about resulting sensitivity or pain.

Auscultation

Another technique is listening, with or without the aid of a stethoscope, to sounds of the temporomandibular joint, to speech defects or abnormalities, or to teeth as they meet in occlusion.

Olfaction

Often overlooked, the sense of smell can help to diagnose some obvious problems (Acute Necrotizing Ulcerative Gingivitis [ANUG] has a characteristic and unforgettable aroma), as well as less obvious problems (people with diabetes who are in ketoacidosis may have a slight fruity or acetone odor on their breath).

FINDINGS

All bits of information obtained in the history and examination process are called findings. Findings may be normal or abnormal, healthy or pathologic.

CHIEF COMPLAINT

This is the reason, usually a symptom or cluster of symptoms, why the patient seeks treatment. It can be urgent, such as acute pain or gross swelling, or minor, such as a small chip on a tooth, which has been present for some time. The chief complaint should *always* be noted and addressed, because it is generally why the patient sought care in the first place.

SYMPTOMS AND SIGNS

All findings can generally be grouped as either *symptoms* (subjective, elicited by history and interview, as described by the patient) or *signs* (objective, often measurable, discovered by examination). (See SOAP below.) Some examples of each are given in the box.

Symptoms:	pain, sensitivity to hot or cold, altered taste, inability to chew or to speak clearly, esthetic complaints
Signs:	redness, swelling, measurable fever, tenderness to palpation, crepitus, bad breath, molar crossbite

Obviously some overlap is possible. A patient may report feeling hot and feverish (symptom) and have a measurable fever of 101.5°F (sign). A patient may report that a central incisor is sensitive (symptom), and it is found to react to an electric pulp test at a very low range, for example, 10 on a scale of 80 (sign).

SOAP

This acronym, often seen in medical and dental progress notes, describes a routine approach to any given problem, and stands for:

Subjective (symptoms elicited from patient – see above)
Objective (signs discovered by examination)
Assessment (analysis of the information – the diagnosis)
Plan (what you intend to do about the problem).

NORMAL, OR RANGE OF NORMAL

Through much of this text I refer to the 'range of normal.' There are a great many findings which, although somewhat atypical or unusual, are still within the range of normal, and the dentist must be on guard to avoid treating what is not disease.

PAIN, THE CARDINAL SYMPTOM

Pain or discomfort is the most common chief complaint, and should always be given weight in the diagnosis. Questions about pain include its **location**, **duration**, **severity**, and **alteration** by temperature, posture, or function.

DIAGNOSIS

Diagnosis is an assessment of the findings which specifies what is happening to a patient and why. There are a number of related terms of interest.

'Snap' diagnosis

Made quickly on the spot, it can be a perfectly good diagnosis, for example, a patient returns 3 days after removal of a lower third molar complaining of pain and a bad taste, and exhibiting inflammation and odorous discharge at the extraction site. This patient *probably* has a 'dry socket' (localized alveolar osteitis), and exhaustive diagnostic tests are not appropriate unless routine treatment does not bring rapid response. A patient who presents with a palatal ulcer and complains that he or she burned the roof of the mouth with hot pizza can be safely diagnosed as having 'pizza burn' – biopsy is not indicated unless the lesion does not resolve within a normal time period.

Tentative or working diagnosis

A little more precise than the 'snap' diagnosis, this type of assessment assumes that the clinical picture 'fits' a given disease state, so that preliminary treatment may proceed, or other diagnostic tests may be selected. An ulceration under a partial denture flange of which the patient has been unaware *may* simply be an inflammatory response to irritation. With that as a tentative diagnosis, the appliance may be adjusted in that area, or the patient instructed to leave it out, and a reevaluation scheduled for a week later. If the ulcer is unresolved at that time, the tentative diagnosis is discarded, and further investigation started.

Differential diagnosis

This refers to the process which, given a set of findings (signs and symptoms), the clinician categorizes that information into data relevant to making a diagnosis, and develops a list of the most likely diseases or disorders consistent with the findings. Given the differential list, the clinician may pose pertinent questions which tend to confirm some possible diagnoses and rule out others. Further tests may then be selected to narrow the field, until a single diagnosis or cluster of diagnoses remains. At that point, additional tests to confirm the diagnosis or differentiate within the cluster are performed, leading to a final definitive diagnosis.

Definitive or final diagnosis

Using the differential process just described, the definitive or final diagnosis is derived, and appropriate treatment rendered. If the disease fails to respond, it may be necessary to backtrack on the differential diagnosis, and try again. In the case of soft tissue diseases, microscopic examination of tissue samples at the cellular level often determines the final diagnosis. Blood dyscrasias or diseases provoking an immune response may be proved serologically. Not all problems can be solved so neatly, however, because the range of abnormal is as wide as that of normal.

Multifactorial (problem list) diagnosis

Dentists often deal with basically healthy individuals, primarily seeking preventive and long-range health maintenance care, and presenting without a specific or urgent chief complaint. Such patients may have multiple dental and oral problems revealed in the course of a comprehensive examination and, although in no immediate danger, will benefit from a 'problem list' diagnosis. This is aimed at addressing the problems so as to provide maximum comfort, function, and esthetics, with the goal of long-term retention of the natural dentition.

TREATMENT PLAN

This is a written plan of treatment which addresses both disease and etiology; it is the end product of data gathering and diagnosis, and it may take one of two forms:

Emergency or immediate treatment plan

This addresses the definitive diagnosis directly, and must generally be instituted at once.

Comprehensive or long range treatment plan

This derives from a problem list diagnosis, and may be safely postponed if necessary, or carried out in stages over time.

PATIENT-ORIENTED DIAGNOSIS/TREATMENT

Also referred to as a humanistic or holistic approach, patient-oriented diagnosis and planning means working from our patients' frame of reference, and involving them in the entire process. Arriving at a rational solution *with* patients, rather than imposing our solution on them, will result in better compliance, rapport, and long-term success. This approach requires the dentist to communicate effectively with patients, to listen and understand their felt needs, and to respond to them. So-called optimal or ideal treatment is only optimal if it fits that patient. Even the best clinical examination, radiographs, and diagnostic casts cannot tell the whole story; we must get to know our patients before we can help choose the optimal treatment specifically for them.

PREVENTION-ORIENTED DIAGNOSIS/TREATMENT

If in our diagnosis we have successfully identified etiologic factors, then they can be addressed in the treatment plan. External causes may be responsible for many systemic diseases (for example, malaria transmitted by mosquito vector). Most dental diseases are, however, behaviorally induced or aggravated; for example, it makes little sense to remove and restore carious lesions without addressing the patient's oral hygiene and diet.

1 BASIC PREMISES

ART AND SCIENCE

We call it the art and science of dentistry. For generations, dentists have struggled with the dichotomy of being artists and craftsmen, and yet scientists as well. In recent times leaders in the profession have struggled to put us on a more scientific plane, urging us to be 'physicians of the oral cavity.' Proposals to merge the dental and medical professions have been seriously considered. Foremost in such proposals is the desire to put dentistry on a more scientific and less empirical basis: to base diagnoses and treatment choices more on science, less on art.

Proponents of this shift have occasionally cast a jaundiced eye over time-tested therapies for their lack of scientific validation. As an example, zinc oxide and eugenol have together been a staple dental material and medicament for as long as anyone can remember. Millions of symptomatic teeth have been relieved, sedative bases and fillings have been placed, and castings have been cemented using this material, all with good long-term clinical results. Now some recent research suggests that a chronic inflammatory response may be induced by zinc oxide and eugenol, and suddenly there is a move to abandon the material, in favor of new materials that may have good scientific rationale, but lack the decades, indeed the generations, of good clinical experience.

In situations in which the essential oil component (eugenol) may interfere with newer cements and bonding agents, this may make sense. On the other hand, materials and techniques that have stood the test of time should not be so quickly exchanged for substitutes, which look good on paper or in short-term clinical use, but lack the degree of clinical experience that many dental products and techniques enjoy.

Silver amalgam is another good example. Under long and intense scrutiny as a result of its mercury component, no material has been studied as closely for potential systemic side effects. Given the consistent clean bill of health that it has received, and its proven clinical advantages including ease of placement, good marginal seal, and durability, it is troubling that so many dentists are moving away from silver amalgam. In its stead, they are employing other materials which are clearly less forgiving, less durable, and whose potential systemic side effects are yet to be determined and may indeed prove more troublesome in the long run than anything ascribed to silver amalgam.

Another example is the widespread use of neutral (CR) splints, orthotics fabricated for the relief (and, in some cases, the diagnosis) of temporomandibular pain disorders (TMD). We don't know why such splints provide such consistent and widespread relief to symptomatic patients, but they do and so consistently that prudent clinicians use them routinely, despite the lack of scientific explanation for their efficacy.

Dentists serve patients well using materials and techniques that have proven themselves with long-term clinical results, even though they lack scientific validation. It's that 'art and science' problem again. If we waited for scientific validation – for a proven explanation of why the devices work – we might never be able to justify the use of many effective clinical tools. Decades of 'unscientific' experience, and the substantial body of reported clinical experience (albeit anecdotal), give us confidence that we have safe and effective therapeutic devices in our hands, and we use them with confidence to help our patients.

On the other hand, newer diagnostics and therapies that lack scientific validity raise serious questions, especially when issues of cost, invasiveness, and irreversibility come into play. How much of our treatment may be 'art', and how much 'science'?

As we prepare to be dentists in the twenty-first century, we struggle to find the right balance in our journey toward excellence. How do we serve our patients best? How do we, at the least, 'do no harm'? How do we practice more scientifically, without losing the artistry and technical excellence that has gained us such respect from the public at large?

This book is written by and for general practitioners in dentistry, who are not afraid to be artists as well as scientists, for whom being labelled a 'fine technician' is a compliment, not an insult, and who put their patients' best interests above all else. It is based on the reality that clinicians must draw on shared experience and intuition as well as data, because the data alone may not always lead to the best treatment choice for a given patient. To understand this, one must accept, or at least understand, some basic premises about the nature of dentistry, and some critical differences between medicine and dentistry.

DENTISTRY AND MEDICINE ARE DIFFERENT

The two disciplines obviously share a common knowledge base, and the oral cavity and related structures can never be treated in isolation from the total person. However, there are some critical differences which must shape and inform our approach to the practice of dentistry, and we need to consider these differences when choosing a model for our patient care.

MOST DENTAL DISEASES ARE SUBSTANTIALLY PREVENTABLE

Both caries and periodontal disease are, on a rudimentary level, the result of bacterial plaque acting upon a susceptible organ, be it tooth or tissue. Bacterial plaques can be effectively controlled with basic home care, that is, toothbrush and dental floss; they can be further suppressed with therapeutic agents such as the various forms of fluoride and chlorhexidine. Host resistance can be altered with fluorides, the application of bonded sealants, and the removal of harmful and contributory factors such as tobacco and frequent dietary sugars, and other fermentable carbohydrates.

Every dentist should know these things, practice them daily, and encourage family and loved ones to do the same. Patients deserve no less, and those patients who are willing to practice preventive dental care with reasonable diligence will have little or no dental disease in need of treatment. Dentists can, have, and continue to 'work themselves out of a job,' through the enthusiastic and consistent practice of preventive dentistry.

MOST DENTAL DISEASES ARE NON-FATAL

Untreated, pulpal and periodontal infections can lead to some painful episodes if acute abscesses arise, and could eventually result in the loss of some or all teeth. This condition is so widespread on a global basis that it often passes for a normal consequence of aging, that is, you get older, you lose your teeth. In developed countries the dental profession has, over the past generation, changed that picture dramatically through the application of fluorides and other preventive methods. This is a source of great pride to us all, but the fact remains that many people all over the world still have uncontrolled dental diseases, and lose many or all their teeth, yet live long and productive lives in spite of this. This should remind us that we in dentistry are not, for the most part, dealing in life and death situations.

If one were to establish a hierarchy of medical and dental procedures, based on which have the greatest potential impact on people's lives and health, the vast majority of procedures carried out day to day in dentistry would be far down the list. This should not discourage or demean us, but it should help us to realize that we are different from the medical profession. Dental care and treatment, other than relief of severe pain and control of acute infection, are essentially elective.

MOST DENTAL TREATMENT IS ELECTIVE

Other than the very rare life-threatening oral disease or lesion, we deal primarily with patients seeking a higher level of quality in their lives, who desire in their oral and dental condition a certain level of comfort, function, and esthetics (often not in that order). They do not see dentistry as a life and death issue, but they value it nevertheless. Our role as practitioners, then, is to help these patients to make informed choices, and to carry out the desired treatment to the best of our ability, whether it involves the ultimate in dental arts and technology to achieve the utmost in comfort, function, and esthetics, or simply making a good temporary 'patch,' to hold things together until the patient is able (or desires) to go further.

DENTAL DIAGNOSIS IS DIFFERENT

Dental diagnosis is generally broader and more multidisciplinary in nature, whereas the medical model generally strives to narrow diagnosis down to a specific disease or syndrome. In the classic medical differential diagnosis model, findings are assessed and, based on knowledge and experience, a list is developed of potential diseases that could account for the findings. Appropriate tests are then performed to rule out some possibles, or confirm others, until the 'definitive' diagnosis is established. This definitive diagnosis is often based on histological or biochemical tests which are specific for the most probable diagnosed condition.

Dentists also employ the differential diagnostic model when assessing, for example, oral lesions or symptomatic teeth. More commonly, however, dentists see patients with a number of problems which may or may not have been symptomatic, and which are often related to caries or periodontal disease – the most common 'diagnoses' that we encounter. Developing a problem list, and then crafting a plan to address the problems in a logical and effective sequence, is clearly a different game from the medical differential diagnosis model.

DENTAL TREATMENT PLANNING IS AN ART

The net effect of all this is seen when choosing a treatment plan for a patient. In the medical model, choices are often informed by data. A patient with constricted coronary arteries can be treated by surgical bypass procedures, by balloon angioplasty, or by drugs and diet. Each of those choices is likely to be accompanied by some reasonably reliable statistical data about long-term survival rates and the morbidity of the procedure; in other words, the risk/benefit equation is calculable, and can be brought to bear in the decision-making process.

As a comparison, a dental patient who has lost posterior support and occlusion may be treated with a removable partial denture, fixed cantilevered bridgework, or implant-supported prostheses. None of these choices has hard data available about the expectation of longevity, or the level of comfort, function, and esthetics expected from one versus another. Our predictions are based on our own experience and various opinions that have been gathered together, not on hard epidemiological data. Even if such data were available (and credible), they are not of much use.

We know that, for any given patient, any of the choices may be highly satisfactory, and any of the choices may be a dismal failure. The success of any option is highly dependent on the technical excellence of the dentist and supporting staff, especially the laboratory technician, and on the ability and willingness of the patient to maintain the healthy oral environment so critical to the viability of any treatment option.

Treatment choices will be strongly influenced by available resources, such as the time and money needed to carry out various options, which are very much the purview of the patient.

TECHNIQUE IS CRITICAL

The physician orders a blood test, a diagnostic procedure, a radiograph. Such data are assessed and analyzed, and a diagnosis is made. Treatment often consists of prescription medications, the success of which is measured by follow-up blood tests, diagnostic procedures, radiographs. Hands-on treatment is most often delegated: a Hickman catheter inserted by the resident, physical therapy carried out by the physiotherapist, and so forth.

The dentist, on the other hand, selects the diagnostics, and then often carries out the tests personally. Treatment is generally not prescribed in the form of pills, or left to ancillary personnel (nurses, therapists, etc), but in most cases it is delivered personally, directly, from the painless local anesthetic injection to the surgical or restorative procedure, to the postoperative or maintenance examination. The most carefully crafted plan is ineffective if the procedures selected in that plan are carried out carelessly, incompetently, or sloppily. The need for 'good hands' in dentistry hasn't changed, and those who would put the dentist 'above the treatment,' delegating treatment to auxiliaries, are missing an important point. In dentistry, *how* you do it is clearly just as critical as *what* you do.

CARE, SKILL, AND JUDGMENT

We are expected to meet a standard of care, skill, and judgment in our treatment of patients, and we, much more so than the physician, are most often directly and solely involved 'hands-on' in delivering that care and treatment, and in meeting that standard.

Care implies giving our patients the respect that they deserve as our fellow human beings, to minimize discomfort, allay fears, empathize, monitor, manage, and in general treat them as you or I would want to be treated. It

further implies attention to detail and concentration to avoid mistakes.

Skill is a variable, and not all practitioners are as gifted as others. We are all obligated to develop and maintain a minimum acceptable level of skills, and even the best dental treatment plan may be compromised by lack of skills on the part of the dentist. Referral to specialists or other dentists can ameliorate this situation, but all dentists must continue to hone old skills and develop new ones as the 'state of the art' advances.

Judgment is the most difficult standard to define, but is often the critical link in successful treatment. How do we determine which patient is and which is not a good candidate for a given treatment? Which medically compromised patient can and which cannot tolerate lengthy appointments and extensive dental treatment? In which patient will a long span bridge succeed mechanically and in which will it fail?

Traditionally, we have depended heavily on experience to help us make such judgments, learning from our mistakes if necessary, or from shared experience (others' mistakes) if possible. One of the purposes of this book is to combine the given wisdom of my teachers and colleagues, add my own experiences, and identify some general principles and common strategies to apply in dental treatment planning. In this way art and science may be joined, bringing aspects of each to bear on dental diagnosis and treatment planning.

THE TREATMENT PLANNING PROCESS

Given these basic premises, let's look at the process that we call dental treatment planning. When a skilled and experienced clinical dentist studies radiographs, diagnostic models, history, and clinical findings to arrive at a diagnosis and create a plan of treatment, it may seem magical. The apparent effortlessness, speed, and insight with which the skilled dentist identifies and deals with issues that others might not even consider has impressed and intimidated many a young dentist.

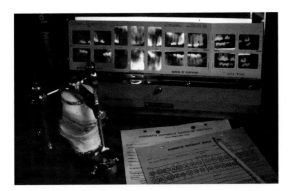

Fig. 1.1

'Tools of the trade' ready for treatment planning to start.

How does one begin to develop such skill, finesse, and wisdom? Age and experience are useful, but effective treatment planning must not wait for old age. Nor is time alone a guarantee; many dentists, rather than accumulating experience over the years, seem to repeat their early mistakes again and again.

The answer lies in the knowledge that treatment planning is not a random, intuitive process practised by the 'gurus' of our profession, but an orderly systematic process which can be broken down into its component parts and studied. Time and experience accelerate the process so that it appears to be a matter of deep insight, but in fact a process is occurring, a routine system that can be analyzed.

This text will identify components of the treatment planning process and develop a number of concepts upon which this process is based. It will identify a number of general principles in the hope of providing any dentist, young or old, with strategies for successful treatment planning (Fig 1.1).

THE ROLE OF THE GENERAL PRACTITIONER

The role of the general practitioner in treatment planning is key. As our knowledge of every aspect of dentistry expands, we are forced to assimilate ever more specialized information. Indeed, the specialist is aptly defined as someone who 'knows more and more about less and less'. As treatment becomes more specialized and compartmentalized, it falls to the general practitioner to 'direct' the play, to assemble the actors, to coordinate and script their roles, and to ensure that each specialized step in treatment is performed in a logical sequence, leading to the overall desired goals. Each specialty area tends to develop its own treatment plan, but the failure to integrate all phases of dental treatment can be disastrous. The general practitioner acts as the director of care and treatment, coordinating the various disciplines (most often delivering a good deal of the care personally). This ensures the proper sequencing, integration, and continuity of care and treatment. An effective dental treatment plan, then, is a general and comprehensive plan, involving the patient first and foremost, directed toward goals established with and for that individual patient by the general practitioner.

THE ROLE OF THE PATIENT

It is absolutely critical to involve the patient in treatment planning, and the earlier this involvement begins the better. The nature of most dental disease, as previously discussed, makes most dental care and treatment elective, and success or failure of dental treatment is primarily in the hands of the patient. The patient is involved in dental treatment planning in a stepwise process:

1. The dentist gathers information about the patient, including not only the clinical dental and oral findings, but also the human factors, which will influence the patient's dental health and the course and outcome of treatment. As the dentist is discovering the patient, the patient is discovering the dentist, establishing (or failing to establish) the confidence and trust necessary to allow treatment to begin. The information gathering process will be explored more fully in Chapters 2–5.
2. The dentist must present the findings to the patient, in terms that the patient can

comprehend. The patient must also be made aware of the etiologic and contributing factors that contributed to the problems, and the need for behavioral changes to prevent further disease. This requires good basic communication and patient involvement throughout the entire process.

3. Together, the dentist and patient establish goals for treatment. Such goals might involve optimal oral health, function, and esthetics to be achieved by stringent home care on the part of the patient, and optimal comprehensive dental treatment provided by the dentist. On the other hand, goals might also be limited to the immediate relief of pain and minimal 'holding' treatment to allow the patient to deal with more pressing life issues than teeth.

There are a number of key issues to address in such a patient-oriented diagnosis and planning model, and I will touch on some of them briefly.

Basic communication

The process by which ideas are put into words (spoken or written), transmitted, received, and finally understood is complex. Without going into the theories involved, let's consider the basics of the communication process as they apply to the dentist–patient situation.

Message

The message must be clear in the mind of the sender. Before presenting a diagnosis or proposed plan, the dentist should have a clear picture in mind, a written outline at hand, and a general idea of how to present the information to this particular patient. If the dentist is unclear on what is to be communicated, there is no hope that the patient will understand.

Common language

The message, whether spoken or written, must be in a common language. Dentists, like most professionals, are steeped in their own jargon , and all too often use terms that the

patient does not understand. Words must be chosen that are clear, correct, and understandable (or defined as you go along). Words should not frighten, inflame, or repulse. Communication aids, such as posters, pamphlets, videos, and the like, need to be simple, clear, and non-technical.

Feedback

Feedback is critical. The only sure way to determine whether the patient has heard you, and comprehends what you have said, is for him or her to repeat it back, in his or her own words. The best way to illustrate is with the following hypothetical conversations between dentist and patient.

Dentist.   Mrs Smith, I'd like to take a minute to explain why your gums are bleeding, and what we feel should be done about it at this time.

Patient.   All right.

Dentist.   Well, it's like this, Mrs Smith: there are certain bacteria in the mouth – germs, you might say – that can act on the foods we eat and form colonies on the teeth and gums. We call these colonies 'plaque', and if they are allowed to remain on the teeth for some time, and are not removed with a toothbrush and dental floss at least once a day, the gum tissues can become infected, swollen, and may bleed easily. This is the first sign of gum disease, which can be very serious. Do you understand?

Patient.   I think so.

Now nothing is inherently wrong with the message this doctor is sending; it is accurate, clear, concise, and the language is fairly simple. What is lacking is feedback. Now consider this conversation:

Dentist.   Now then, Mrs Smith, from what you've seen, heard, and read so far, and from what we have shown you in your own mouth, can you tell me what you think is causing your gums to bleed?'

Patient. Well, I see now that I haven't been flossing regularly, and your hygienist showed me areas where I wasn't getting to the plaque very well with my brush, and those are the places where I'd noticed most of the bleeding.

Dentist. And what do you think all that means?

Patient. I watched the video, and looked at this brochure the hygienist gave me, and I'm afraid I may have this gum disease. Does this mean I'm going to lose my teeth?

Note that both conversations arrive at about the same place, and either may prove to have been an effective communication. Only the second conversation verifies receipt of the message, however, and demonstrates through *feedback* that the message has been received and understood.

Listening

Listening is required. We cannot expect patient feedback if we don't shut up and listen. Patients give us messages on two levels: the literal message and the underlying, unspoken message. We must try to hear and attend to both. An example of an underlying message is seen in this exchange:

Dentist. I see it has been 5 years since your last dental visit. How did it get to be so long?

Patient. I don't like dentists.

Taken literally, this statement doesn't make sense, and it can be rather off-putting to the dentist. What the patient may really be saying is 'I have had bad experiences with dentists in the past,' or 'I am afraid that the dentist may do something painful and/or unpleasant.' If we take that statement literally, we may get sidetracked into a fruitless discussion. We must listen to statements such as 'I don't like dentists,' or 'I can't afford to spend any money on my teeth,' and attempt to find the hidden message.

Patients may bring their anxieties about dental treatment into the communication, expressing them openly ('I am really afraid of the needle') or more often masking them with hostility, or even a manic joviality. Effective listening allows and encourages the patient to communicate, and gives us the opportunity to consider both the literal message and the emotional components of our patient's response.

Setting

The setting is important. Patients may react to the operatory and its association with dental procedures, and do better in an office or consultation area. On the other hand, modern dental operatories can be designed and decorated to reduce visual threats, and every effort should be made to conceal instruments and delivery systems when talking before treatment.

Communication aids

Patients may benefit from carefully selected pamphlets, posters, albums, or video presentations. Simplicity is the key here, because many aids on the market offer too much information, that is, the illustrations have so much detail that the patient is overwhelmed. As appealing as full color, anatomically correct depictions may be to the dentist's trained eye, simple line drawings or schematics may be more effective for most patients.

Patient involvement in the examination

This is one of the most effective ways to communicate and lay the groundwork for later discussion of diagnosis and presentation of treatment plans. Chapter 2 deals with the initial patient interview, and establishing the dentist–patient relationship. The following strategies are effective in getting the patient involved from the outset.

Verbalize the findings

As the examination proceeds the dentist should say out loud what is being examined, and what is being found. An assistant records the findings, and may 'cue' the examiner to the next step in the examination. Most important, the findings should be in lay terms. We say 'cavity' not 'caries', 'bruise' not 'hematoma', 'gumline' not 'marginal gingivae.' When there is no simple lay term for a finding, then the examiner must stop and briefly explain the term that is used. The purpose of verbalizing is to help the patient understand the clinical findings better, not to impress or confuse.

When a finding is noted that is unusual, significant, or pathologic, the patient should hear this, and be shown what the examiner is describing (see below).

Verbalizing the findings gives patients an appreciation of what the examination is covering, and gets them involved in the diagnosis at the very outset.

Show the findings

Show patients what you see in their mouths: a good mirror works fairly well; a magnifying mirror with a light source is better. An intraoral video camera can be a very effective tool to demonstrate intraoral findings. Color printouts of captured video images can go home with them.

Once diagnostic casts have been obtained they can be used to show patients the problems and conditions that are in need of attention. It is sometimes useful to allow patients to take their models home with them after you have discussed the findings that they present. The more opportunities given to patients to self-discover problems in their own mouths, their own dentition, the easier is the dentist's job in presenting diagnosis and treatment proposals.

SETTING GOALS

We can draw all kinds of roadmaps for dental care and treatment, but we need to know where the patient wants to go, and for that we need to establish goals that have been agreed upon. Formal training in dental school may produce dentists who see the goal of 28 teeth in good occlusion and alignment as the holy grail. Esthetics, the appearance of the mouth, is often considered as an accessory to that goal. Patients, on the other hand, lacking the benefit of years of dental education, may not know (or much care) how many teeth they have, as long as they are getting along 'OK.'

Without an appreciation of the curves of occlusion, canine protection, bone levels, or incipient caries, they may simply seek a comfortable mouth and attractive smile. Four very simple questions might be posed, and goals established on the basis of the patient's answers. These are in the order of most patients' priorities.

How will they look?

Is the patient satisfied with the appearance of the teeth: the alignment, the shape and the color? Beauty is in the eye of the beholder, and many patients seek the 'whitest teeth money can buy' to the chagrin of the dentist striving for a beautiful but 'natural' that is, 'real,' appearance. On the other hand, many patients are quite content with teeth that the dentist perceives as disfigured, and in need of 'improvement' through bleaching, bonding, veneers, etc. A large diastema may be a source of embarrassment to one patient, a point of pride in a family trait to another. Goals for esthetics can vary greatly, then, from the desire for perfectly straight and pearly white, to just 'covering up the black spots.'

How will they work?

Can the patient speak, chew, and swallow comfortably, without undue difficulty? Can the patient confidently take on tough foods without fear of teeth cracking, or dental work coming loose? Functional goals once again are individual. Some partially edentulous patients are perfectly content to go through life without most of their posterior teeth, whereas other patients are greatly perturbed by the loss of just one posterior tooth, and demand prosthetic replacement at the earliest opportunity!

Will they be healthy?

This question concerns patients' ability and willingness to care for their teeth, but it also addresses the ease with which this may be done. Severely crowded teeth, open contact areas allowing food impaction, or rough poorly contoured contacts that prevent floss from passing through easily will inevitably lead to future dental disease. Missing and tipped teeth, deep bites, hypertrophic tissues, and complex dental restorations that are inaccessible to reasonable hygiene are all examples of health issues that the dentist and patient need to consider when setting treatment goals. Any existing conditions that now compromise health, or are likely to compromise health in the future, need to be addressed.

How long will they last?

Dental care and treatment is, or can be, long term. How long is obviously related to the type of treatment selected, what materials are used, and, most importantly how well the patient maintains the work. We have all seen treatment fail in the presence of uncontrolled disease or excessive functional forces. We have also seen what can happen when optimum dental treatment meets rigorous daily home care and regular professional maintenance. Esthetics, function, and health can be maintained for decades. One of the satisfactions of a career in dentistry is to see healthy patients, whose dental care and restorations have provided them 10, 20, 30 years of esthetic, functional, and healthy service and are still going strong.

These four simple questions can form the basis for mutual goals between dentist and patient. Some patients will come to us seeking the utmost in esthetics, function, and health, with time and money being no object. Most patients in the real world, however, seek one or more of these goals, but within a 'budget.' They put dental care in a hierarchy with all their other needs and wants, and we need to reach a compromise that will allow us to treat them safely, with positive benefits, at a level that they can accept. Some patients are more concerned with esthetics, less with function or health. Our responsibility is to show patients how those issues are interrelated, and offer approaches and alternatives that address them all. This is where strategic dental treatment planning starts.

THE PATIENT INTERVIEW

The patient interview is usually the first and often the most important step in effective diagnosis and treatment planning. It is clear that the impressions formed by the patient early in the initial interview can have a huge impact on the patient's acceptance of the dentist, and the dentist's credibility with the patient. Lose the patient now, and all the technology, all the expertise, all the excellence in the world will not salvage the relationship.

There are excellent texts and reference works on patient interviewing, communication, and behavior, some of which are cited at the end of this chapter.[1,2] Certain key issues are so critical to the process, however, that they must be briefly addressed here.

THE DOCTOR–PATIENT RELATIONSHIP

To the extent that they are of legal age and mentally competent, patients should be treated as our partners in dental care and treatment. Given the degree to which dental disease is related to behavior, any other model is irrational. If we accept that effective dental care involves the control of dental and oral diseases, as well as the long-term daily maintenance of the oral cavity, including our restorations and prostheses, then success of such care is primarily in our patients' hands. Furthermore, in a traditional fee-for-service arrangement, patients are not only in control of the outcome, they are also ultimately responsible for paying for it.

Given that, we must from the very outset treat our patients as partners, communicating with them on their level, rather than from above. This does not mean that we relinquish our position as trained and licensed professionals, but it does demand that we treat patients as we would wish to be treated, as fellow human beings, deserving of all the respect and dignity that we would wish for ourselves in the same position. Here are some key issues to consider in establishing that relationship.

- Meet and greet the patient at eye level, either both standing or both seated in a comfortable, non-threatening setting. Modern dental operatories can (and should) conceal dental handpieces and other instruments that may be disturbing or distracting to the new patient (Fig 2.1).

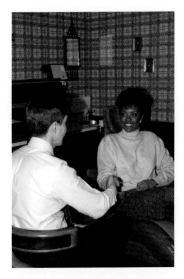

Fig 2.1

Meeting the patient on an even playing field, at eye level, in comfortable surroundings.

- Introduce yourself (or be introduced) and, although you may be comfortable offering your first name to the patient, you should not, in most cases, address the patient by their first name until invited, or until the relationship has had time to develop. This is especially true when addressing older patients for the first time.
- Early in the initial interview, often at its outset, you should pose an open-ended question to the patient that frames the relationship that you hope to establish. The question goes something like this: 'Mrs Brown, how may I help you?' or 'Mr Green, what can I do for you?' or 'Ms White, what brings you to see me today?'
- Listen to your patients, really listen. Whatever motivated them to seek care, or specifically to select you as a dentist must be understood and respected. They may be dentally well informed and articulate, as was one young man whose chief complaint was a 'chipped buccal cusp on number three.' Or they may have little or no understanding of their various problems or what might be done about them, in which case education may have to precede and accompany therapy. In either case, allowing and encouraging our patients to tell us why they came is a good way to find out where they are at the outset of the doctor–patient relationship. We must go to them, appreciate our patient's point of view, and start the relationship there.
- Understand the level of trust that our patients need to have in us. For most people, the dental environment is at best somewhat uncomfortable and, at worst, terrifying. We used to think that that would change, with fluoride and preventive dentistry reducing or eliminating entirely the need for many dental procedures in childhood, and with the actual realization of 'painless' dentistry. We supposed that most patients, particularly young adults, would have less anxiety, never having experienced painful or frightening dental treatment in the past.

For some, this is indeed the case. But current research is suggesting, much to our chagrin, that there remains a broad, culturally based level of dental fear and anxiety even among people who have had no unpleasant dental experiences; this has to be dealt with one patient at a time.

Perhaps other concerns about cost, appearance, and so forth are also involved here. More likely, the fact that dentists invade patients' personal space, working right in the head, so close to where we 'live,' is what makes apprehension unavoidable. Given that, we have to appreciate the tremendous trust that our patients place in us, to use needles, drills, and all types of sharp and blunt instruments in their tender and vulnerable oral cavities.

- Allow the patient to feel 'in control.' To accept the invasion of personal space, our patients must feel in control at all times, so that if they feel pain or need to close or clear their mouth, they know that you will stop. Look them in the eye and tell them so. 'If this is uncomfortable, or you need me to stop, just raise your hand.' 'Please tell me if this bothers you and I will stop.' 'Let me know if you feel any of this and we'll stop and give you more anesthetic.'

A gentle touch on the forearm or a pat on the shoulder, accompanying these reassurances, helps to secure 'permission' from the patient to proceed. The dentist must then be trustworthy, and allow the patient to call 'time out.' In some situations, this will undoubtedly make for prolonged treatment time. It also cements the doctor–patient relationship with a strong bond of trust, and can pay great dividends in the long run. As trust builds, the need for 'time outs' often decreases. For some patients, however, checking out their 'parachute' is a ritual at every appointment and we need to permit and even encourage patients to test their control of the situation.

When patients praise their dentists, it's seldom related to the integrity of their margins, although over time patients do come to value long-lasting and trouble-free dental work. More often, however, the statement that 'my dentist doesn't hurt me,' relating to a painless anesthetic technique, good anxiety and pain management, and continual monitoring of patient comfort, for example 'How are we doing Ms White?', attests to a bond of trust which comes from putting the patient in control.

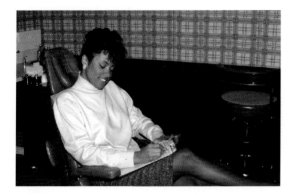

Fig 2.2

Most patients understand the need to complete 'paper-work'. A courteous request, with an explanation of why the information is needed, makes the task less onerous.

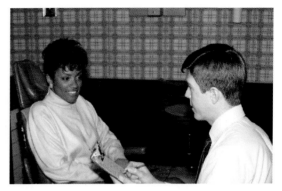

Fig 2.3

Reviewing the written history with the patient is critical.

THE INTERVIEW PROCESS – TOOLS OF THE TRADE

Most dentists employ some kind of pre-printed form or questionnaire to assist in information gathering. These forms can be useful tools, and save time by allowing patients to complete them before the appointment or before the interview (Fig 2.2).

Avoid questionnaires that are unnecessarily intrusive or lengthy, or you may alienate or antagonize patients before you ever meet them. Labelling the form 'CONFIDENTIAL' and including some explanation of why the information is being requested may help, along with a courteous and apologetic presentation when the form is given to the patient such as 'we know it's a bother to fill out forms, but we want to be sure we get your information right, and treat you safely.'

Just as important as careful selection and presentation of questionnaires is their sensitive use to frame the interview. If the doctor appears to ignore the information that the patient has just spent time and effort writing down, it can compromise the interview.

Thank patients for completing any forms and questionnaires, and take time to peruse them. Refer to them again in the interview process, to probe, to clarify, and to document additional information.

Finally, be aware that the information provided by patients on questionnaires is not always accurate, or complete. Nothing takes the place of a careful one-on-one interview to elicit critical information from patients, especially when it is sensitive or potentially embarrassing in nature (Fig 2.3).

Given these premises, let's consider the baseline data necessary to diagnose and plan quality comprehensive dental treatment.

BASIC DEMOGRAPHIC INFORMATION

The dentist needs to know the patient, for both business and legal reasons. In addition to name, address, and telephone number, etc, a personal profile of the new patient is useful to find the common ground necessary to establish communication and to initiate the relationship. At the least, the following demographic information should be obtained and recorded:

- Patient's full name, and how he or she prefers to be addressed, for example, Mrs, Ms, first name, etc. If the name is unusual, a phonetic spelling to assist in correct pronunciation at the initial interview can be very helpful.

- Address and telephone number(s).
- Age, sex, and race. Although this information is routinely included in patient questionnaires, it may be more prudent to house it in the medical history instead of the demographic form, emphasizing its need for legitimate patient care purposes.
- Occupation.
- Marital status.
- Party to contact in case of emergency.
- Third party involvement, if any, such as private insurance, Government benefit programs, and the like.
- Responsible party: when dealing with a minor child, or legally disabled adult, it is critical to ascertain who can give consent for treatment, and who will be responsible for payment of fees. Divorce, remarriage, and all the complications of modern family life can make this question at once both difficult and absolutely essential to answer before proceeding very far.

In addition, a personal profile is useful, and can help structure the new patient interview. Areas to be explored may include the following:

- Referral source: how did the patient happen to choose you or your practice for dental care? Referrals from close friends or relatives obviously imply a higher level of trust than, say, simply finding your name in the telephone book.
- Attitude: how does the patient react to you and the dental setting? Is the patient apprehensive, hostile, and noncommunicative, or relaxed, friendly, and outgoing?
- Desires for treatment: what is the patient interested in doing or having done about his or her mouth and teeth? Has the patient considered comprehensive dental treatment that might prevent so-called 'emergency' situations?
- Family history: do the patient's parents have their own teeth? What dental problems seem to be common among the patient's family members?
- Oral habits: does the patient smoke? What other potentially harmful oral habits does the patient admit?
- Socioeconomic status: what is the patient's present lifestyle and how will it influence

dental treatment planning? Do not prejudge any patient's willingness and/or ability to afford good dental care. Socioeconomic status and lifestyle may affect the dental 'IQ' of the patient, however, and consequently the level of communication at which we must start the interview.

DENTAL HISTORY, INCLUDING CHIEF COMPLAINT

Our patients' past experiences with dental problems and dental treatment will have a strong influence on the developing doctor–patient relationship. At the least, the following information should be obtained and recorded:

- Chief dental complaint: what prompted the patient to seek care at this time? This may be as general as 'I think I'm due for a check-up' or as specific as 'I lost a filling on my upper front tooth.' Whatever it is, the chief complaint needs to be addressed, even if it is a minor issue in the overall course of events.
- Present dental illness, that is, history of the chief complaint: when did it first arise and how has it progressed up to the present?
- Past dental problems: what dental conditions, diseases, pain, or dysfunction has the patient experienced in the past?
- Past dental treatment: what types of treatment has the patient received in the past? How does the patient feel (subjectively) about the dental care and treatment encountered up to now?

Exploring the issue of past dental treatment may trigger lengthy recitations of unhappy experiences, dissatisfaction with previous dentists, and past dental care. There is no point in arguing with what may sound like unfair criticisms, nor is there a need to agree with even the most plausible complaints when we are not privy to all sides of the story.

Simply acknowledging the patient's feelings and empathizing (without necessarily agreeing) are sufficient. 'I can understand how you feel' is preferable to 'you must have had a terrible dentist!' for obvious reasons.

Implicit in this history is the need to assess the patient's level of dental anxiety or fear, so those issues can be effectively confronted and dealt with by the dentist and the dental team. A standardized instrument, such as the Corah Dental Anxiety Scale[3,4] may be employed, or the dentist may explore these issues during the course of the initial interview (Fig 2.4).

Score ....   Name ....   Date ....

A. If you had to go to the dentist tomorrow, how would you feel about it?
☐ 1. I would look forward to it as a reasonably enjoyable experience.
☐ 2. I wouldn't care one way or the other.
☐ 3. I would be a little uneasy about it.
☐ 4. I would be afraid that it would be unpleasant and painful.
☐ 5. I would be very frightened of what the dentist might do.

B. When you are waiting in the dentist's office for your turn in the chair, how do you feel?
☐ 1. Relaxed.
☐ 2. A little uneasy.
☐ 3. Tense.
☐ 4. Anxious.
☐ 5. So anxious that I sometimes break out in a sweat or almost feel physically sick.

C. When you are in the dentist's chair waiting while he gets his drill ready to begin working on your teeth, how do you feel?
☐ 1. Relaxed.
☐ 2. A little uneasy.
☐ 3. Tense.
☐ 4. Anxious.
☐ 5. So anxious that I sometimes break out in a sweat or almost feel physically sick.

D. You are in the dentist's chair to have your teeth cleaned. While you are waiting and the dentist is getting out the instrument which he will use to scrape your teeth around the gums, how do you feel?
☐ 1. Relaxed.
☐ 2. A little uneasy.
☐ 3. Tense.
☐ 4. Anxious.
☐ 5. So anxious that I sometimes break out in a sweat or almost feel physically sick.

Fig 2.4

The Corah Anxiety Scale is one tool to measure and confront patient's fears. Using the scale: the questionnaire, or its updated version[4] (which removes gender references and modifies item 'D' to include dental hygienists) is scored by adding the total score for the four items, responses 'a' to 'e' valued 1 to 5 respectively. A score of 20 indicates very high anxiety, whereas a score of 4 would indicate no anxiety. If the patient scores 12 or less and doesn't mark 'e' on any item, no follow-up is recommended; however, any 'e' response even if the total is 12 or less should be noted and followed up verbally, to identify and deal with that concern. If the patient scores 13 or 14, suggesting an anxious patient, they should be asked about their dental experiences with an emphasis on what you can do to make them most comfortable. Again, any 'e' response should be noted and followed up verbally, to identify and deal with that concern. A score of 15 or higher suggests a highly anxious patient. A digression from the interview is indicated to explore the source of the anxiety, encouraging the patient to recount and confront old experiences, to admit fears, and to suggest ways to relieve anxiety about future care.

Dental History

What is your main problem/reason for coming? ....

Who referred you to us? .... Any concerns about dental treatment   *Yes / No*

How do you feel about the condition of your teeth? ....

How do feel about your past dental experiences? ....

....

Do you now, or have ever had, (check if yes)

☐ Clicking or popping in jaw   ☐ Any missing teeth   ☐ Root canal treatment
   joint   ☐ Bleeding Gums   ☐ Bridgework or partial
☐ Clenching or Grinding, day   ☐ Toothaches   dentures
   or night   ☐ Bad Breath   ☐ Gum Surgery, or non-
☐ Pains in or near the ear   ☐ Pain in Chewing   surgical treatment—root
☐ "TMJ" splint, or other types   ☐ Canker Sores   planing
   of treatment   ☐ Orthodontic treatment
☐ Other sore or painful areas   (braces)
   in mouth   ☐ Regular dental check-ups

When was your last dental visit? ....   Did you have x-rays at that time?   *Yes   No*

Have you been instructed on how to brush and floss?   *Yes   No*

How often do you brush? ....   Times per day/week

If so, When and By Whom? ....   When, usually? .... Type of brush: hard / soft

What kind of toothpaste? ....   Do you use dental floss?   *Yes / No / Occasionally*

Dietary History

Do you eat or drink between meals during the day?   *Yes   No*   In the evening?   *Yes   No*

Does your diet include:

☐ Chewing gum   ☐ Sugar in coffee/tea   ☐ Soft drinks, soda, fruit juice
☐ Coookies/pastry   ☐ Hard candy   ☐ Breath mints or cough
☐ Candy bars   ☐ Lifesavers   drops?

Thanks again for taking time   .... / .... / ....
to complete this form!   today's date   signature

Fig 2.5

The dental and dietary histories: note that the patient's chief complaint (reason for coming) is addressed first, and an opportunity given for the patient to express subjective concerns about dental condition and past experiences. The check boxes are clusters, with the left column serving as a 'TMJ' screening, the center column looking for current complaints and symptoms, and the right column addressing past dental treatment, leading into questions about the last dental visit. The patient's home care is assessed, and the dietary history serves as a quick screen for sugars in the diet.

- A checklist of past and/or present dental problems is useful both to ascertain the patient's previous dental history, and as a screen for current problems which may have yet to be diagnosed. The example shown in Fig 2.5 has a number of 'screening' items for temporomandibular disorders, as well as dental and periodontal problems.
- Dietary profile: excessive amounts or high frequency of intake of fermentable carbohydrates in the diet are clearly major factors in dental caries. At the systemic level, good general health demands a healthy and balanced diet.
- Oral hygiene habits: what is the patient's daily oral hygiene regimen? How often does the patient brush, and what type of toothbrush is used? Does the patient use dental floss and, if so, how often? What other oral hygiene devices does the patient use?

MEDICAL HISTORY

The importance of an adequate medical history before dental treatment cannot be exaggerated. For the patient's health and well-being, and for the dentist's protection, a thorough medical history must be obtained and regularly updated. Contemporary concerns with widespread communicable and infectious diseases, and with an aging population, many of whom are taking multiple medications for a variety of ailments, make this aspect of data gathering even more critical.

There is no single answer to the question of 'how much is enough?' when taking a medical history. It is necessary to balance the interests of time and energy with our need to gather critical information. Histories that are overly intrusive or cumbersome in their length and detail may frustrate or annoy the patient, even to the point of their withholding critical information. Histories that fail to identify illnesses or conditions that clearly impact on dental treatment can put both patient and dentist at risk. In any event, when a written history form or questionnaire is used, it is absolutely essential to review it verbally with the patient, restating critical questions and clarifying positive responses or non-responses.

There are clearly a number of medical issues that must be addressed in the dental environment; these include, but are not necessarily limited to, the following:

PATIENT'S GENERAL HEALTH

When was the last physical examination or doctor visit, and what were the findings? Is the patient currently under treatment for any medical condition? Has the patient been hospitalized recently (in the past 2–5 years), and for what reason? Who is the patient's physician (or physicians)? This is often a good point at which to obtain vital signs, generally including pulse, temperature, respiration, and blood pressure (Fig 2.6).

What drugs or medications (prescription or nonprescription) is the patient currently taking? Answers to these questions, if adequately explored with the patient, can give a fairly clear picture of the patient's general health status.

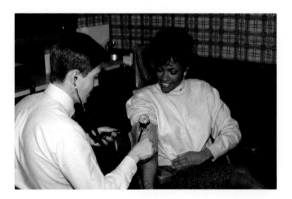

Fig 2.6

Vital signs, including blood pressure, are obtained and recorded.

The issue of medications is particularly critical, because an ever-growing percentage of the population is taking one or more (and often many more) drugs on a daily basis. Some of these may be prescribed therapeutics for acute and chronic illnesses, such as oral agents for the control of non-insulin-dependent diabetes, or nonsteroidal antiinflammatory drugs for chronic inflammatory diseases; some are preventive in nature such as prescription cholesterol-lowering agents, or non-prescription low-dose daily aspirin; some are health- promoting agents obtained over the counter such as vitamins, herbal preparations, or nutritional supplements.

The potential for drug interactions among the many agents being ingested is always present, and when we add potentially stressful dental procedures, and additional prescription or nonprescription medications given in the course of dental treatment to the mix, the pharmacologic situation becomes even more complex. Finally, the patient may not always tell us about all of the drugs being taken, in some cases because they are illegal or involve issues of abuse. Likewise, compliance with prescribed drug regimens is not generally good, and so some of what the patient tells us about their medication regimen may be truer in theory than in practice.

ALLERGIES AND SENSITIVITIES

Has the patient had a reaction to a drug, medication, or anything else (foods, pollens, insect bites, etc)? If so, what type of reaction was it? It is important to differentiate a severe anaphylactic allergy to penicillin, for example, from 'heartburn and gas' caused by an erythromycin compound. Latex allergies are a significant and growing problem, given the widespread use of latex gloves and dams in dental treatment.

SYSTEMIC DISEASES

A number of systemic conditions have dental implications. Damaged heart valves may create a risk of endocarditis if seeded by oral microorganisms. Diabetes may compromise a patient's ability to fight dental infection, or to heal properly after dental surgery. Active tuberculosis presents a risk to the dentist and auxiliary personnel, and cocaine use may precipitate severe reactions to local anesthetics with vasoconstrictors. (Please refer to the sources cited for far more comprehensive discussion of this general topic.) For purposes of this discussion, the systemic diseases and conditions in the box, grouped by system, are appropriate to the dentist's medical history.

Endocrine:	arthritis, diabetes, thyroid problems
Respiratory:	asthma, tuberculosis, shortness of breath
Cardiac:	heart disease, rheumatic fever, heart murmur, heart valve problems, pacemaker, high blood pressure, chest pains, swollen ankles
Blood:	abnormal bleeding, anemia, transfusions, fatiguability
Gastrointestinal/genitourinary:	jaundice, hepatitis, liver disease, contact with HIV or AIDS virus, sexually transmitted disease, kidney disease
Central nervous system:	epilepsy, fainting spells, nervous disorder/psychiatric care

Get Acquainted Questionnaire: Confidential

So that we may treat you safely and effectively, please answer all questions fully. Thank you.

Name .... Age ....

Date of Birth .... / .... / ....

UPDATES: W/INITIALS
.... / .... / ....
.... / .... / ....
.... / .... / ....
.... / .... / ....
.... / .... / ....

(office use only)

Medical History

When was your last physical exam? .... Reason for exam? ....

Are you seeing a physician at this time? *Yes / No* If so, for what? ....

Physicians's name .... Party to notify in case of emergency ....

Please list any medications (prescription or non-prescription) you are taking, and what they are for:

....

....

....

....

Are you allergic, or do you react to anything (drugs, food, etc.) *Yes/No* If so, what? ....

....

....

Do you now, or have you ever had: (check if yes)

☐ Arthritis
☐ Diabetes
☐ Thyroid Problem
☐ Asthma
☐ Tuberculosis
☐ Heart Problems/ murmur
☐ Rheumatic Fever
☐ Heart Valve Problems

☐ Pacemaker
☐ High Blood Pressure
☐ Pain in Chest on exertion
☐ Swollen Ankles
☐ Abnormal Bleeding
☐ Anemia
☐ Blood transfusion
☐ Fatigue Easily

☐ Jaundice
☐ Hepatitis
☐ Liver Disease
☐ Contact with AIDS virus
☐ Venereal Disease
☐ Epilepsy
☐ Fainting Spells
☐ Nervous disorder/ Psychiatric Care

☐ Are you allergic to latex?
☐ Malignancy or Tumor
☐ Radiation Therapy
☐ Artificial Joint
☐ Do you smoke? How much? /day
☐ History of alcohol/drug use or abuse
☐ (female) Is there any chance you could be pregnant?

Fig 2.7

The medical history can be compact, while addressing many critical issues. The check box items in the first three columns are arranged by system: endocrine, respiratory, cardiac, blood, gastrointestinal/genitourinary (GI/GU), and central nervous system (CNS). The right-hand column addresses history of malignancy, joint replacement, habits (tobacco, alcohol, other drugs), and pregnancy potential.

Get Acquainted Questionnaire: Confidential

So that we may treat you safely and effectively,
please answer all questions fully. Thank you.

Name .... Age .... Date of Birth .... / .... / ....

UPDATES:	W/INITIALS
.... / .... /	....
.... / .... /	....
.... / .... /	....
.... / .... /	....

(office use only)

Medical History

When was your last physical exam? .... Reason for exam? ....

Are you seeing a physician at this time? *Yes / No* If so, for what? ....

Physicians's name .... Party to notify in case of emergency ....

Please list any medications (prescription or non-prescription) you are taking, and what they are for:

....

....

Are you allergic, or do you react to anything (drugs, food, etc.) *Yes/No* If so, what? ....

....

Do you now, or have you ever had: (check if yes)

- ☐ Arthritis
- ☐ Diabetes
- ☐ Thyroid Problem
- ☐ Asthma
- ☐ Tuberculosis
- ☐ Heart Problems/ murmur
- ☐ Rheumatic Fever
- ☐ Heart Valve Problems
- ☐ Pacemaker

- ☐ High Blood Pressure
- ☐ Pain in Chest on exertion
- ☐ Swollen Ankles
- ☐ Abnormal Bleeding
- ☐ Anemia
- ☐ Blood transfusion
- ☐ Fatigue Easily
- ☐ Jaundice
- ☐ Hepatitis

- ☐ Liver Disease
- ☐ Contact with AIDS virus
- ☐ Venereal Disease
- ☐ Epilepsy
- ☐ Fainting Spells
- ☐ Nervous disorder/ Psychiatric Care

- ☐ Are you allergic to latex?
- ☐ Malignancy or Tumor
- ☐ Radiation Therapy
- ☐ Artificial Joint
- ☐ Do you smoke?
  How much? .... /day
- ☐ History of alcohol/drug use or abuse
- ☐ (female) Is there any chance you could be pregnant?

Dental History

What is your main problem/reason for coming? ....

Who referred you to us? .... Any concerns about dental treatment *Yes / No*

How do you feel about the condition of your teeth? ....

How do feel about your past dental experiences? ....

....

Do you now, or have ever had, (check if yes)

- ☐ Clicking or popping in jaw joint
- ☐ Clenching or Grinding, day or night
- ☐ Pains in or near the ear
- ☐ "TMJ" splint, or other types of treatment

- ☐ Other sore or painful areas in mouth
- ☐ Any missing teeth
- ☐ Bleeding Gums
- ☐ Toothaches
- ☐ Bad Breath

- ☐ Pain in Chewing
- ☐ Canker Sores

- ☐ Root canal treatment
- ☐ Bridgework or partial dentures
- ☐ Gum Surgery, or non-surgical treatment—root planing
- ☐ Orthodontic treatment (braces)
- ☐ Regular dental check-ups

When was your last dental visit? .... Did you have x-rays at that time? *Yes   No*

Have you been instructed on how to brush and floss? *Yes   No*

How often do you brush? .... Times per day/week

If so, When and By Whom? .... When, usually? .... Type of brush: hard / soft

What kind of toothpaste? .... Do you use dental floss? *Yes / No / Occasionally*

Dietary History

Do you eat or drink between meals during the day? *Yes   No*   In the evening? *Yes   No*

Does your diet include:

- ☐ Chewing gum
- ☐ Coookies/pastry

- ☐ Candy bars
- ☐ Sugar in coffee/tea

- ☐ Hard candy
- ☐ Lifesavers

- ☐ Soft drinks, soda, fruit juice
- ☐ Breath mints or cough drops?

Thanks again for taking time   .... / .... / ....
to complete this form!   today's date   signature

Fig 2.8

Patient questionnaires can be many pages long. This example is condensed to a single page. Note the specific box for updates (upper right).

ISSUE OF PAST DISEASES, CONDITIONS, AND TREATMENT

The following issues may have significant dental implications:

- Malignant and/or non-malignant tumors.
- Radiation therapy.
- Artificial or prosthetic joints.
- Use/abuse of tobacco, alcohol, narcotics, or other illicit drugs.
- Other past medical conditions, especially those requiring hospitalization and/or surgery.
- Pregnancy issues: female patients must be queried as to pregnancy, not only whether they know themselves to be pregnant, but whether there is any potential that they could become so. We may need to prescribe drugs the safety of which is not established in pregnancy, or drugs that are clearly contraindicated, and the patient may not be cognizant of an unplanned or early pregnancy.

The example medical questionnaire shown in Fig 2.7 is a reasonable and adequate history form, but, as with any pre-printed questionnaire, it would still require verbal review to be fully effective. You will note that it clusters certain items to establish a systematic review. It also includes documentation of subsequent updates over time.

Combined on a single page, the medical, dental, and dietary histories provide a compact instrument for information gathering (Fig 2.8). Without a doubt, a history form may be considerably more extensive than suggested here, and each clinician is entitled to his or her own opinions as to the breadth and depth of the history. Geographic locale, type of clinic and patient population, and the practitioner's own judgment will shape the medical history; what is offered here are minimum guidelines for a typical general dental practice.

Just as important as a thorough initial history and review is the regular review and updating of the information. The dates of such reviews, and the initials of the person documenting such updates, are critical, both for obvious medico-legal reasons and to help cue the dentist and dental team to perform the function on a regular basis.

Finally, the importance of verbal review and reiteration cannot be overstated. The potential for patients to forget, confuse, or omit important information is considerable, and can put both patient and practitioner at risk.[5,6]

REFERENCES

1. Chambers D, Abrams R, *Dental Communication*. OHANA GROUP: Sonoma CA, 1992.
2. Milgrom P, *Treating Fearful Dental Patients: A patient management handbook* Reston Publishing Co. Reston, VA, 1985.
3. Corah NL, Development of a dental anxiety scale. *J Dent Res* 1969; **45**:569.
4. Ronis D, Hansen C, Antonakos C, Equivalence of the original and revised Dental Anxiety Scales. *J Dent Hygiene* 1995; **69**:270–2.
5. Sampson E, Meister F, The importance of verbally verifying a health history. *Wisconsin Dent Assoc J* 1981; **1**:15–17.
6. McDaniel T, Miller D, Jones R, Davis M, Assessing patient willingness to reveal health history information. *J Am Dent Assoc* 1995; **126**:375.

RADIOGRAPHS

RADIOGRAPHS IN THE COMPREHENSIVE EXAMINATION

Radiographs are indispensable in dental diagnosis and treatment. Much of the information obtained with a radiograph is unobtainable any other way. Dental radiographs assist in discovering pathology and non-pathologic abnormalities, and in confirming normal healthy conditions. With current technology and technique, radiographs are a safe and cost-effective tool in dental diagnosis and treatment.

TYPES OF DENTAL RADIOGRAPHS AND THEIR APPLICATION

Intraoral films

- The standard *periapical* (PA) film is the most common and versatile radiographic tool in dentistry. With it, we can image an entire tooth or several teeth, including the apex and periapical region. PA films can be used for an emergency assessment (usually one or two films), or regional surveys, or a full mouth survey (Figs 3.1 and 3.2).
- Turned horizontally and held with a cardboard sleeve or adhesive tab, the *bite wing* film is probably the most frequently used radiograph in dentistry. It can clearly demonstrate proximal caries and interproximal periodontal bone levels, as well as many other findings of clinical crown and crestal bone (Fig 3.3).

  Turned vertically with an adhesive or mechanical film holder, a *vertical bite wing*

film can be used to visualize periodontal bone levels in advanced periodontitis, or post-periosurgical patients, which may not be covered by the normal horizontal bite wing. Figure 3.4a illustrates an acceptable bite wing film which nevertheless fails to demonstrate bone crest in the maxillary molar region. The vertical bite wings (Fig 3.4b) demonstrate the bone level despite significant periodontal bone loss.
- The *occlusal* film offers broader coverage to assess bone trauma and pathology away from teeth such as cysts, stones, etc (Fig 3.5).

Extraoral films

- Much of the head and facial skeleton is displayed on *panoramic* films which are useful in screening situations to assess trauma (especially mandibular fractures), demonstrate cysts, and locate third molars and other notable findings or conditions that are not in the usual range of PA films. Panoramic films can be used instead of PAs for patients who do not tolerate intraoral films well. Definition of detail is not as good, however, and some panoramic formats are non-diagnostic in the anterior region (Fig 3.6).
- Temporomandibular joint films, including transcranial, tomograms, and corrected tomograms, produce images of the condyle and fossa of varying quality (Fig 3.7). Computed tomography (CT) can produce highly detailed images of bony structures, but both the cost and the radiation dose are high. Soft tissue derangements are *not* demonstrable with any of these films. Arthrography, with injection of contrast

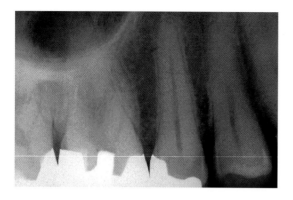

Fig 3.1

The standard single periapical radiograph.

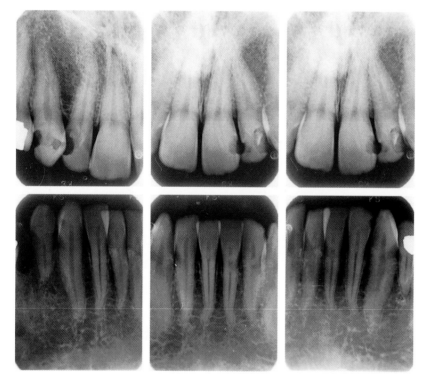

Fig 3.2

Six anterior PAs provide a wealth of information regarding both coronal and apical conditions in this patient's mouth.

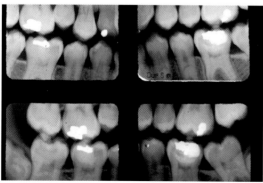

Fig 3.3

Standard double bite wing films.

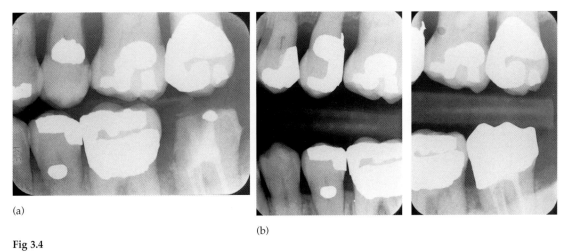

(a)

(b)

Fig 3.4

(a) Standard bite wings of patient's left posterior, losing the crestal bone in the maxilla. (b) Turned vertically, the crestal bone is demonstrated.

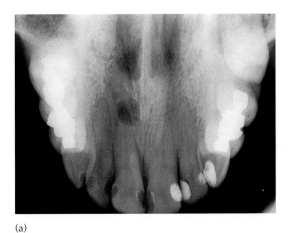

(a)

Fig 3.5

(a) An occlusal film, maxillary anterior. (b) Here standard PA films are used as occlusal films in a child, with similarly good results.

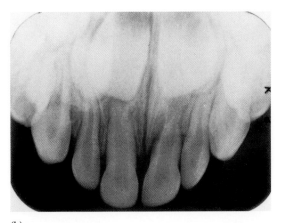

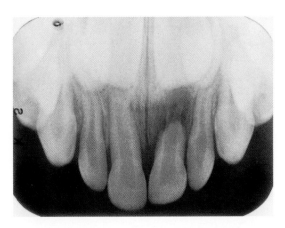

(b)

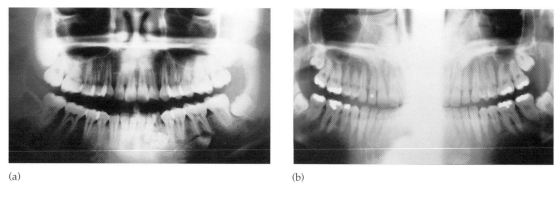

(a)   (b)

Fig 3.6

(a) Panoramic radiograph; (b) with some panoramic technology, the image is split at the midline.

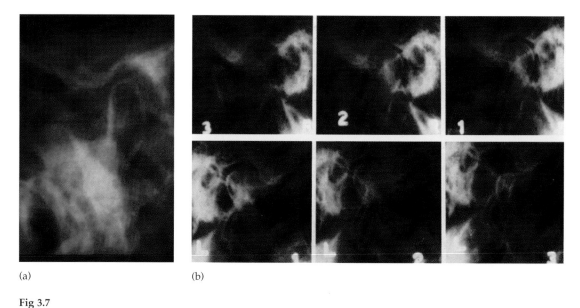

(a)   (b)

Fig 3.7

(a) The head of the condyle is imaged in the glenoid fossa in this transcranial view. (b) Transcranials of both joints in closed, rest, and open positions.

media into the joint space(s), is definitive of soft tissue derangement, but somewhat invasive (Fig 3.8). Magnetic resonance imaging (MRI) can demonstrate both bone and soft tissue joint components and, although non-invasive, is quite costly, time-consuming, and often difficult to interpret (Fig 3.9).

- Skull projection films, taken at various angles, can demonstrate specific areas and problems. Most common in dentistry is the lateral or frontal cephalometric film, used to diagnose orthodontic problems and to predict growth patterns (Fig 3.10).
- Bone scans employing radioactive isotopes, which accumulate in areas of rapid bone

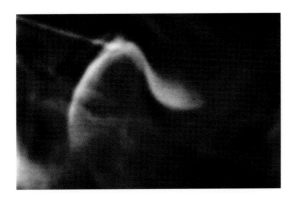

Fig 3.8

Radio-opaque die injected into the joint space helps define soft tissue joint components in this temporo-mandibular joint arthrogram.

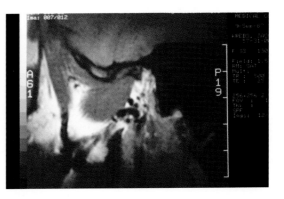

Fig 3.9

Magnetic resonance imaging of the joint and fossa region.

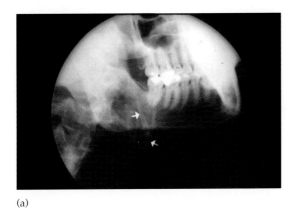

(a)

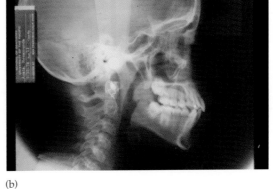

(b)

Fig 3.10

(a) Oblique extraoral view of mandible. (b) Lateral skull projection, suitable for cephalometric analysis.

metabolism (either osteoblastic or osteo-clastic), can point to bone pathology such as osteomyelitis in various areas of the head and neck. Such scans are extraoral in that the film is not placed in the mouth. The patient becomes the radiation source, however, as the isotopes collect and decay in affected regions.

SELECTION AND USE

How many?

The extremely low radiation dosage employed in dental radiography, especially when combined with collimation and protective leaded drapes and collars, provides a high

The recommendations in this chart are subject to clinical judgement and may not apply to every patient. *They are to be used by dentists only after reviewing that patient's health history and completing a clinical examination. The recommendations do **not** need to be altered because of pregnancy.*

Patient Category	Child — Primary Dentition (prior to eruption of first permanent tooth)	Child — Transitional Dentition (following eruption of first permanent tooth)	Adolescent — Primary Dentition (prior to eruption of third molars)	Adult — Dentulous	Adult — Edentulous
New Patient* *All new patients to assess dental diseases and growth and development*	Posterior bitewing examination if proximal surfaces of primary teeth cannot be visualized or probed	Individualized radiographic examination consisting of periapical/occlusal views and posterior bitewings *or* panoramic examination and posterior bitewings	Individualized radiographic examination consisting of posterior bitewings and selected periapicals. A full mouth intraoral radiographic examination is appropriate when the patient presents with clinical evidence of generalized dental disease or a history of extensive dental treatment		Full mouth intraoral radiographic examination *or* panoramic examination
Recall patient* *Clinical caries or high-risk factor for caries***	Posterior bitewing examination at 6-month intervals *or* until no carious lesions are evident		Posterior bitewing examination at 6- to 12-month intervals *or* until no carious lesions are evident	Posterior bitewing examination at 12- to 18-month intervals	Not applicable
No clinical caries and no high-risk factors for caries**	Posterior bitewing examination at 12- to 24-month intervals if proximal surfaces of primary teeth cannot be visualized or probed	Posterior bitewing examination at 12- to 24-month intervals	Posterior bitewing examination at 18- to 36-month intervals	Posterior bitewing examination at 24- to 36-month intervals	Not applicable
Periodontal disease or a history of periodontal treatment	Individualized radiographic examination consisting of selected periapical and/or bitewing radiographs for areas where periodontal disease (other than nonspecific gingivitis) can be demonstrated clinically		Individualized radiographic examination consisting of selected periapical and/or bitewing radiographs for areas where periodontal disease (other than nonspecific gingivitis) can be demonstrated clinically	Individualized radiographic examination consisting of selected periapical and/or bitewing radiographs for areas where periodontal disease (other than nonspecific gingivitis) can be demonstrated clinically	Not applicable
Growth and development assessment	Usually not indicated	Individualized radiographic examination consisting of a periapical/occlusal or panoramic examination	Periapical *or* panoramic examination to assess developing third molars	Usually not indicated	Usually not indicated

* Clinical situations for which radiographs may be indicated include:

A. *Positive Historical Findings*
1. Previous periodontal or endodontic therapy
2. History of pain or trauma
3. Familial history of dental anomalies
4. Postoperative evaluation of healing
5. Presence of implants

B. *Positive Clinical Signs/Symptoms*
1. Clinical evidence of periodontal disease
2. Large or deep restorations
3. Deep carious lesions
4. Malposed or clinically impacted teeth
5. Swelling
6. Evidence of facial trauma
7. Mobility of teeth
8. Fistula or sinus tract infection
9. Clinically suspected sinus pathology
10. Growth abnormalities
11. Oral involvement in known or suspected systemic disease
12. Positive neurologic findings in the head and neck
13. Evidence of foreign objects
14. Pain and/or dysfunction of the temporomandibular joint
15. Facial asymmetry

16. Abutment teeth for fixed or removable partial prosthesis
17. Unexplained bleeding
18. Unexplained sensitivity of teeth
19. Unusual eruption, spacing or migration of teeth
20. Unusual tooth morphology, calcification or color
21. Missing teeth with unknown reason
22. Serial assessment of previous surgical site

**Patients at high risk for caries may demonstrate any of the following:

1. High level of caries experience
2. History of recurrent caries
3. Existing restoration of poor quality
4. Poor oral hygiene
5. Inadequate fluoride exposure
6. Prolonged nursing (bottle or breast)
7. Diet with high sucrose frequency
8. Poor family dental health
9. Developmental enamel defects
10. Developmental disability
11. Xerostomia
12. Genetic abnormality of teeth
13. Many multisurface restorations
14. Chemo/radiation therapy

Fig 3.11

Current guidelines for 'How often?'. (This chart has been adapted and reprinted with permission from Eastman Kodak Company.)

ADA—American Dental Association
AGD—Academy of General Dentistry
AAOMR—American Academy of Oral and Maxillofacial Radiology
AAOM—American Academy of Oral Medicine
AAPD—American Academy of Pediatric Dentistry
AAP—American Academy of Periodontology
FDA—United States Food and Drug Administration

degree of safety and confidence. The dentist may have to educate patients in this area. The most common radiographs used in dentistry are also very cost-efficient. Therefore, the answer to 'how many?' is 'enough,' that is, we must obtain a sufficient number of good quality radiographs to make accurate diagnoses. This is a professional, ethical, and legal standard of care. On the other hand, we must also take care not to take more radiographs than are needed simply to fill up slots on the mount. Radiographs should always be based on diagnostic need, rather than any routine protocol.

Example 1.   An 18-year-old male patient is seen as an emergency after a blow to the chin (sports accident). There is swelling and bruising on lip and chin, and two lower incisors are very loose. What radiographs are indicated?

Answer.   As this is an emergency and not a fully comprehensive examination, only the areas of immediate concern need to be imaged. This would include PA views of the loosened anterior teeth, and panoramic or other extraoral images of the mandible to diagnose or rule out fracture either at the site of the trauma or elsewhere within the mandible. The condyles need to be imaged, because the neck region is the thinnest portion of the bone, and most at risk of fracture.

Example 2.   A 57-year-old new female patient (missing all bicuspids and molars) needs general dental care, including upper and lower distal extension partial dentures. What radiographs are indicated?

Answer.   A combination of panoramic film and anterior PAs to image the teeth and surrounding bone will provide good coverage. As an alternative to the panoramic film, holding devices of various types can be used to image posterior edentulous areas.

Example 3.   A 34-year-old fully dentulous male with numerous visible carious lesions and fractured teeth is seen for a new

patient examination. He recalls having bite wing radiographs a year or so ago. What radiographs are indicated?

Answer.   The presence of active dental disease calls for current and accurate diagnostic data. A full mouth series, including periapicals of all teeth and double bite wings, is indicated.

How often?

Frequency is another issue involving both cost and exposure. Here again routine protocols (bite wings every 6 months) based solely on time interval are not acceptable. Current guidelines, developed by a panel of experts representing the ADA, AGD, AAOMR, AAOM, AAPD, AAP, under the sponsorship of the FDA are outlined in Fig 3.11.

Example 1.   A 12-year-old boy with eight proximal carious lesions visible on radiograph will be placed on 6-month recalls for examination, cleaning, and fluoride. When would you next take bite wing radiographs?

Answer.   As a result of the high caries rate and likelihood of undetectable incipient caries, follow-up bite wings at the 6-month recall are indicated. Based on findings at that time, continued monitoring at 6–12 month intervals may be indicated.

Example 2.   A 40-year-old new female patient has no pathology or abnormality visible in full-mouth radiographs. No dental treatment is needed, other than routine cleaning. When would you next take a full series of radiographs?

Answer.   Assuming that regular check-ups reveal no pathology, and no symptoms arise, this patient could easily go 3–5 years or more before another full series is taken.

Example 3.   A pregnant 24-year-old female patient is seen on emergency with an acute dental abscess. She agrees to endodontic therapy, and two additional appointments are scheduled. What radiographs would you take?

Answer.   Using appropriate shielding, there is no contraindication to dental radiographs in pregnancy. This clinical situation calls for periapical diagnostic and measurement films appropriate to endodontic therapy. Sensitivity to patient concerns and careful education may be required to allay fears.

The general operative principle in the selection and use of dental radiographs is to obtain whatever films are necessary for diagnosis and treatment planning consistent with radiation safety and cost-effectiveness. All dental radiographs must meet minimum standards for quality, that is, they must be 'diagnostic' films, properly aligned, exposed, and processed.

Inadequate radiographs can seriously compromise dental and oral diagnosis, and lead to inappropriate or untimely treatment.

The reader is encouraged to consult the many excellent reference works for specific details regarding dental radiography.

Digital radiography, employing a radiation-sensitive receiver in place of the X-ray film, can produce digital images on a computer monitor almost instantaneously. It has the advantage of lower radiation exposure as a result of the great sensitivity of the receiver, and having images available immediately is a great convenience and time saver. Applications in endodontic treatment and surgery, especially for measurement and assessment of work in progress, are obvious. Drawbacks at this time include the high cost of the technology, difficulty in archival storage which requires considerable computer capacity, and problems from the medicolegal standpoint. As digital images can be altered without a trace, their use as evidence can be questioned. These problems may well be addressed with advances in technology in years to come.

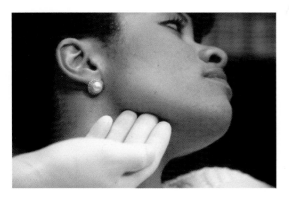

Fig 4.4

Submandibular lymphatics may be palpated against the inferior border of the mandible.

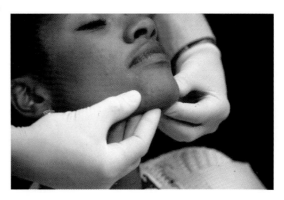

Fig 4.5

Bilateral palpation proceeds anteriorly to the submental lymphatics.

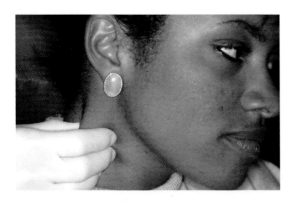

Fig 4.6

The patient should be in a relaxed, upright position to palpate along the sternocleidomastoid muscle. The superficial cervical lymphatics may be found anterior to this muscle.

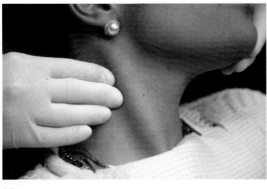

(a)

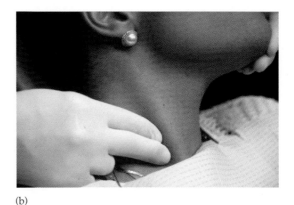

(b)

Fig 4.7

(a) The deep superior cervical lymphatics may be palpated against the upper sternocleidomastoid muscle. (b) The deep inferior cervical lymphatics may be palpated against the lower sternocleidomastoid muscle.

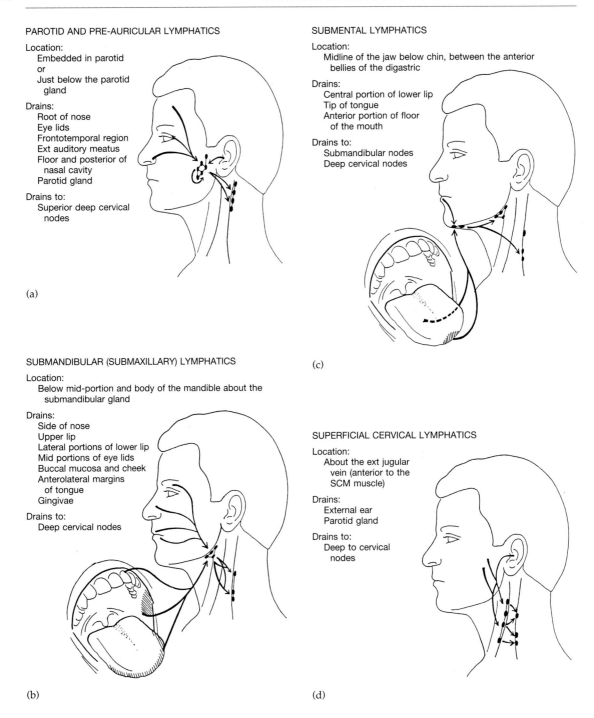

PAROTID AND PRE-AURICULAR LYMPHATICS

Location:
    Embedded in parotid
    or
    Just below the parotid
        gland

Drains:
    Root of nose
    Eye lids
    Frontotemporal region
    Ext auditory meatus
    Floor and posterior of
        nasal cavity
    Parotid gland

Drains to:
    Superior deep cervical
        nodes

(a)

SUBMENTAL LYMPHATICS

Location:
    Midline of the jaw below chin, between the anterior
        bellies of the digastric

Drains:
    Central portion of lower lip
    Tip of tongue
    Anterior portion of floor
        of the mouth

Drains to:
    Submandibular nodes
    Deep cervical nodes

(c)

SUBMANDIBULAR (SUBMAXILLARY) LYMPHATICS

Location:
    Below mid-portion and body of the mandible about the
        submandibular gland

Drains:
    Side of nose
    Upper lip
    Lateral portions of lower lip
    Mid portions of eye lids
    Buccal mucosa and cheek
    Anterolateral margins
        of tongue
    Gingivae

Drains to:
    Deep cervical nodes

(b)

SUPERFICIAL CERVICAL LYMPHATICS

Location:
    About the ext jugular
        vein (anterior to the
        SCM muscle)

Drains:
    External ear
    Parotid gland

Drains to:
    Deep to cervical
        nodes

(d)

Fig 4.8

The regions and structures, both extraoral and intraoral, drained (afferent) by the various lymphatics, and where they drain to (efferent), on their way to the jugular trunk. Swollen and/or tender nodes can then be traced back to potential sites of infection, inflammation, or, more rarely, neoplasms. (a) Parotid and preauricular lymphatics; (b) submandibular (submaxillary) lymphatics; (c) submental lymphatics; (d) superficial cervical lymphatics.

DEEP SUPERIOR CERVICAL LYMPHATICS

Location:
    Course of the carotid artery and int jugular
      vessels (behind SCM muscle)

Drains:
    Back of Neck
    Occipital region of scalp
    Portions of ext ear
    Post and central portions:
      Tongue
      Palate
      Nasopharynx
      Nose
      Larynx
      Upper esophagus

Drains to:
    Jugular trunk

(e)

DEEP INFERIOR CERVICAL LYMPHATICS

Location:
    Inferior portion of course
      of carotid artery and
      int jugular vessels

Drains:
    Back of neck
    Lower portion of
      occipital scalp
    Superior anterior
      chest wall

Drains to:
    Deep jugular trunk

(f)

Fig 4.8 *continued*

(e) deep superior cervical lymphatics; (f) deep inferior cervical lymphatics.

The head and neck lymphatic systems

The lymphatic system consists of: a capillary network which collects lymph in organs and tissues; collecting vessels that convey lymph to the bloodstream; lymph nodes which are filters in the path of collecting vessels; lymphatic organs, such as the tonsils and aggregate lymphatic nodules; and the spleen and thymus.

Lymph is a transparent, colorless or slightly yellow, watery fluid resembling blood plasma, but more dilute. White blood cells (lymphocytic type) are found floating in the fluid, increasing in number after the passage of the lymph through the nodes. Lymph drainage of the head and neck returns to the bloodstream via the **jugular trunk**. On the right side, this trunk ends in the junction of the internal jugular and subclavian veins. On the left side, it joins the thoracic duct, which

---

Critical factors in assessing a mass or swelling

Size: estimate the dimensions in millimeters, and note whether the mass or swelling is solitary or multiple.

Consistency: describe the swelling as either hard (like a pebble), firm (like tensed muscle tissue), or soft (fluctuant) like a water balloon.

Duration of enlargement: this must come from the patient's history.

Mobility: when manipulated, the swelling may be fixed, rooted to underlying and surrounding tissue, or freely movable, able to be 'rolled' under the fingers.

Tenderness: the patient's reported response to palpation whether painful, tender, or non-tender should be elicited.

Location: unilateral findings are more likely to represent pathology than bilateral swellings.

also terminates near the junction of the internal jugular and subclavian veins. The diagrams in Fig 4.8 represent the lymph node chains and clusters which are palpated in the routine systematic approach. Note the structures and regions which each cluster drains (afferent), and where each then drains to (efferent).

Palpable lymphatics may provide clues to diagnosis of oral and perioral disease, extra-oral disease (neck and/or chest), or actual lymph system disease. Bear in mind that not all palpable masses in the head/neck are lymph glands/nodes. Part of the differential diagnosis of findings from palpation involves the consideration of other possible sources. Consider the anatomy of the region (thyroid gland, salivary glands, muscles, etc) and recall the potential for anomalies (thyroglossal duct cyst, branchial cleft cyst, etc) in the development of the region.

Causes of lymph node enlargement

By far the most common cause for swellings of the lymph tissues are inflammatory or infectious processes, which could include the following:

* Chronic nonspecific lymphadenitis arising from upper respiratory infections, dental infections, tonsillitis–pharyngitis, and stomatitis or dermatitis.
* Acute nonspecific lymphadenitis developing from similar causes, or as a result of severe pyogenic or nonpyogenic infections caused by viruses, spirochetes, and/or rickettsiae (e.g. mumps, herpes zoster, herpes simplex, erythema multiforme, parasites, etc).
* Specific infections, such as tuberculosis or infectious mononucleosis.

Far less commonly, swellings of the lymph tissues represent metastatic tumors to the lymph nodes, with a primary lesion either in the region drained by the node or at a remote primary site.

The least common cause or source of lymph node enlargement is primary neoplasms of the lymph system. These may include diseases such as lymphoma, lymphosarcoma, reticular cell sarcoma, Hodgkin's disease, and leukemia.

It is important to remember that the normal lymph node is *not* palpable; it is soft, compressible, and freely movable. The first principle of oral diagnosis is to observe and describe deviations from normal; therefore we must *know* what is normal, *recognize* findings (including palpable masses) that are abnormal, *analyze* the abnormality, and *refer* for consultation and biopsy when indicated.

The lips

The lips (Fig 4.9) are observed and palpated bilaterally and bimanually, and reflected to reveal the mucosa.

The labial and buccal mucosa

The labial and buccal mucosa (Fig 4.10) is observed and palpated, including the parotid region to determine salivary flow.

The tongue

The tongue (Fig 4.11) is examined: the dorsum, the lateral aspects (requiring careful retraction with 2 × 2 gauze), and the ventral aspect and lingual frenum.

The floor of the mouth

The floor of the mouth (Fig 4.12) is observed and palpated, bimanually, using a finger or thumb under the chin for resistance. The medial aspect of the retromolar area deserves careful attention.

The hard palate

The hard palate (Fig 4.13) is observed and palpated, extending distally back to the soft palate.

The soft palate/pharynx

The soft palate and pharynx (Fig 4.14) are observed, completing the soft tissue examination.

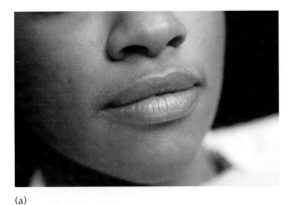

(a)

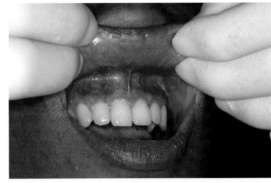

(b)

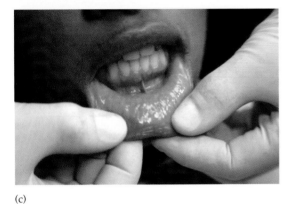

(c)

Fig 4.9 (a–c)

The lips are inspected, palpated bimanually and bilaterally, then reflected to reveal and inspect the labial mucosae.

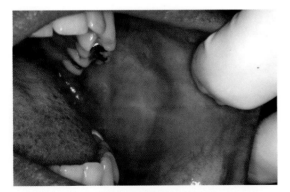

Fig 4.10

Buccal mucosa, including the parotid duct, and typical linea alba. Care should be taken not to obscure tissue with finger or mirror used to retract the cheek.

PERIODONTAL EVALUATION

The periodontal examination is a logical continuation of the soft tissue evaluation.

Factors to be considered in the periodontal examination:

Color
Surface consistency or texture
Contour of marginal gingivae
Keratinized gingiva and papillae
Clefts
Frenum pulls
Mucogingival involvement
Mobility
The 'big three' periodontal findings:
Inflammation, bleeding, and/or
pockets deeper than 3–4 mm

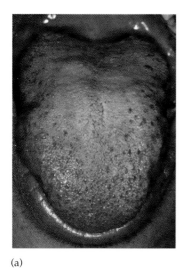

(a)

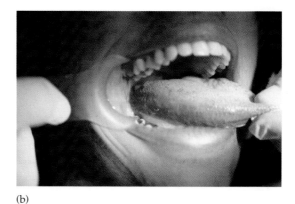

(b)

Fig 4.11

The tongue presents a wide range of normal in its size, shape, and surface character. The dorsum should be examined and palpated back to the circumvallate papillae, the lateral aspect back to the foliate papillae (lingual tonsils). Retraction of the tongue is absolutely necessary in order to visualize this area, which presents a relatively high incidence of oral malignancy. The ventral aspect is appreciated for the lingual frenum, typical varicosities, and submandibular salivary ducts.

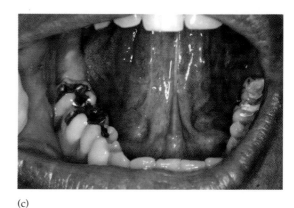

(c)

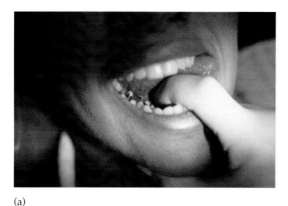

(a)

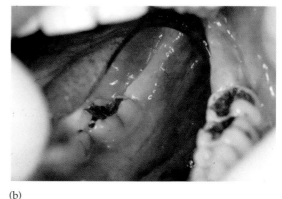

(b)

Fig 4.12

(a) The floor of the mouth is palpated bimanually, with an opposing thumb or finger braced under the chin, appreciating salivary glands and the muscular floor of the mouth. (b) Careful visual inspection of the floor on either side of the tongue should include the medial aspect of the retromolar area, because of the relative incidence of oral malignancy in this area, and the difficulty of direct visualization (this image is reflected in a mirror).

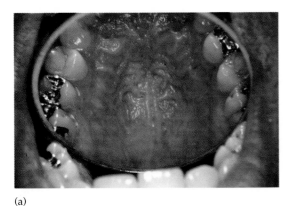

(a)

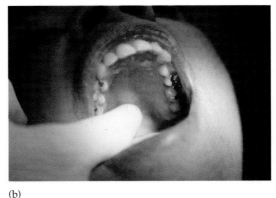

(b)

Fig 4.13

(a) The hard palate is examined as are all soft tissues, for color, surface texture or consistency, swellings, nodes, or lesions. (b) Palpation should extend back to the soft palate, noting consistency, and any report of pain or tenderness to palpation.

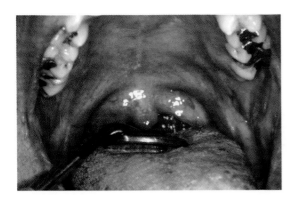

Fig 4.14

The soft palate, uvula, and pillars of the fauces (and tonsils, if not removed) are examined. The tongue should be depressed and the patient asked to say 'ahh,' to observe the posterior pharyngeal wall and complete the intraoral soft tissue examination.

The periodontal examination is carried out visually (Fig 4.15a) to obtain clinical and radiographic findings, and with a periodontal probe (Fig 4.15b,c). A new generation of electromechanical probes, some connected to computers for automatic charting, offers a potential improvement in accuracy, consistency among examiners, and ease of recording. The most critical issue is simply to use probe depths regularly to assess improvement or deterioration over time. Slight discrepancies between examiners or probes are offset by repeated assessments over months and years.

Whether a full six-point recorded probing is done, or a screening examination such as the Periodontal Screening and Recording (PSR) protocol is employed in its stead, all teeth must be assessed, because local periodontal disease or defects can appear in an otherwise healthy dentition (Fig 4.16).

After more than a quarter of a century of efforts on the part of dental educators to instill the importance of a thorough periodontal examination into dentists in training, and a similar number of years in which the US malpractice litigation scene has seen many cases of failure to diagnose or treat periodontal disease adequately, one would think that dentists would have gotten the message. Unfortunately, the basic examination just described, combined with appropriate information and advice to the patient, is still not a routine procedure in many general dental offices. It is, however, the standard of care in dentistry today, and there is no good excuse for failure to carry it out.

ORAL HYGIENE ASSESSMENT

The presence of plaque, calculus, and stain on teeth can be a critical finding, because plaque is the primary etiologic agent of both caries and periodontal disease. Hence, the patient's

daily oral hygiene regimen, its relative effectiveness or lack of same must be accurately assessed in the comprehensive examination (Fig 4.17). Many dentists perform their new patient examinations after a scaling/polishing by the dental hygienist. Although this makes for better visibility in some cases, it sometimes creates a false sense of well-being, in that the mouth may appear cleaner (and therefore healthier) than is the case.

A qualitative measure such as slight, moderate, or heavy may be used, or a more quantitative method such as the Oral Health Progress Record or OHPR (Fig 4.18) may be preferred. The OHPR uses a simple criterion-based scoring of key indicators of the patient's oral health and home care. It plots those scores by date, giving an immediate visual impression of patient improvement or deterioration over time. It provides a check-off for preventive measures taken, and

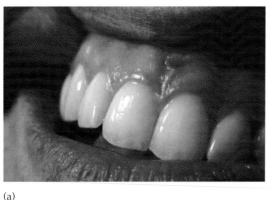
(a)

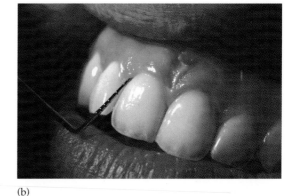
(b)

Fig 4.15

(a) The normal healthy periodontium. (b) Careful probing is done parallel with long axis, around each tooth, with measurements taken at six points (mesial, mid, and distal points on buccal and lingual aspects). (c) A variety of probes is available, including the curved furcation probe (bottom). The critical issue is consistency from examination to examination, so that improvement or worsening can be accurately assessed.

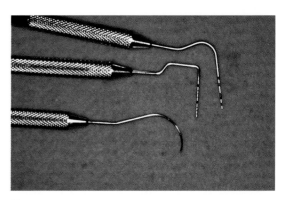
(c)

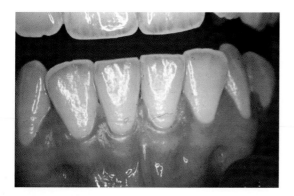

Fig 4.16

Another example of healthy appearing periodontal tissues.

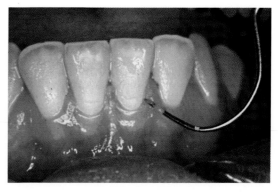

Fig 4.17

This is the same 'healthy' periodontium shown in Fig 4.16 before scaling and polishing. Note the plaque which has been harvested on the explorer, and the telltale bleeding elicited by gentle contact. This is where periodontal disease begins, and it is where it can most effectively be stopped.

counseling given, which is again visible at a glance. Without having to go back through progress notes or multiple re-evaluation forms, the patient's general oral health status and progress over time can be seen at once and are clearly documented.

As human behavior does not change easily or quickly, multiple follow-up assessments are essential to track the patient's ability and/or willingness to establish and maintain good oral hygiene on a regular basis.

DENTAL EXAMINATION

Despite the many efforts to broaden the focus of dentistry to oral medicine and the oral cavity as it relates to general systemic health, clinical dentistry is still basically about teeth. If we dentists are not so focused, our patients' expectations will often lead us there. In fact, much of what we do in terms of systemic assessment, soft tissue diagnosis, and periodontal and functional treatment in the end relates back to the teeth, their function, appearance, and retention. The risk entailed in

downplaying the tooth orientation of past generations of dentists is that we may fail to maintain the standards of dental care that have earned our profession the high esteem of the public we serve. So we strive to seek a happy medium, putting the dental examination in its proper context within the comprehensive examination.

The dental examination should include a charting of the teeth, existing restorations, carious lesions, and defective restorations. The charting of missing teeth and existing restorations serves three main functions. First, it serves to separate the current dentist's treatment and restorative care from that done by previous practitioners, should misunderstandings arise over failed restorations or symptomatic teeth. Second, treatment planning is aided greatly by a graphic chart including existing restorations, because radiographs may not reveal the buccolingual extent of existing restorations, which might require a crown in one case, or a simple class II restoration in another. Third, and most important, a complete and accurate charting of teeth and dental restorations can be invaluable in the event of a tragedy – fire, plane crash, or foul

CRITERIA FOR ORAL HEALTH PROGRESS SCORING

PLAQUE
- 0 Plaque free—no observable plaque with disclosant
- 1 Slight plaque—five teeth or less (is using floss)
- 2 Slight plaque—six teeth or more (generalized)
- 3 Moderate to heavy plaque (generalized)
- 4 Gross plaque and debris—no evidence of brushing or any oral-hygiene efforts

STAIN/CALCULUS
- 0 None
- 1 Very slight—lower linguals or upper buccals only
- 2 Moderate—requiring definite scaling and polishing
- 3 Heavy—requiring cavitron or multiple sittings

TISSUE (BLEEDING)
- 0 No observable inflammation or bleeding with probe or floss*
- 1 Slight inflammation, some bleeding with probe or floss*
- 2 Generalized inflammation, bleeding, with *pockets* measuring 3 mm or more
- 3 Periodontal disease

PROGRAM ACCEPTANCE
- 0 Patient is enthusiastic, volunteers information, uses disclosant at home
- 1 Receptive, interested, will respond to questions readily
- 2 Skeptical, but communicative
- 3 Disinterested—noncommittal or refuses preventive services

*Probe or floss interproximally five teeth: mesial interproximal nos. 3, 6, 13, 18, 27

(a)

date:										
PLAQUE	0 1 2 3 4	0 1 2 3 4	0 1 2 3 4	0 1 2 3 4	0 1 2 3 4	0 1 2 3 4	0 1 2 3 4	0 1 2 3 4	0 1 2 3 4	0 1 2 3 4
STAIN/ CALCULUS	0 1 2 3	0 1 2 3	0 1 2 3	0 1 2 3	0 1 2 3	0 1 2 3	0 1 2 3	0 1 2 3	0 1 2 3	0 1 2 3
TISSUE (BLEEDING)	0 1 2 3	0 1 2 3	0 1 2 3	0 1 2 3	0 1 2 3	0 1 2 3	0 1 2 3	0 1 2 3	0 1 2 3	0 1 2 3
PROGRAM ACCEPTANCE	0 1 2 3	0 1 2 3	0 1 2 3	0 1 2 3	0 1 2 3	0 1 2 3	0 1 2 3	0 1 2 3	0 1 2 3	0 1 2 3

NEW CARIES
DISC
P & P
TBI
FLS
DIET

FILM:
KIT
BRUSH
'D' TABS

COMMENTS

(b)

date:	3-5-95	3-12-95	4-26-95	7-1-95	1-8-96	7-15-96	7-27-96			
PLAQUE (0–4, circled = score)	(3)	(2)	(1)	(2)	(1)	(3)	(0)	—	—	—
STAIN/ CALCULUS (0–3, circled = score)	(3)	(0)	(0)	(1)	(1)	(2)	(0)	—	—	—
TISSUE (BLEEDING) (0–3, circled = score)	(2)	(1)	(0)	(1)	(1)	(2)	(0)	—	—	—
PROGRAM ACCEPTANCE (0–3, circled = score)	(2)	(1)	(1)	(1)	(1)	(1)	(0)	—	—	—
NEW CARIES	YES	—	—	—	—	YES	—			
DISC	✔	✔	✔	✔	✔		✔			
P & P	✔					✔				
TBI	✔	REV	REV	✔	REV	✔	REV			
FLS	INTRO	✔	REV	✔	REV	✔	REV			
DIET		✔								
FILM:	P&P	TRIGGER FOODS								
BRUSH	✔					✔				
'D' TABS			✔				✔			
COMMENTS	ABILITY GOOD DIGEST REPRINT		MUCH IMPROVED			PT. HAS HAD PROBLEMS AT HOME RE-EMPHA- SIZED PREV. SET UP FOR ADD'L APPT.				

(c)

Fig 4.18

(a) Criteria for scoring the Oral Health Progress Record. These criteria are easily learned by auxiliary staff (hygienists and assistants), and allow for regular monitoring of a number of oral health indicators. The criteria are written so that, in general, a score of '0' or '1' indicates excellent to good oral health, a score of '2' indicates borderline problems, and a score of '3' or higher signifies a definite problem in that area, requiring further evaluation or intervention. (b) The OHPR (Oral Health Progress Record) uses a criterion-based scoring assessment for Plaque (the patient's level of daily home care), Stain/Calculus (accretions on the teeth requiring professional help in removal), Tissue (Bleeding), which is an approximation of a periodontal diagnosis (the actual diagnosis and classification being the dentist's responsibility), and Program Acceptance, which is a neutral way of describing the patient's attitude toward oral and periodontal health counseling. Scores are recorded and displayed graphically over time, and check-off boxes indicate preventive procedures done and instructions given on each visit. (c) This example, adapted from an actual patient record, illustrates the use of the OHPR. Immediate improvement from first to second visits (one week) is seen, with continued improvement at 6 weeks. Scores remain in an acceptable range over the next two recalls (3 months, then 6), but clearly fall at the next 6-month recall. A follow-up 2 weeks after that indicates a successful intervention and excellent patient response.

play. In many cases positive identification of human remains can be made only through dental records, and incomplete or poorly kept records may deny a bereaved family or police authorities the positive identification they so badly need.

Diagnosis of carious lesions and defective restorations is often colored by clinical judgment. It is critical to develop a routine and standard approach to your examination technique, so that the same criteria are always used in gathering data. The judgment of when and whether to restore/replace can then be based on individual patient situations. For example, a very slight stick on a pit or margin might call for restoration in a patient with many carious lesions and contributing factors present, whereas the same finding might call only for a 'watch' to be placed on an otherwise caries-free mouth. All dentists make these clinical judgments, but it is critical that dentists be consistent within their own practice.

It is usually helpful to examine the teeth twice, the first time accounting for all teeth by their numbers, nos 1–32, and charting existing restorations. The second time around, carious lesions, defective restorations, improper contacts, contour, and problems of cleaning are noted and charted. The explorer is the primary tool for assessing tactile changes in the enamel or dentin indicating caries, or in determining the integrity of restoration margins. Different configurations of explorers are useful (Fig 4.19) to access all surfaces of the teeth. It is critical that explorers be uniformly sharp, so that the desired consistency in findings is assured. Using a few factory sharp instruments for examination only, and 'retiring' them to general use once they have been dulled or resharpened, is an effective way to keep consistency in the dental examination. Clinicians may differ in what they consider restorable caries or defective margins on probing, but it is critical to maintain individual consistency even within those differences.

Both visual and tactile caries assessment depend on having a dry tooth. The air syringe is an indispensable tool in the dental examination, because saliva can easily mask a pit or a margin in need of probing (Fig 4.20).

The dental examination should also include assessment of excessive mobility (Fig 4.21), abnormal pulpal response (Fig 4.22), and abnormalities in size, shape, or color of teeth. In addition to electronic vitality testing, thermal testing by the application of hot or cold, percussion, and having the patient bite on flexible wedges, etc, it is very important carefully to elicit patient symptoms to complete the dental examination. The use of multiple signs and symptoms in arriving at a conclusion about pulpal pathology will be illustrated in Chapter 6.

Finally, consider that both caries detection and treatment are entering a new phase in dental practice. Newer technologies on the horizon may increase our sensitivity to early caries just as new therapies may allow us to arrest and even remineralize such caries nonoperatively. When caries or defective restorations are detected there continues to be a need for clinical judgment about how best to address the problem; this is dependent on the stage of the lesion itself as well as on the patient's overall dental health, diet, ability/willingness to carry out intensive home care measures, and availability for regular follow-up visits.

These clinical judgments will continue to be made individually, as no two lesions are alike, no two patients alike, and indeed, no two clinicians.

FUNCTIONAL EVALUATION

The functional evaluation has to do with how the components of the oral facial complex, that is, the teeth and associated tissues, work together. It can be divided into three separate but related areas: the occlusion, the temporomandibular joint and related musculature, and the myofunctional components, that is, tongue, lips, and speech.

THE OCCLUSION

Occlusion is assessed on a number of accounts.

The static relationship of maxilla to mandible, usually assessed by its Angle Classifi-

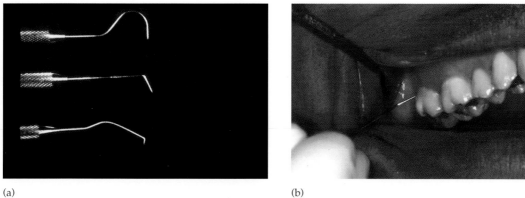

(a)   (b)

Fig 4.19

(a) Different explorers are preferred by various clinicians. It is useful to keep different configurations on hand for special situations that may require them. (b) Beginning the dental examination, distobuccal, upper right posterior.

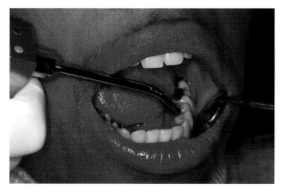

Fig 4.20

Drying the teeth is critical for both visual and tactile examination of pits and margins.

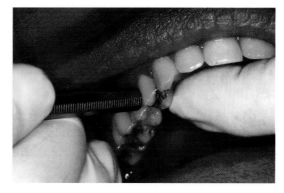

Fig 4.21

Mobility is best determined with a hard object such as a mirror handle on at least one side of the tooth, to avoid false impressions of movement resulting from examiner's finger tissues being compressed.

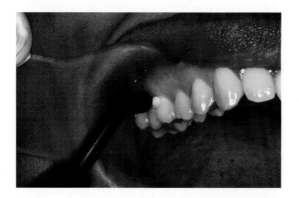

Fig 4.22

Pulp testing, whether with electronic impulses, heat, or cold, is generally carried out when patient history or radiographic findings suggest a problem. No current test is definitive by itself. Diagnosis of pulpal pathology is nearly always made from a number of signs and symptoms.

cation (I, II (division 1–2), and III), should always be noted (Fig 4.23). The overbite and overjet in anterior teeth are observed and recorded. The relationship of centric relation (CR, retruded position, hinge position) to centric occlusion (CO, intercuspal position, maximal occlusal contact) should be determined (Fig 4.24), particularly if there is significant discrepancy between the two. Inability to locate or retrude the patient's teeth/mouth into a hinge position may also be significant.

The dynamic occlusion is appreciated, assessing lateral and protrusive function, noting which teeth are in contact in those movements, on both working and balancing sides (Fig 4.25).

The loss of space through either supereruption or loss of vertical dimension must be recorded, especially in cases where teeth are missing, to complete the occlusal assessment (Fig 4.26).

THE TEMPOROMANDIBULAR JOINT AND RELATED MUSCULATURE

Examination of the temporomandibular joint, taken here to include assessment of the joint itself, and its related musculature, starts with measurement of the range of motion on opening and lateral excursions (Fig 4.27). Measures in millimeters are useful, but it is also acceptable to relate range of motion to individual anatomy: the patient can attempt to open wide enough to fit their three finger-widths between incisors, which approximates the range of normal. In lateral excursion, if the patient can slide the teeth side to side over the width of the upper central incisor or more, they are again in normal range. During opening, any significant deviations are noted.

Palpation of the joint directly over the glenoid fossa or via the external auditory meatus (Fig 4.28) during movement may reveal subluxations, crepitus, or discrete clicking or popping indicative of dysfunction or incoordination of the joint complex.

Palpation of the major muscles of mastication may elicit reports of pain or tenderness to the palpation which can be significant (Fig 4.29). Other muscles of mastication and muscles of the head and neck may also be palpated.

Finally, patient symptoms must again be considered, such as joint pain, earache, ear noise, headaches, pain in chewing, or other symptoms potentially indicative of temporomandibular disorders.

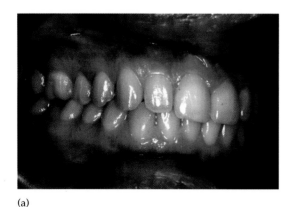
(a)

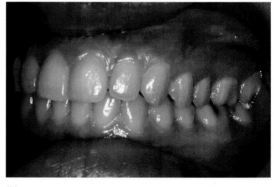
(b)

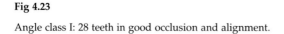

Fig 4.23

Angle class I: 28 teeth in good occlusion and alignment.

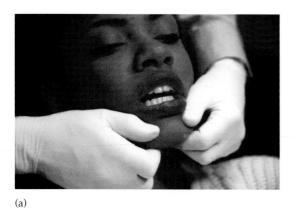

(a)

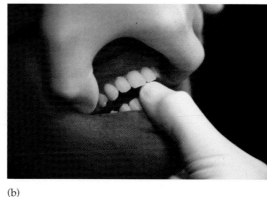

(b)

Fig 4.24

(a) Cradling the mandible from behind, the patient's jaw is 'eased' into a retruded (hinge) position (Dr Peter Dawson's method). (b) Using examiner's right thumbnail as a 'ramp', and interposing left finger and thumb slightly between posteriors, to help 'de-program' the habitual path of closure, retruded (hinge) position is readily located.

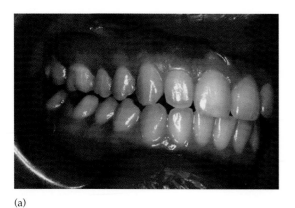

(a)

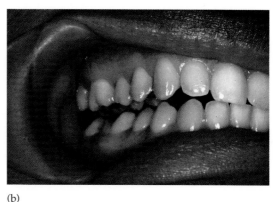

(b)

Fig 4.25

(a) The right working side occlusion is observed in right lateral excursion, the first few millimeters being the most significant, as that is the normal functional range in chewing strokes. (b) In left excursion, any balancing contact or interference on the right side is noted. The process is repeated for the patient's left side as well.

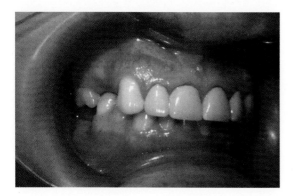

Fig 4.26

This patient had recently had six upper anterior crowns placed. Unfortunately the posterior occlusion, compromised by a combination of supereruption and overall loss of vertical dimension, was not addressed.

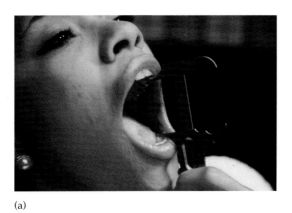

(a)

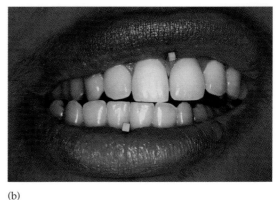

(b)

Fig 4.27

(a) Range of motion vertically – interincisal dimension on full unassisted opening – can be measured in millimeters or in finger-breadths. (b) Lateral range of motion sometimes requires cueing the patient to open slightly, allowing canines to clear, or a tongue blade or flat metal object (such as the bar of a vernier caliper) may be placed between anterior teeth for them to slide on. The green wedges shown here are just to illustrate midlines.

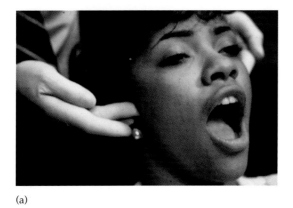

(a)

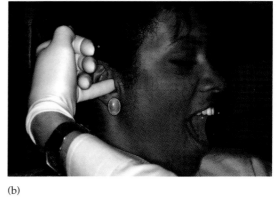

(b)

Fig 4.28

(a) Bilateral palpation of the joint during opening. The fingers are placed over the joints, and will fall into the glenoid fossae as the condyles translate forward in opening. With teeth slightly apart, ask the patient to move left and right to appreciate joint function in lateral excursions. (b) Subtle joint vibrations can sometimes be appreciated better by palpating via the external auditory meatus. Again, simultaneous (bilateral) palpation is desirable.

Myofunctional analysis

Myofunctional analysis includes the following: tongue function, especially in swallowing; lip function as to noxious habits, weak perioral musculature, incompetence in closure, etc; and any impediment or abnormality in speech.

Specific observable findings include tongue range of motion (ability to reach upper

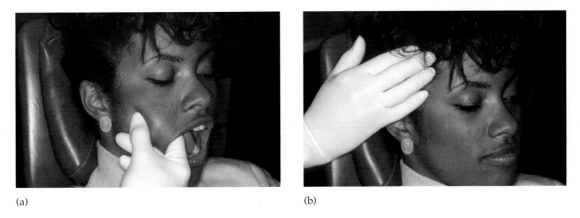

(a)   (b)

Fig 4.29

(a) Palpation (bimanual) of the masseter muscle. (b) Palpation (bilateral) of the temporalis muscles.

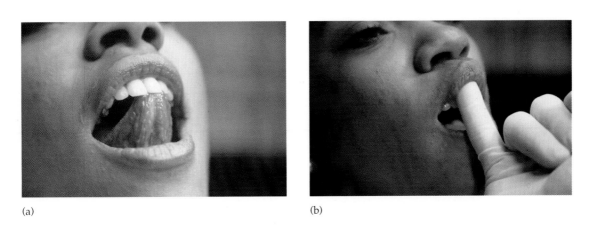

(a)   (b)

Fig 4.30

(a) The patient is asked to open slightly, then attempt to touch the upper teeth with the tongue (minimum range of normal), then to reach the tongue to cover first upper, then lower lip (preferable range of normal). (b) The examiner places the last (little) finger under the upper lip in a passive way, and asks the patient to tense the lip so as to pull it back off the examiner's finger. Normal lip muscle tone can accomplish this, weak upper lip muscles may not.

incisors with tongue) and upper lip strength (ability of patient to pull the upper lip down and off examiner's finger) (Fig 4.30).

5 OTHER DIAGNOSTIC CONSIDERATIONS

MODIFICATIONS FOR PEDIATRIC AND GERIATRIC PATIENTS

The routine systematic approach discussed so far applies to typical adult patients. There are some obvious modifications necessary when working with very young or very old individuals, which include the following:

PEDIATRIC CONSIDERATIONS

The major added emphasis in the pediatric oral examination is in the area of growth and development, keeping in mind that we can often intercept problems, remove harmful influences, and encourage positive factors if we recognize them early enough. These factors should be evaluated and considered carefully.

Space management

If crowding is suspected, a mixed dentition space analysis should be carried out. This will help predict whether there is sufficient arch length for the unerupted permanent teeth between erupted permanent incisors and erupted permanent 6-year molars. Just as pertinent here is an arch width assessment, using Schwartz's or Pont's indices. Although there is considerable debate over the potential for increasing arch width in the mandible, the maxilla offers great opportunity for expansion with various techniques and appliances, and relieving a constricted maxilla or deep anterior overbite may allow fuller development of the mandible.

Maxillo/mandibular relationship

Here again, it is possible at an early age to intervene and often correct a class II or class III before it becomes an established trait. In the early mixed dentition, about age 6–7, you can use a quick analysis based on deciduous second molar position (Fig 5.1).

Airway assessment

As it is absolutely critical to proper growth and development, upper airway competency, or the ability to breathe with the mouth closed should be determined. This can be done quickly in a number of ways, including observation of a forcible inhale with the mouth closed. The nares should flare. If they constrict, suspect a problem. A cold mirror placed under the nose will fog during nasal breathing. You can see differences in volume from one nostril to the other.

An unusual but effective test is to place your hand gently but firmly over the mouth (after explaining thoroughly to the child and parent the purpose of the exercise) and simply monitor whether the child can breathe comfortably through the nose for 2 minutes. This will help distinguish the 'habit' mouth breather from the true impeded airway mouth breather. Remove your hand if the child exhibits any distress.

If you suspect a significant airway problem further evaluation may be done with lateral head plate radiograph (cephalometric radiograph), and/or in consultation with a pediatrician or ear/nose/throat specialist. Allergies can play a major role, as can anatomic problems (deviated septum, impacted turbinates,

If upper and lower 'e's are in a flush terminal plane relationship,

Most will go into Class I (because the lower 'e' is larger than the upper, and if space allows, the lower six year molar will drift mesial more than the upper.)

Some will go into Class II (if space does not allow normal mesial drift, or heredity and other influences predispose to class II)

None will go into Class III

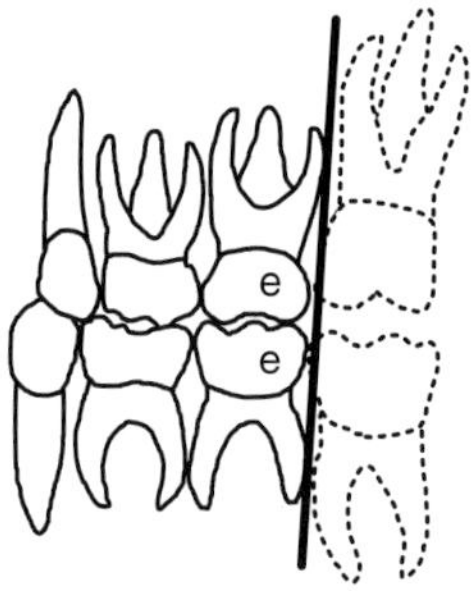

If lower 'e' is mesial to upper,

65% will go into Class III
35% will go into Class I

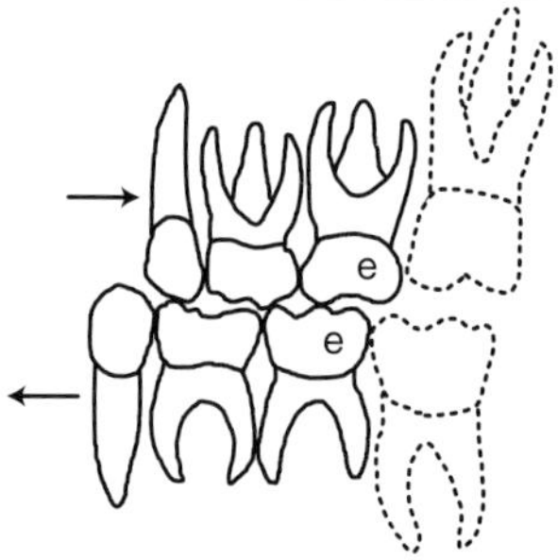

If upper 'e' is mesial to lower,

Expect to get 100% Class II

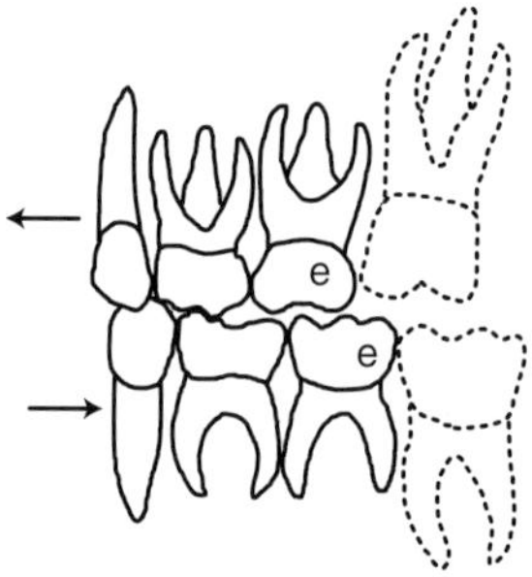

Fig 5.1

Deciduous second molar position just before eruption of first permanent molars can help predict their eventual Angle classification. Note especially the high tendency to class III when lower 'e' is mesial to upper, and the near certainty of permanent class II molar relationship when upper 'e' is mesial to lower.

enlarged adenoids, etc). Mouth breathing can have devastating effects on the growth, development, function, and health of the dentition. It must not be ignored.

Habits

Oral habits such as finger/thumb/pacifier or blanket sucking will alter normal growth and development and should be assessed. Also consider lip and cheek involvement, as the same biting or sucking habits will impact on the dentition. Sleeping with the hand under the face, or other postural habits, should also be investigated if abnormalities are observed.

Functional assessment

Look for tongue thrust or infantile swallow patterns (Fig 5.2), weak upper lip, poor lip competence (lips not closed at rest), and hyperactive mentalis during swallow. Test for normal tonicity and range of motion of:

- Upper lip – can patient curl it around and under upper teeth so the vermilion border disappears? Can patient exert normal force on examiner's finger under the upper lip?
- Tongue – can patient reach upper incisors with mouth open? Can patient extrude tongue down and over lower lip? Can patient place tip of tongue on rugae behind upper incisors, close lips, breathe nasally, and swallow easily with tip of tongue not moving forward? You can use a small orthodontic elastic on the tip of the tongue to determine this, but be prepared for some patients with incorrect swallows to swallow the elastic.

Finally, keep in mind that many of these pediatric findings are interrelated. It doesn't matter whether open bites produce tongue thrusts or the other way around as long as you recognize that there is a problem to be dealt with. The general practitioner who sees young patients *must* recognize problems of function, growth, and development, and be prepared to treat them or refer to others who will.

GERIATRIC CONSIDERATIONS

A growing segment of the population, elderly people are becoming more important to dentistry, especially as many more of them are retaining some or all of their teeth. If these patients are going to keep their teeth for a lifetime, then we must be aware of the dental problems unique to the aged, and deal with them effectively.

A geriatric oral examination should follow the same basic approach as any other adult examination, but with special emphasis given to the following:

Recession, root caries, erosion/abrasion/abfraction

Gingivae recede naturally with age, and management of the exposed root surface becomes critical in the dentate geriatric patient (Fig 5.3).

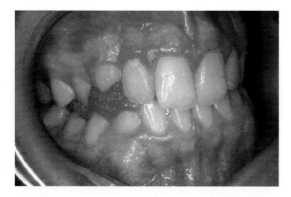

Fig 5.2

This lateral tongue thrust swallow creates functional as well as esthetic problems, and must be taken into account in any treatment plan.

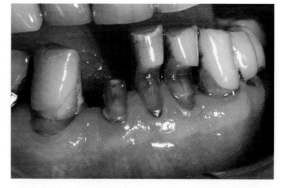

Fig 5.3

Loss of tooth structure at the gumline can be related to abrasive stresses (hard toothbrushing), chemical erosion (dietary acids or low oral pH), flexural stresses concentrated in the area (abfraction), and caries. Often these factors act in combination in the elderly patient.

Salivary flow and consistency

Age should not in itself diminish salivary secretions. More likely the daily intake of multiple medications among aged patients – any or all of which can reduce the amount or change the consistency of saliva – is responsible for significant problems in this area.

Oral hygiene limitations resulting from age or physical impairment

Common conditions such as arthritis or failing eyesight can reduce a patient's ability to remove plaque and maintain oral health. The general effects of aging will often compromise daily home care significantly.

Cracked teeth, non-vital teeth

Over time, simple wear and tear take its toll on the teeth, especially teeth already weakened as a result of earlier caries and multiple restorations. Loss of vital pulp tissue, even when asymptomatic, may leave teeth more susceptible to fracture.

Missing teeth, loss of vertical dimension, or arch space caused by tipping, supereruption, or flaring

These findings, common to many elderly patients, present special challenges in dental treatment planning. Considerable attention will be given to these situations in later chapters of this book (Fig 5.4).

Existing prostheses – fixed and/or removable

Such devices are more likely to be found among the elderly population, and we must note the age, condition, and fit of the existing

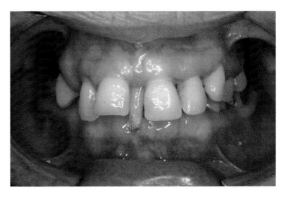

Fig 5.4

Loss of posterior support, even if not total, can result in compromised vertical dimension and complicate any dental treatment planning.

prostheses, and assess their potential for future service (prognosis), while considering the age and tolerance for treatment of the individual patient. Some people are good candidates for new full or partial dentures at an advanced age. Others – whose general systemic health is severely compromised, who are not able to tolerate much treatment, and who are not complaining about their existing prostheses (or lack thereof) – may be better off left alone.

Limitation of temporomandibular joint, secondary to osteoarthritis

Although arthritic temporomandibular joints are often seen radiographically without apparent symptoms, we must be aware of this problem, because limited opening can complicate both daily home care and dental treatment.

Considerations in the examination of edentulous or partially edentulous patients

The examination of these patients should include special notice of the following items:

- Vibrating line
- Tori
- Incisive papilla
- Type of ridge
- Retromolar pad
- Genial tubercle
- Relationship of arches
- Nasal spine
- Zygomatic arch
- Mental foramen
- Floor of mouth
- Nature of fornix
- Position, size, and tonus of tongue.

Surgical procedures may be indicated for the following:

- Bony spines
- Tori, exostoses
- Hyperplastic tissue
- Unerupted teeth
- Frenula
- Lesions
- Retained roots
- Severe undercuts.

OTHER DIAGNOSTIC CONSIDERATIONS

There are several other considerations that may come into play in the comprehensive examination, depending on the individual patient's situation. Some of the most common 'other' considerations are the evaluation of existing appliances, appropriate laboratory aids, diagnostic casts, diagnostic wax-ups, and photographs. Let's look at each, briefly and in turn.

EXISTING APPLIANCES

Patients may be wearing full or partial prostheses, orthodontic retainers, orthotic splints, or other intraoral appliances (Fig 5.5). All such devices should be assessed for the following.

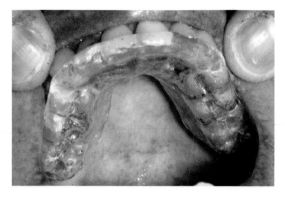

Fig 5.5

Patients of all ages may be using intraoral appliances whether they are prosthetic or therapeutic, such as this hard night guard employed to control bruxism.

Age

When was the appliance first placed? Have there been previous appliances placed? Has the appliance been altered, relined, or modified by a dentist or the patient?

Condition

Is the appliance intact, or have portions (clasps etc) been broken? Is it cracked? Does it show signs of wear, discoloration, or other deterioration?

Fit

Does it adapt well to the teeth and/or tissue? Does it harmonize with the occlusion? Is it comfortable to the patient? Does the patient wear the appliance and, if so, how much or how often?

Condition of the supporting tissue, the teeth, and ridge

What is the relationship of the oral structures to the appliance? What is the condition of

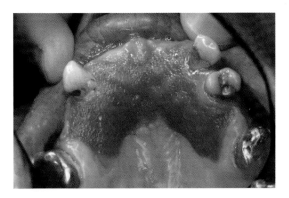

Fig 5.6

Severe erythematous reaction to a partial denture base material.

those structures in terms of health and disease? To what extent is the appliance contributing to that health or disease (Fig 5.6)?

Replacement of the appliance, or discontinuation of use, may need to be considered, depending on the results of this assessment. Judgments must often be made weighing the usefulness of the appliance in providing function, comfort, esthetics, or therapeutic benefit against its potential for harm.

LABORATORY AIDS

These generally fall into three categories: specific dental aids, systemic (medical) aids, and instructional or motivational aids.

Specific dental aids

These include, but are not limited to, the following:

- Biopsy/cytology of suspicious oral lesions. Although these provide accurate diagnostic information, they can be somewhat invasive and are quite likely to alarm the patient. Generally then, biopsy should not be performed unless suspicion of malignancy is high.
- Vital staining of suspicious oral lesions. A good example is the use of toluidine blue, marketed as OraScan and OraTest (Fig 5.7) which can be a valuable and non-invasive tool for screening suspicious lesions. Research demonstrates good diagnostic validity for this agent, and it may well become a standard tool for soft tissue diagnosis.
- Bacteriologic cultures may be especially useful as more bacteria become resistant to common antibiotics. Culture and sensitivity tests can ensure the selection of appropriate and effective antibiotics in cases of persistent or life-threatening oral/dental infections.
- Surface smears testing for *Candida albicans*, spirochetes, or other specific suspected non-bacterial organisms are available.
- DNA probes are being developed and marketed to identify specific infective organisms in periodontal pockets in order to select antibiotic regimens.
- Determination of fluoride level in non-fluoridated water supplies should be done when treating patients from birth to the age of 12, in order to select appropriate levels of supplemental fluoride for maximum caries prevention.
- There are many other tools and techniques, including various electronic and computer-related devices, which may be employed in the comprehensive examination, and they can be of some value in the diagnostic process.

    Unfortunately, many of the devices on the market lack solid research evidence of their validity, and may provide data that lack specificity and/or sensitivity, or that can be obtained more efficiently (and cheaply) by other, usually simpler means. Using such devices may not be contraindicated, but when significant fees are charged for measures and tests that are not scientifically validated, a real ethical problem arises.

The dentist should always choose diagnostics and treatments, the scientific validity and cost effectiveness of which have been well established.

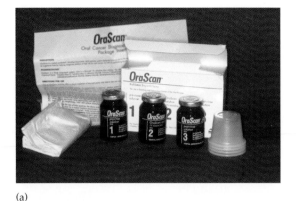

(a)

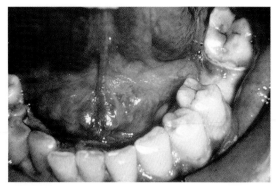

(b)

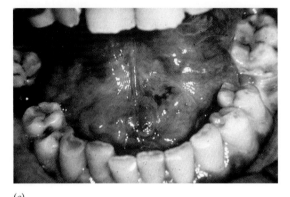

(c)

Fig 5.7

(a) Toluidine blue dye rinse is preceded by an acetic acid (vinegar) rinse to cleanse the mouth, and followed by another acetic acid rinse to clear the dye where it has not become affixed into a surface neoplasm. (b) A small red lesion in the floor of the mouth calls for further investigation. (c) Toluidine blue dye is strongly retained by the lesion, raising strong suspicions of malignancy. This lesion would be considered for biopsy and histologic evaluation.

Systemic (medical) aids

These include, but are certainly not limited to, the following:

- Immune assay hepatitis testing to determine, among other things, the patients' present hepatitis status, whether they have been exposed to, infected with, are immune to, or are carriers of various forms of the disease.
- HIV testing, which becomes critical in the event of a needle stick or other exposure to potentially bloodborne pathogens.
- Wasserman test for active syphilis, again as a protective measure when the patient's history is positive.
- Urinalysis screening for a number of systemic conditions, including the presence of sugars in the urine, a possible indication of diabetes.

- Glucose tolerance test, often used when urinalysis is positive, and which can diagnose diabetes more definitively.
- Blood count: in the routine hematology screen the complete blood count usually includes red blood cell count (RBC), hematocrit (Hct), hemoglobin (Hgb), white blood cell count (WBC), a differential white blood cell count (DIFF), blood smear for cell morphology, and a thrombocyte or platelet count.[1]

This is by no means an exhaustive discussion of currently available medical laboratory tests for various systemic conditions. Other texts (see Bibliography) address systemic medical laboratory tests and values in detail. I would advise caution in this area, however. As such tests are used for the detection and diagnosis of systemic problems not exclusive to the oral cavity, it is advisable to involve the patient's physician early in the diagnostic process. The reasons are twofold: first, the selection, ordering, and interpretation of such tests falls into the realm of medicine and, although the dentist may be both clinically competent and legally entitled to prescribe and interpret many of these tests, referral to a physician early in the process would reflect positively on the dentist's judgment if there are any medical or legal problems at a later date. Second, the very number and complexity of medical tests have mushroomed in recent years and will certainly continue to do so. Many physicians find it difficult to keep abreast of changes in medical technology. The dentist, who already faces the challenge of keeping abreast of developments in dentistry, is not likely to be able to keep up with internal and general medicine as well. Thus, if systemic problems are suspected on the basis of the history and/or oral examination, a physician might be in a better position to select the medical laboratory tests that are the most appropriate, current, scientifically valid, and time- and cost-effective. Dentists should be able to access information about medical laboratory tests and understand the implications that the results may have on dental disease and treatment.

Instructional or motivational aids

These have been employed in dentistry to help patients visualize their oral and dental disease processes, and motivate the necessary behavioral changes to control them.

- Caries activity tests of various types have long been used, with the current generation possessing a degree of scientific validity not always present in the past.
- Phase contrast microscopy is a visual tool that allows the patient to see the organisms present in the plaque, in hopes that the 'yuck' factor will encourage better brushing and flossing.
- Many other tests have come and gone from the marketplace that clearly lacked scientific validity, and which, if used to generate

fees, were most probably unethical. Various nutritional analyses, including bogus hair and nail analysis, resulting in the prescription (and outright sale) of vitamins and other supplements, are some outrageous examples of this practice.

DIAGNOSTIC CASTS

Diagnostic casts (study casts, study models) are very useful tools in the 'other' category, and have a wide range of applications in dental diagnosis and treatment planning. In many cases, they are as indispensable as dental radiographs. What follows is a brief discussion of diagnostic casts, how they may be related to one another (maxillomandibular) and to a temporomandibular joint analog (articulator), and some typical applications they have in the dental treatment planning.

Types of casts and bases

- 'Immediate:' if casts are needed in a hurry, impressions can be made with quick-setting irreversible hydrocolloid (alginate) impression material and poured in a quick-setting plaster or stone. Snap-Stone is an exceptionally fast material for this purpose. Useful casts for diagnosis, patient education, or even appliance fabrication can be produced in 10–15 minutes (Fig 5.8).
- Diagnostic: although the same impression material may be used, speed is not of the essence in producing a truly diagnostic set of casts. Carefully mixed alginate impression material (with few air bubbles) is used to make good impressions capturing full detail and anatomy. These impressions are poured in a vacuum-mixed, dimensionally accurate plaster or stone. This is the most common type of cast used in dental diagnosis and treatment planning (Fig 5.9).
- High accuracy: casts of exceptional detail and accuracy may be required in some situations, and may be produced by the use of reversible hydrocolloid or one of the

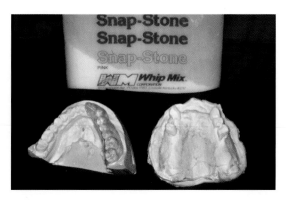

Fig 5.8

A 'quick' cast can be used to fabricate a 'pull-down' shell for temporary fabrication (left) or to produce an 'immediate' treatment partial denture following extraction (right).

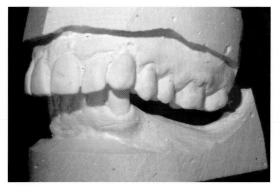

Fig 5.9

Quality diagnostic models have a great many uses in dental diagnosis and treatment planning.

many elastomeric impression materials (silicon, polyether, polyvinyl siloxane, etc). Poured in an improved stone (die quality), the resulting cast offers an extremely faithful reproduction of the oral hard and soft tissues impressed.

Depending on the intended use of the diagnostic casts, the bases developed for them may take a number of forms:

- Arbitrary: simply trimmed to eliminate gross excess and to permit viewing of the impressed area, arbitrary bases are most commonly seen. Such bases should not be so thick as to make the casts difficult to manipulate, or so thin as to be easily broken. Bases should not be left so broad as to complicate storage or mounting, or trimmed so closely as to lose portions of the duplicated teeth and tissue to the model trimmer.
- Orthodontically trimmed: bases can be made more useful if they are orthodontically trimmed. Once the casts are grossly trimmed (arbitrarily), they are articulated by hand or with a wax wafer bite, and placed together on a model trimmer (Fig 5.10). The distal aspects of both upper and lower model bases are then trimmed until

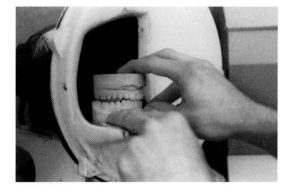

Fig 5.10

Trimming the distal aspect of articulated models will facilitate hand articulation of these orthodontically trimmed models.

both are flush with the grinding wheel. The result is that such casts can be placed back down on a flat surface and, when brought together, they will be immediately re-articulated in occlusion. This technique is especially useful when casts are not going to be mounted on an articulator, or when missing teeth and/or malocclusion makes their articulation by hand problematic.

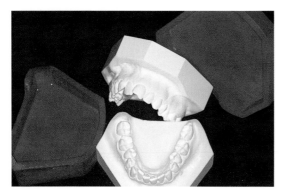

Fig 5.11

Orthodontic-quality model bases and the tray formers employed to produce them.

- Base formers: casts intended for display or archival purposes may be made more uniform and attractive in appearance through the use of base formers. In this technique, the casts are initially poured without a base, but with retention loops or plaster lobules to secure a second pour. The cast is then set into freshly mixed plaster or stone in the former, and the resulting bases are sharp and uniform (Fig 5.11). Upper and lower bases can be oriented so that the backs are flush when the casts are articulated, just as they are in orthodontically trimmed casts.
- Split casts: another modification of a cast base is the split cast, in which the initial base is kept thin and indexed with 'V' grooves. A separating medium is applied, and a second pour of a contrasting color stone is added to the base. Trimmed flush and separated, the split cast is useful in mounting to various 'check bite' articulators using wax records of various maxillomandibular relationships (Fig 5.12).

Relating the diagnostic casts

Casts may be related to one another and/or to an articulator simulating the temporomandibular joint apparatus. Models can often

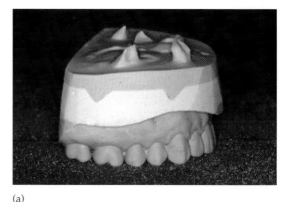

(a)

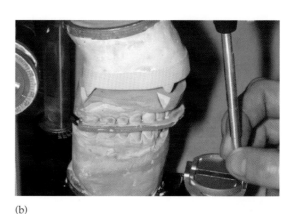

(b)

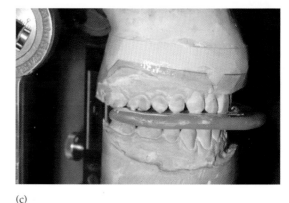

(c)

Fig 5.12

(a) Split casts use contrasting stone to allow separation, and later reunion. (b) After initial mounting, split casts are separated, and protrusive and/or lateral records are firmly related to the occlusal surfaces of the models. (c) Articulator elements are manipulated until the split casts reunite, producing an analog of temporomandibular joint movements.

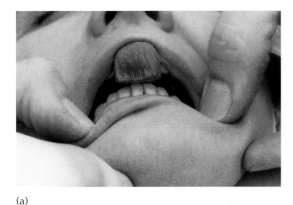

(a)

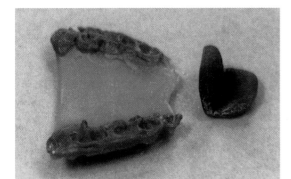

(b)

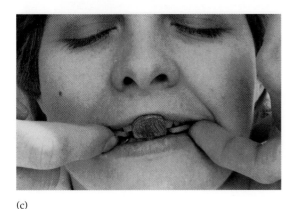

(c)

Fig 5.13

(a) Anterior acrylic jig is seated over upper anteriors; lower anteriors then contact on inclined plane tending to retrude the mandible into a centric relation (RP) position. (b) Centric relation corrected wax record showing anterior cut away for jig. (c) Wax record being tried in mouth with jig in place.

be simply articulated by hand, provided that centric occlusion is well established, and does not differ greatly from centric relation. Casts can be marked, or trimmed orthodontically, to record this relationship. If missing teeth or malocclusion makes the relationship difficult, an interocclusal bite registration, made of wax or elastomeric bite material, should be taken in the mouth to be used later to approximate the casts. This record can be critical to the dentist's assessment of the occlusion, and should be made carefully. The bite may be in centric occlusion (IP), with teeth brought together through the bite medium into full closure, or it may be at a slightly open vertical, with mandible retruded to centric relation (RP, hinge position). This type of bite is preferable in cases where CO and CR do not coincide, and can be combined with a hinge axis location to replicate and study the discrepancy.

Obtaining such a retruded record is made easier with the fabrication and use of an anterior acrylic 'jig' (Fig 5.13), fabricated from cold cure acrylic molded directly onto upper incisors (it is helpful to lubricate the teeth/tissue first). After hardening, the jig is trimmed, smoothed, and contoured so that it provides an inclined ramp for lower anteriors to contact in the retruded position, with the posterior teeth held just slightly apart. This assists in positioning the mandible in its retruded position, and can be used while taking the bite recording by cutting away the anterior section of the bite wafer. The bite is then taken with the patient making light contact on the jig, the wax or other recording material being dead soft and thereby reducing or eliminating any reflex proprioceptive shifting of the mandible into habitual centric.

Casts can be studied more easily by mounting them on an articulator. Arbitrary mountings are generally used on simple-hinge articulators, or on non-plaster articulators such as the Galetti (Fig 5.14). Arbitrary mountings can also be used with semiadjustable instruments such as the Whip-Mix. However, a more accurate emulation of the occlusion can be obtained by use of a transfer bow to capture the patient's approximate hinge axis and its relationship to the maxillary teeth (Fig 5.15).

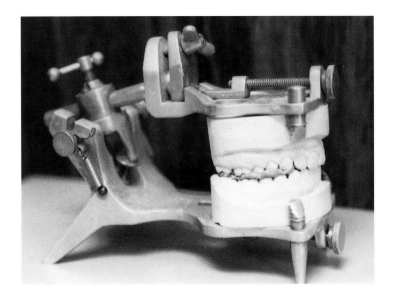

Fig 5.14

Casts are clamped to upper and lower members of this Galetti articulator.

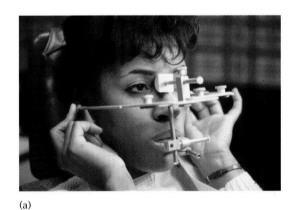

(a)

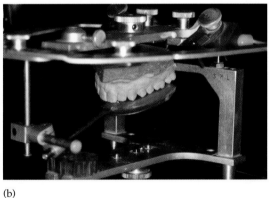

(b)

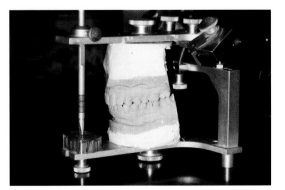

(c)

Fig 5.15

(a) The transfer bow of this Whip-Mix articulator uses ear plugs and Frankfort plane indicator to orient the maxillary model to condylar analogs. (b) The bow is brought to the articulator, oriented parallel to the floor, and the maxillary model is set into the wax bite. (c) Using a centric relation bite record, the mandibular cast is then related to the maxillary to complete the process.

Accurate articulation of diagnostic casts

Both diagnostic casts and working models require accurate articulation to be of the greatest use to the dentist and technician. In ascending order of sophistication and accuracy, the following are some alternative methods for relating casts to each other and to the articulator:

- The centric occlusion bite record with arbitrary hinge axis location.
- The centric relation bite record with arbitrary hinge axis location and transfer. If one is going to use a transfer bow to relate the maxillary cast to the articulator, the bite record might as well be taken in retruded (CR, RP) position without tooth contact so as to provide some indication of discrepancies. Methods of establishing an arbitrary hinge axis include, but are not limited to, the following:
  - palpation of condylar head in opening movements, and approximating hinge axis by that palpation
  - location of a point 10–11 mm anterior to the tragus of the ear along a line from the tragus to the canthus of the eye
  - relating hinge position to the external auditory meatus, either directly, using ear 'plugs' on a transfer bow (such as the Whip-Mix illustrated in Fig 5.15), or manually drawing the tragus anteriorly, and putting an arbitrary mark just anterior to the meatus.
- The centric relation bite record with actual location of hinge axis by means of a bow attached to the mandible, with fine pointers over the approximate hinge location. The bow and pointers are adjusted until retruded opening/closing of the mouth rotates about a singe point, which is then marked indelibly for transfer reference. This is the truest approximation of the hinge position and, when combined with a semi- or fully adjustable articulator capable of accepting lateral records, an excellent analog is created.

- The centric relation bite record with use of a fully adjustable articulator is certainly the most sophisticated approach in relating casts. This articulator employs pantograph tracings or multiple check-bites to emulate mandibular movements in the fossa, including Bennett shift. This articulator is also fairly specialized, time consuming, and in most cases impractical for day-to-day diagnosis and treatment planning.

DIAGNOSTIC WAX-UPS

Diagnostic wax-ups, a further application of diagnostic casts, are used in diagnosis and treatment planning in a number of ways. Alterations can be made to casts to represent proposed changes in tooth size, shape, or position. Such wax-ups assist in planning treatment options, presenting plans and options to patients, and communicating with laboratory technicians. Fig 5.16 illustrates the use of wax-ups to plan the esthetics and function of an anterior fixed bridge. Another application of diagnostic wax-up is also illustrated (Fig 5.17).

PHOTOGRAPHS

Clinical photographs taken with a 35mm camera or specially adapted Polaroid camera, or digital images obtained with intraoral video equipment, can be valuable in diagnosis and planning, in documentation of care, and in case presentation. The illustrations throughout this book provide a great many examples of the use of clinical photographs.

REFERENCE

1. Bricker S, Langlais R, Miller S, *Oral diagnosis oral medicine and treatment planning*. Lea & Febiger: Philadelphia, PA, 1994.

Fig 5.16

Using a diagnostic wax-up to solve esthetic and functional restorative problems. (a) This 18-year-old man traumatically avulsed central incisors some years previously. Pontic space is insufficient for normal size central incisors, the right lateral incisor is rotated, and the right canine is in end-to-end contact with the lower. (b) Diagnostic casts are articulated and teeth prepared as for abutment crowns. (c) A diagnostic wax-up is developed that is both functionally and esthetically acceptable. (d) The wax-up is duplicated, and a plaster model made, which is the precursor of the clinical prosthesis.

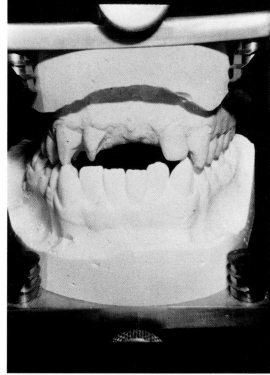

(b)

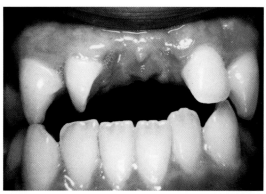

(a)

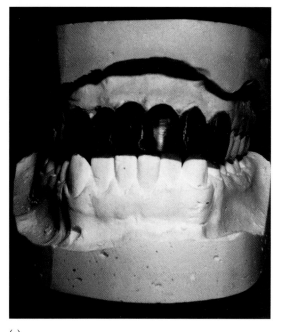

(c)

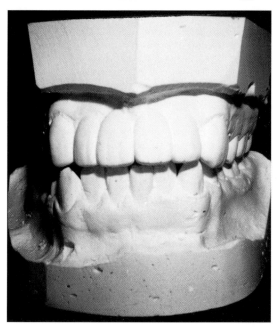

(d)

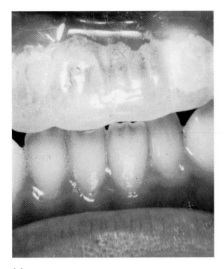

(e)

Fig 5.16 *continued*

(e) A celluloid 'pull-down' shim is fabricated to serve both as a guide for reduction in the preparation, and as a former for the temporary bridge. (f) The clinical prosthesis, a porcelain fused to gold fixed bridge, demonstrating the addition of canine lateral guidance to the working side group function, anterior group function in protrusive, and modification of the original steep canine disclusion into anterior group function in left lateral. (g) An acceptable esthetic and functional result has been achieved with the use of a pre-treatment diagnostic wax-up.

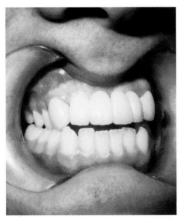 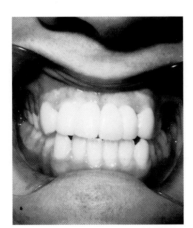 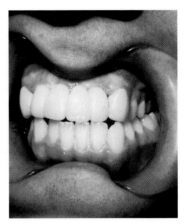

(f)

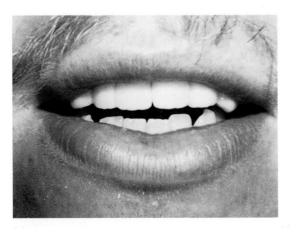

(g)

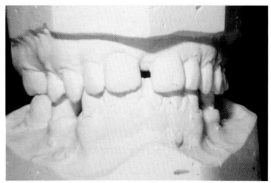

(a)

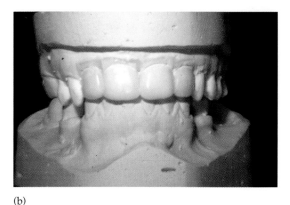

(b)

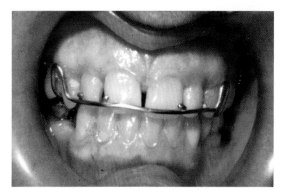

(c)

Fig 5.17

(a) Anterior esthetics can be pre-planned with the use of a diagnostic wax-up. Here a proposed diastema closure is complicated by wide central incisors and narrow lateral incisors. (b) The diagnostic wax-up anticipates a combination of orthodontics to distribute space among the incisors, followed by bonded restorations on all four incisors. This approach is carried out on the diagnostic casts before the start of clinical treatment, both to allow the patient to see and approve the projected result, and to assist the clinician in carrying out the treatment. (c) Removable orthodontic appliance in place, partially closing diastema space and distributing excess space among incisors.

DIAGNOSIS

The essence of diagnosis is identifying precisely what is happening and why; it is not, as is too often assumed, assigning a technical or scientific name to a clinical picture. Although we sometimes do assign such names when making a diagnosis, it is critical that we keep the entire picture in mind when selecting treatment. So many dental patients present with multiple interrelated problems that a single diagnosis may not lead to the appropriate treatment.

Take the medical diagnosis of 'acute appendicitis.' Beginning with the complaint of acute abdominal pain, a process of differential diagnosis is used to rule out other possible diagnoses, and make the appendicitis diagnosis definitive. The sequence might begin with palpation revealing exquisite tenderness over the lower left quadrant, fever, and malaise. Blood tests including white blood count might point to bacterial infection, and a radiograph or other imaging could confirm a greatly enlarged appendix.

Once this diagnosis is established, some very specific treatment options present themselves, such as aggressive antibiotic therapy and appendectomy. The diagnosis is finally confirmed histologically when the offending appendix is studied, first grossly and then under the microscope.

Compare this with the diagnosis of 'moderate periodontitis.' Beginning with a complaint of bleeding gums, some of the same differential process may occur (ruling out blood dyscrasias, for example) but the clinical appearance of periodontal tissues, measurement of pocket depths around the teeth, and radiographic evidence of bone loss quickly confirm the diagnosis.

Treatment options are not, however, immediately suggested by the diagnosis alone.

We wouldn't even consider making specific treatment recommendations unless we know a great deal more about the extent, past history, and contributing factors to the disease, unless we know more about the patient's general health and ability/willingness to participate in treatment, and unless we assess the occlusion and existing restorations or prostheses.

Diagnosis in dental practice must then address both the differential diagnosis of a specific disease or lesion, and the multifactorial or problem list model which is often more appropriate in general dentistry. We will consider both models, with examples offered for purposes of illustration.

DIFFERENTIAL – MEDICAL MODEL

In this model, the patient presents with certain signs and symptoms. The practitioner elicits the chief complaint, its history (present illness), and a general history as well (symptoms). A careful examination of the patient documents all pertinent signs. From the data collected, a clinical picture is developed of the patient's disease which can be compared with similar pictures of known disease states. An algorithm, or decision tree, is often used to narrow the possibilities to a more workable differential group. Further tests are selected to rule out some, and confirm other, possible diagnoses. Skill and experience on the part of the practitioner may make it possible to narrow the field more rapidly, reducing the number (and cost) of tests required to make a definitive diagnosis.

This model is pertinent in certain areas of dental diagnosis. Discrete soft tissue lesions are diagnosed in this manner, as is acute dental pain. Signs, symptoms, and history are assembled to form the clinical picture. An astute dentist may even be able to differentiate an acute serous pulpitis from an acute purulent pulpitis, based on the signs and symptoms. In such a case, however, the medical model may not serve to determine appropriate treatment.

We know that acute pulpitis is irreversible and requires either extraction or endodontic treatment. The choice of treatment, however, depends on a multitude of factors such as the patient's general dental condition, attitude, ability to pay, and desire for treatment. The strategic value of the tooth in question, its periodontal status, and how it relates to the overall dentition will all impact on treatment choices.

Nor does the medical model always serve in etiologic assessment. An acute pulpitis may have a specific bacterial etiology, which could be confirmed by culture. But how did the infective organism reach the pulp? If via a carious lesion, then dental caries is the actual etiology. Remembering that caries is very much behaviorally related, then lack of effective plaque control may be the real culprit, perhaps abetted by a high sugar diet. Envision three painful teeth each diagnosed as having acute pulpitis. A second molar may have been

cariously invaded. A first premolar in traumatic occlusion as a result of lack of canine or anterior guidance may have developed an infrabony periodontal defect, leading to bacterial invasion through accessory canals in the furcation. A central incisor, devitalized by a traumatic injury many years previous, may have become host to an opportunistic microbe during a transient bacteremia. It is necessary to supplement the medical model with other intellectual approaches, other strategies to determine what is happening and why. These other approaches are designed for oral health maintenance, rather than oral disease management. They apply to the many diseases and disorders, often chronic, often asymptomatic, which represent a large part of the typical dental practice. Given that, let's consider some examples of how the medical model does apply in dentistry, using case histories and some of the possible diagnostic algorithms available.

RED LESION

This patient (Fig 6.1a) presents with multiple red vesicular lesions. Using the algorithm for red lesions (Fig 6.2) we differentiate the condition as generalized rather than solitary, and as

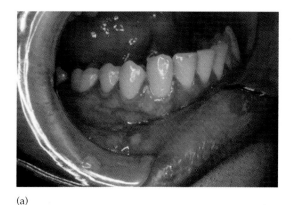

(a)

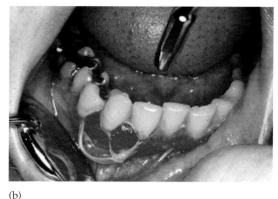

(b)

Fig 6.1

(a) Multiple red vesicular lesions. (b) Epithelium sloughs easily. In this case, a blast of air demonstrates a positive Nikolsky's sign.

exhibiting other clinical signs. Vesicle formation is evident, which leads to differentiation by a positive Nikolsky's sign (Fig 6.1b), and the final differential cluster of pemphigus, and benign mucous membrane pemphigoid or BMMP.

Another patient presents with a small solitary red lesion in the floor of the mouth

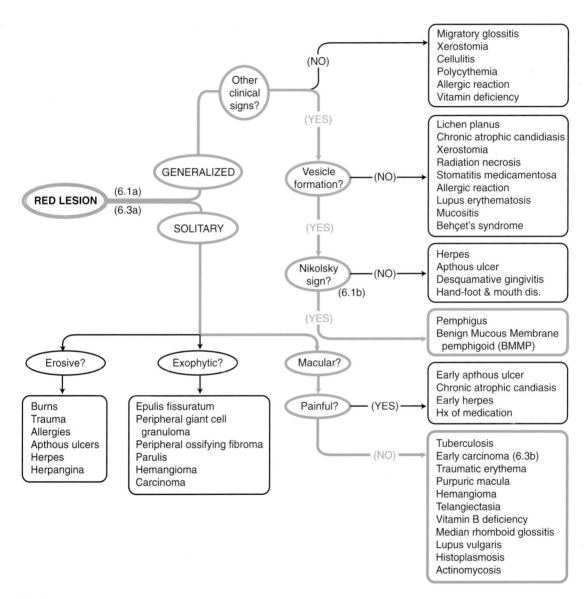

Fig 6.2

Algorithm for red lesions. First differential: generalized versus solitary. The differential lists (in boxes) in all the algorithms presented are arranged in approximate order of likelihood, for example, a generalized pattern of red surface lesions and no other clinical signs is more likely to be migratory glossitis (first of the differentials), than polycythemia, allergy, or vitamin deficiency. Note: there are many such algorithms for differential diagnosis, and no single schema is the 'right' one. Likewise, diseases may not always present in such as way as to fit neatly into a given scheme.

(Fig 6.3a) which, again using the algorithm, we describe as macular, rather than erosive or exophytic. Being non-painful to palpation, we find a large cluster of possibilities from which to differentiate. In the absence of any systemic findings suggesting tuberculosis, potential for malignancy is tested with toluidine blue (see Chapter 5, page 66–67). Retention of the dye in the lesion (Fig 6.3b) gives a tentative diagnosis of early carcinoma, which would be confirmed through biopsy.

WHITE LESION

These two patients (Fig 6.4) present with white surface lesions. Using the algorithm for white lesions (Fig 6.5) we find that neither lesion can be wiped off with gauze, and both mucosal surfaces appear keratotic, not normal, abraded, or ulcerated. Both are flat, but the upper lip lesion is clearly thickened, whereas the lesion in the floor of the mouth is more plaque like. Note that the algorithm

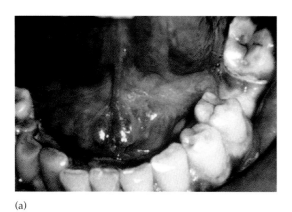

(a)

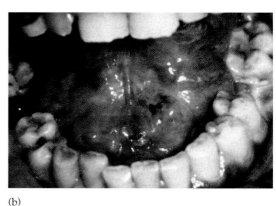

(b)

Fig 6.3

(a) A solitary flat (macular) lesion in the floor of the mouth. (b) Being non-painful, and lacking any systemic indication of tuberculosis, the lesion is stained with toluidine blue, producing a strong positive result, suggesting a malignancy. Biopsy confirms squamous cell carcinoma.

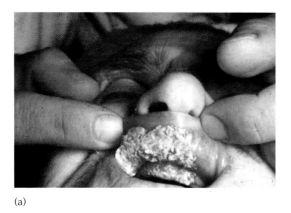

(a)

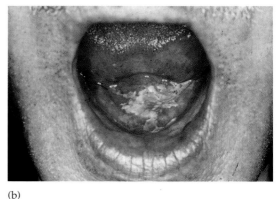

(b)

Fig 6.4

(a) This white lesion does not wipe off with gauze. The surface is keratotic and flat, but thickened rather than plaque like. White sponge nevus is the histologic diagnosis. (b) Another non-wipable white lesion, flat and keratotic, but not elevated. This plaque-like lesion was described histologically as 'clinical leukoplakia,' without malignant changes.

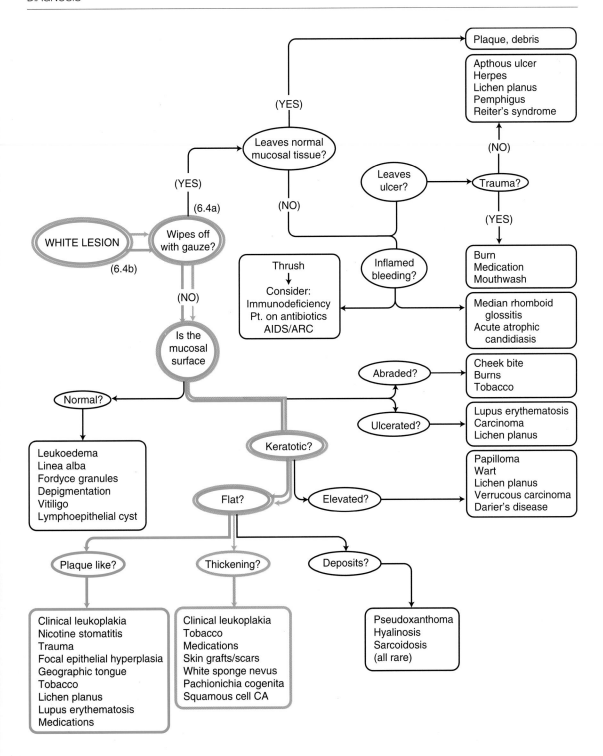

Fig 6.5

Algorithm for white lesions. First differential: wipable versus non-wipable.

offers a number of possible diagnoses, and they often overlap. On histological examination, the lip lesion was determined to be a white sponge nevus, whereas the floor of the mouth was described histologically as clinical leukoplakia.

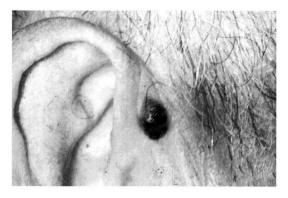

Fig 6.6

This pigmented (blue, brown, black) lesion was solitary and non-palpable. Histologic diagnosis of 'compound nevus' ruled out malignancy.

BLUE (BROWN, BLACK) LESION

This pigmented lesion (Fig 6.6) is both solitary and non-palpable. Using the algorithm for pigmented lesions (Fig 6.7) we find a cluster including various nevi and ephelis (freckle). Based on the clinical picture, the presumptive diagnosis is a nevus, which subsequently was histologically diagnosed as a compound nevus.

ORAL ULCER OR FISSURE

This lesion in the floor of the mouth (Fig 6.8a) is clearly an ulcer, which the patient had noticed recently for the first time a few weeks after insertion of a relined lower full denture.

Using the algorithm for oral ulcers/fissures (Fig 6.9) we note that the ulcer is well circumscribed, which offers a number of possible options, the most likely of which is trauma, confirmed by a 10-day follow-up after relieving the denture, showing complete resolution of the lesion (Fig 6.8b).

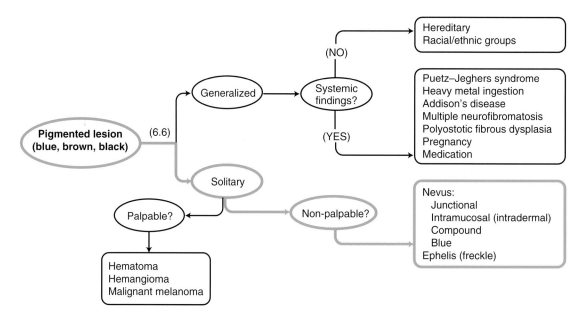

Fig 6.7

Algorithm for pigmented lesions. First differential: generalized versus solitary.

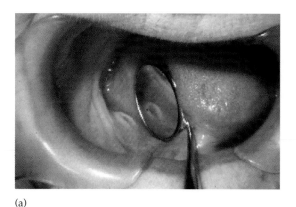 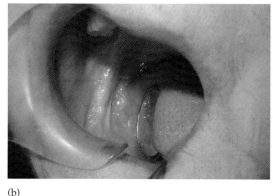

(a)   (b)

Fig 6.8

(a) An ulcer in the posterior floor/lateral tongue region. Differentiated as an ulcer rather than a fissure or erosive lesion, and as a new feature, which is well circumscribed. (b) Suspecting a traumatic etiology, the lower denture is adjusted and worn sparingly for a week or two. Resolution of the lesion confirms trauma as the diagnosis.

HEAD AND NECK – NODES OR SWELLINGS

This swelling in the floor of the mouth (Fig 6.10a) is palpated, and found to be soft and fluctuant. The patient reported tenderness to palpation, and a rapid onset of the swelling, which the patient notices most at mealtimes. Using the algorithm for head and neck swellings (Fig 6.11), we find a presumptive diagnosis of blocked salivary duct, in the submandibular region. This may often be confirmed with a radiograph revealing salivary calculi (Fig 6.10b).

TOOTH PAIN

Dental pain must often be differentially diagnosed. This patient (Fig 6.12a) presents with upper right molar pain solicited primarily by biting, and occasionally by cold. The pain is initially unpleasant but tolerable, and generally passes quickly. A periapical radiograph was unremarkable, and both teeth numbers 2 and 3 had sound conservative occlusal amalgam restorations. Using the algorithm for tooth pain developed by de Guzman and Frick (Fig 6.13) we begin with a presumption (and hope) of reversible pulpal

hyperemia, and start to rule out a number of factors. The following factors were assessed: selective biting pain – none elicited clinically; defective restoration/open margin/caries – none found. There was no history of thermal hypersensitivity, no exposed dentin, and restorations had been present and asymptomatic for many years. The patient did exhibit some wear facets, and slight reaction to percussion was elicited.

The teeth were minimally adjusted to relieve occlusion and symptoms abated for some time. Within 2 months, however, severe unsolicited pain was arising in the same area, resulting in medical assessments for possible trigeminal neuralgia or even brain tumor. When those results came back negative, the patient returned to the dental office, where again no clear clinical signs were evident. As an investigative measure the amalgam restorations were removed from teeth nos 2 and 3, and only then was a fine fracture line evident in the pulpal floor of no. 2, running mesial to distal through the center of the tooth. No movement or separation at the fracture line was apparent.

With a new diagnosis of cracked tooth, a temporary acrylic crown was placed to immobilize the fracture, and the symptoms abated over night! After 6 weeks, impressions

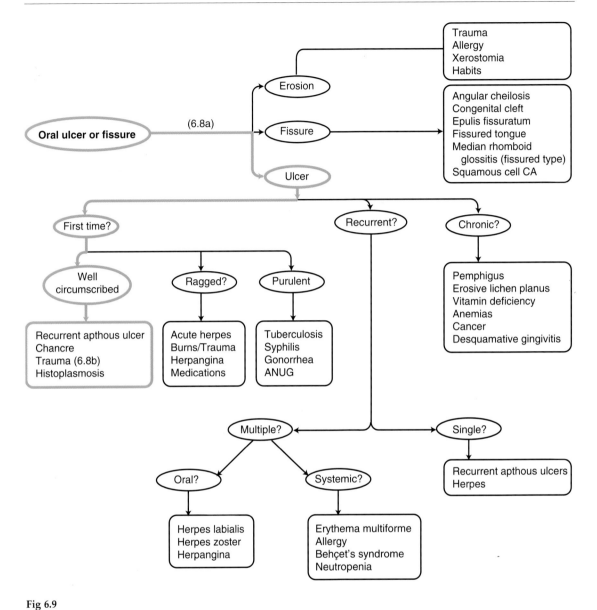

Fig 6.9

Algorithm for ulcers/fissures. First differential: ulcer versus fissure versus erosion. Ulcers are further differentiated by chronicity, that is, new, recurrent, or chronic. If 'first time' ulcers do not resolve but become chronic, malignancy becomes a differential to rule in/out.

were made, and a cast crown was fabricated and then cemented (Fig 6.12b). Endodontic therapy was considered inevitable, but deferred pending the return of symptoms. The tooth remained fully functional and asymptomatic for 6 years. At that time, the crown became debonded revealing that the fracture had clearly worsened, as the two sides of the tooth were movable across the fracture line. The prognosis now being hopeless, the crown was nevertheless recemented with the recommendation that the

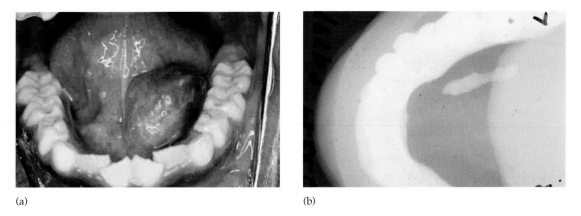

(a)   (b)

Fig 6.10

(a) Swelling in the floor of the mouth palpates as soft and fluctuant, with pain/tenderness reported by the patient. (b) Both timing (rapid onset associated with mealtimes) and location suggest a salivary gland problem, and this mandibular occlusal film confirms a blocked submandibular salivary duct with a large stone visible on radiograph.

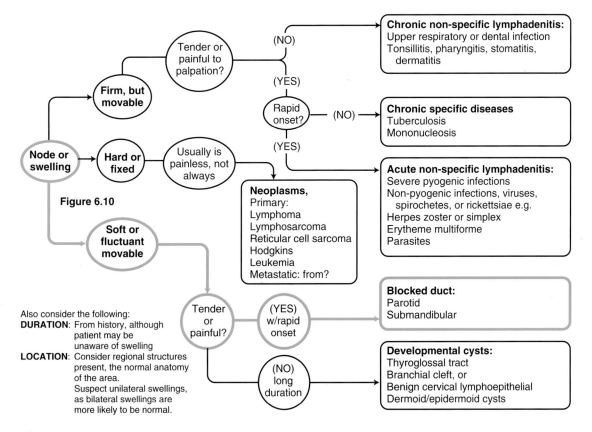

Fig 6.11

Algorithm for head and neck swellings. First differential: consistency on palpation – firm but movable, hard and fixed, soft/fluctuant and movable. Note that hard, fixed swellings may represent neoplasms and must be carefully assessed.

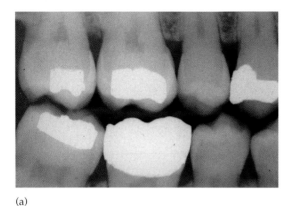

(a)

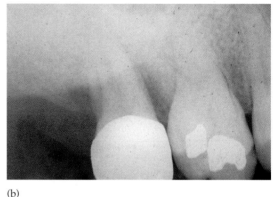

(b)

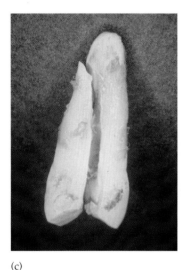

(c)

Fig 6.12

(a) Bite wing radiograph of right posterior (December 1993) revealing no caries or other radiographic pathology. Pain symptoms progressed, with lancinating facial pain radiating over the right face and temple. Medical assessment ruled out tic douloureux and tumor, leading back to the dental office for another look. Exploratory excavations of nos 2 and 3 revealed a crack running mesial–distal in the pulpal floor of no. 2. (b) Eight months (December 1994) after the cracked upper second molar was crowned to immobilize the fracture, the tooth remained asymptomatic and radiographically within normal limits. Anticipated endodontic therapy had not been necessary, and watchful waiting continued. (c) Although the tooth in question remains in function as of this writing, its fate is sealed, and it will probably look like this specimen, which is included here for illustration.

tooth be extracted when symptoms arose. The tooth is still in service at this writing (7 years after initial diagnosis) but its fate is clearly sealed, as suggested by Fig 6.12c.

PROBLEM LIST – DENTAL MODEL

In this model, the patient may present with a chief complaint, and we may use a differential process to identify the cause or source, but we go further, fully examining and assessing the orodental conditions present to develop a problem list – or multifactorial diagnosis.

Some of the factors in that list may relate back to the patient's presenting complaint, some may not. In some cases, there may not be a specific presenting complaint, or some minor concern of the patient is the catalyst in seeking a dental 'check-up.' A comprehensive examination using a routine systematic approach is then used to assess the dental patient thoroughly, and to develop a list of findings that need attention.

The goal of the problem list is to identify all conditions that require treatment in order to establish and maintain good oral and dental health, as well as those conditions that will impact significantly on how we will treat the

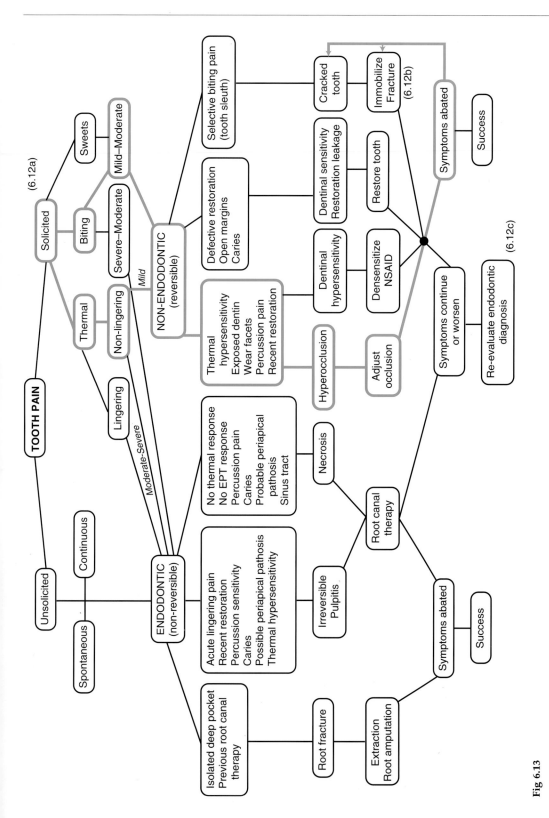

Fig 6.13

Algorithm for tooth pain. First differential: solicited versus unsolicited. This algorithm does not address radiographic findings, because any clear apical or lateral radiolucency on radiograph is highly suggestive of late-stage irreversible pulpitis. The algorithm suggests treatment options and, as illustrated by the case history cited, is subject to re-evaluation as clinical findings change. (Drs de Guzman and Frick, 1996).

patient (such as allergies to common dental therapeutic agents, requirements for premedication, compromised response to infection, and the like).

To develop such a list the clinician must 'know the normal,' and recognize deviations from the norm. Those deviations must be accurately described, and then analyzed as to their significance. This process is applied throughout each step of the comprehensive examination, and what emerges is a multifactorial diagnosis, or a list of problems arising in each of the general areas covered in the examination. Let's consider these areas, and look at the possible diagnoses that may be made in each of them.

GENERAL SYSTEMIC DIAGNOSIS

From our general appraisal and medical history, a thumbnail sketch should be made of the patient's general systemic condition. This general diagnosis should include any findings that may have significance in dental or oral conditions, or in dental treatment. The following are some typical examples of general systemic diagnoses:

These thumbnail sketches summarize and highlight the comprehensive medical history and general appraisal, and should encapsulate those findings that are likely to impact on dental treatment. In many cases the general systemic findings may contain nothing of dental significance and will not be a factor in our diagnosis. In other cases the complexity and severity of a patient's systemic problems may preclude any or all but the most urgent dental treatment. Where there is an impact, systemic findings will influence dental treatment in one of the following three ways:

Direct influence

Diabetes may affect the severity of periodontal disease, or loss of salivary flow may predispose to increased caries. In both examples, the general systemic problem directly impacts on dental disease and treatment. Less obvious might be a case of severe arthritis inhibiting a patient's plaque control, thereby aggravating plaque-related dental diseases.

- Normal healthy 30-year-old woman with an allergy to penicillin and gastric intolerance to aspirin and erythromycin.
- An 18-year-old man, a brittle diabetic on daily injectable insulin. Rather obese; his diet is not well controlled. Appears apathetic and is difficult to engage in communication.
- Severely debilitated 68-year-old man with history of lymphatic cancer. Has had chemotherapy and irradiation of head and neck. His attitude is positive and he is concerned about both appearance and function of his teeth.
- A 53-year-old woman who is menopausal, on estrogen replacement therapy, and who smokes heavily (2 packs/day). She is rather defensive and emotional, has a history of frequent headaches for which there is no established etiology.
- Normal healthy 82-year-old woman with history of arthritis, controlled fairly well with aspirin (8–12 tabs/day). Some hypertension noted with blood pressure recorded at 180/100.

Indirect influence

A history of mitral valve prolapse or an allergy to a commonly used dental therapeutic agent influence dental treatment indirectly, that is, they require a response on our part (prescription of prophylactic antibiotic; avoidance of the allergen, or selection of an alternative therapy) but they do not impact directly on the actual dental diagnosis or treatment.

Reverse influence

Some general systemic findings may actually be the result of dental or oral disease. Headache, earache, and associated head and neck symptoms may arise from occlusal or temporomandibular disorders. Sore throat may be secondary to pericoronitis around a partially erupted third molar. A persistent sinus infection may be linked to chronic pulpitis in an upper molar.

The extent to which a systemic finding will influence dental treatment often depends on what type of treatment is contemplated. Bleeding disorders, haemophilias of various types, may not be significant if one needs simple operative dentistry but would be a critical indirect influence if multiple extractions are indicated.

Since we don't establish a plan of treatment until the diagnosis is fully developed, the general systemic diagnosis should include any findings that may have direct, indirect, or reverse influence on dental treatment.

SOFT TISSUE DIAGNOSIS

From our examination of the external head and neck, lymph chain palpation, and the intraoral soft tissue examination, any significant findings are noted. This would include, but not be limited to, the following:

- Lesions
- Swellings or nodules

- Asymmetry
- Abnormal color or surface texture
- Pain or tenderness to palpation.

If the findings and their history are readily explainable and fairly innocuous, for example, a palatal ulcer that the patient tells us is a result of eating hot pizza, we may not even include them in our summary soft tissue diagnosis. Findings that may be significant because of their clinical appearance and history, for example, a unilateral swelling in the floor of the mouth which comes and goes, should be briefly summarized. The following are examples of soft tissue diagnoses that correspond to some of the examples cited in the discussion of differential diagnosis above (see Figs 6.1–6.11):

- Multiple vesicular erythematous lesions of the mucosa and gingivae, positive Nikolsy's sign, tentative diagnosis: likely pemphigus or BMMP (see Fig 6.1).
- White irregular surface lesion in the floor of the mouth, non-wipable with gauze, painless, keratotic, plaque like, needs reassessment and possible biopsy (see Fig 6.4b).
- Small (1 cm diameter) painless, well circumscribed ulcer in right posterior floor/lateral tongue. Patient had been unaware of it. Adjust denture and reassess in 7–10 days (see Fig 6.8a).
- Soft fluctuant swelling with tenderness in left floor of mouth and submandibular lymphatics, of recent onset. Radiograph confirms sialolith as source of 'ranula' (see Fig 6.10).

Significant soft tissue findings may demand immediate attention (for example, suspected malignancies), or may be watched and re-evaluated over time (for example, fibromas and the like). In many cases soft tissue abnormalities may be related to other factors in the diagnosis (for example, lymphadenopathy related back to oral infection/inflammation).

PERIODONTAL DIAGNOSIS

The periodontal diagnosis is intentionally separated from the rest of the soft tissue findings because of its significance and high incidence. At its conclusion, the careful and exhaustive periodontal evaluation should produce a periodontal diagnosis which, like other factors in the problem list, gives a clear picture of the patient's status. It is necessary to be very specific in our terminology so as to describe exactly the periodontal situation present. 'Gingivitis' has a definite meaning, especially as differentiated from 'periodontitis.' These terms are further modified to refine the diagnosis. Acute versus chronic, local versus generalized, slight, moderate, and advanced, are just a few modifiers applied to the patient's periodontal condition. The following are some partially illustrated examples of typical periodontal diagnoses:

- Normal healthy periodontium and alveolar bone with slight local recession – upper molars (Fig 6.14a,b).
- Chronic generalized moderate periodontitis, with generalized 15–20% horizontal bone loss and local severe infrabony defects lower posterior (Fig 6.14c,d).
- Chronic generalized gingivitis, with bleeding and hypertrophic tissue interproximally, 4–5 mm pockets posterior, with aggravated frenum pull lower midline between teeth 24 and 25 (Fig 6.14e).
- Chronic periodontitis, less significant considering patient's age (68 years), less than 25% bone loss generalized, with slight mobility lower anterior teeth (Fig 6.14f).
- Advanced severe periodontitis, with gross bone loss, 8–12 mm pockets scattered throughout, prognosis poor to hopeless (Fig 6.14g,h).

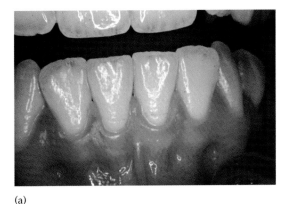

(a)

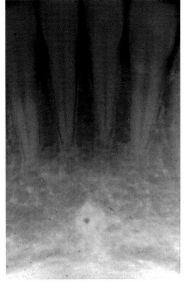

(b)

Fig 6.14

(a) Healthy periodontal tissues: good color, architecture, and surface textures. Papillae are high and tight. (b) Radiograph supplements and confirms findings of healthy normal periodontium and bone.

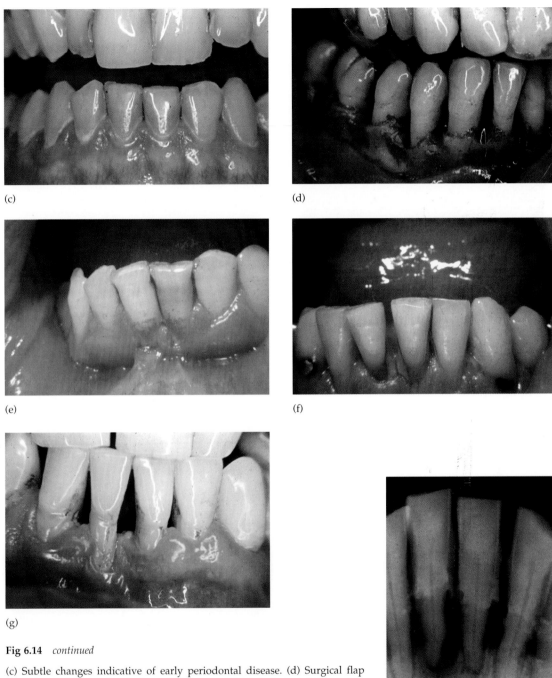

(c)

(d)

(e)

(f)

(g)

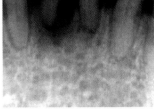

Fig 6.14 *continued*

(c) Subtle changes indicative of early periodontal disease. (d) Surgical flap accessing and illustrating the bony defects present. (e) Periodontal disease can be aggravated by many contributing factors. In this example the lower midline frenum complicates the problem. (f) Moderate chronic periodontitis, with changes in color, architecture, and surface texture. (g) Advanced periodontitis, well beyond the state at which treatment can be predictably effective. (h) Radiograph supplements and confirms the diagnosis, and demonstrates severe bone loss.

(h)

Periodontal diagnoses can be supplemented with case classification indicators, such as the American Academy of Periodontology (AAP) schema. Such classifications can be useful, but the specific descriptive summary diagnosis is preferable, because periodontal conditions present so many variations that a single classification is often inadequate to plan treatment.

Type 0
No to slight bleeding upon probing
No pockets over 3 mm in depth
Mobilities of less than 0.5 mm
No furcation involvements

Type I
Most pockets 1–3 mm but with an occasional 4 mm pocket
Slight bleeding upon probing
Mobilities of less than 0.5 mm
No furcation involvements

Type II
Most pockets 1–3 mm but with some 4–5 mm in depth
Moderate bleeding upon probing, and more generalized than type I
Most mobilities normal, but with some class Is recorded
No furcation involvements, or only grade I furcations noted

Type III
Pockets depths are generally 3–5 mm with possibility of some 6–10 mm
Generalized bleeding upon probing
Mobilities of 1 to 2 are recorded
Grade I with possibility of grade II furcations present

Type IV
Pockets depths are generally 3–6 mm with possibility of some 7–12 mm
Generalized bleeding upon probing
Mobilities of 1 to 2 and 3 are present
Grade I, II, and possibly III furcation involvements recorded

---

DENTAL DIAGNOSIS

Dental diagnosis can be simplified if you consider that teeth which are not normal and healthy can be classed as diseased (generally caries or pulpitis), dysfunctional (malformation, occlusal attrition, erosion/abrasion, fractures, or faulty restoration), or disfigured (intrinsic or extrinsic stain, developmental defect, discolored, or otherwise non-esthetic restoration).

Diseased teeth

Diseased teeth may have hard tissue lesions affecting enamel, dentin, or cementum, lesions of the pulpal tissue, or both (Fig 6.15). Caries is the most common dental disease, and is often surface specific, with certain organisms and environmental factors acting on different tooth surfaces or at different times in life. Our enhanced understanding of the etiology and epidemiology of dental caries is leading to more effective and selective management of the disease. Early pit or surface lesions as well as incipient radiographic lesions may be considered for intensive fluoride therapy, or other modalities aimed at arrest or even recalcification.

Nevertheless, our diagnostic assessment, whether tactile, radiographic, or chemical (caries disclosants), must be scrupulous, because nonoperative approaches, if unsuccessful, can allow significant progression of the lesions. Having seen large carious lesions develop under well-placed pit and fissure sealants, and having seen barely visible subgingival radiographic caries advance to near pulpal exposure in less than 18 months, I would urge caution in the nonoperative management of caries. Unless patients are able to be dependably recalled, and are highly compliant in their daily maintenance regimen, it can be a very risky strategy when compared with conservative operative dentistry.

What remains true is that a clean tooth will not decay, and good oral hygiene combined with good diet (low frequency and amounts of fermentable carbohydrates), supplemented with multiple fluoride uses (incorporated in drinking water or supplements as the teeth

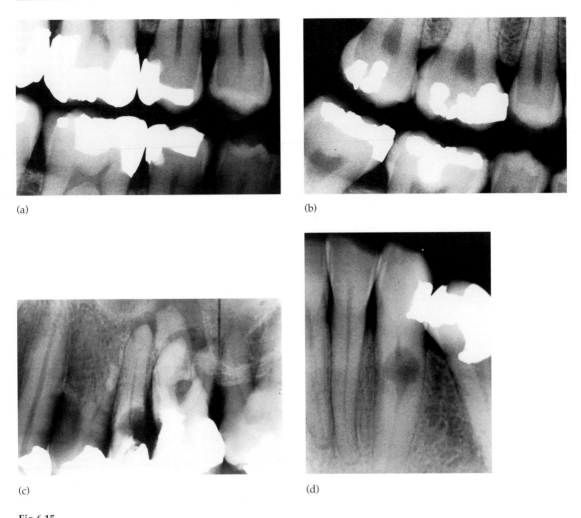

Fig 6.15

(a) Disruption of enamel between upper premolars may be incipient or arrested caries. In fact, the area has not changed in radiographic appearance in 29 years! (b) Frank carious lesion distal of lower first molar, with clear dentinal involvement. Distal of upper first molar may be incipient or arrested. (c) Rather severe caries, upper second premolar (and elsewhere). (d) Internal resorption involving lower canine.

form; added to toothpaste; applied topically both in office and in home use as a gel or rinse) can control or eliminate dental caries in most patients' mouths.

The only other common hard tissue disease is resorption, either internal or external. Although predictable in some cases (re-implanted avulsed teeth, trauma from surgical manipulation, orthodontic movement, impacted adjoining teeth), many cases of internal and external resorption are unexplained.

Soft tissue disease in teeth involves the pulp and, although there are myriad histologic and clinical differentials, the only meaningful distinction is whether the pulpal disease is reversible or irreversible. Some clinical pictures are unmistakable, and give us immediate confirmation of irreversible pulpal disease. These include apical radiolucencies with other positive clinical findings, draining fistulas traceable back to an apical or lateral lesion, and exquisite pain elicited/aggravated by heat but relieved by cold. Other scenarios, particularly those in which significant clinical or radiographic signs are either lacking or inconsistent, may be more difficult to assess. Pain is an important symptom, but it is subjective, and its perception varies from patient to patient.

Palliative treatment, including application of desensitizing agents and sedative restorations, relief of occlusion, and a short course of anti-inflammatory drugs will often relieve symptoms indefinitely, and avoid costly and irreversible treatments such as root canal therapy or extraction. Such palliative treatment can also be used as a diagnostic tool. A pulp that remains symptomatic in spite of multi-mode palliative treatment can be eliminated, one way or another, with a higher level of confidence in the diagnosis of 'irreversible' pulpitis.

Almost 30 years of practice has convinced this clinician to give teeth a chance. One can always extract or attempt endodontic therapy if palliation fails. I have personally seen hundreds of cases in which initial patient complaints of moderate to severe pain, sometimes unelicited, have been resolved with palliative measures, and those teeth have remained functional and asymptomatic for decades.

This is a personal clinical bias and not a universal truth, and many excellent clinicians argue for preemptive endodontic treatment of symptomatic teeth. Every dentist should approach this question with another: 'How would I proceed if this were my tooth?' Every dentist, keeping Hippocrates in mind, should remember 'Primum, non nocere' or 'First, do no harm.'

This discussion must not conclude without considering non-vital but asymptomatic teeth. If such teeth are discovered in the course of examination and diagnosis, but are not directly involved in complex restorations, such as fixed or removable prosthetics, simple surveillance may be all that is indicated. If such teeth are to be involved prosthetically, or if the consequences of subsequent pulpal problems would complicate or compromise overall treatment, then preemptive endodontic therapy (or even extraction) may be required.

Not all abnormal teeth demand treatment. Many teeth with calcified pulps, with over-large pulp chambers (suggesting pulp pathology affecting the ongoing production of secondary dentin), teeth with apparent long-standing direct pulp caps or partial pulpotomies, teeth with short or otherwise inadequate endodontic fills, and discolored, nonresponsive teeth have all functioned for decades without treatment. Indeed, attempting to treat such teeth is itself a risk, because failure of treatment or complications arising from and during treatment may result in the loss of what had been a functional and asymptomatic tooth! Both patient and dentist may have reason to ask 'why did we do that?,' and the answer had better be good.

Endo-perio lesions

Any discussion of pulpal disease must consider the 'endo-perio' question – the occasional relationship of pulpal disease to periodontal disease. The pulp and periodontium communicate at the apex of the tooth, via accessory canals that can occur almost anywhere on the root surface, or from the pulp chamber into a furcation on a multi-rooted tooth. Three possible scenarios must be considered when there are both pulpal and periodontal findings on a given tooth:

1. Lesions may be discrete and unrelated – neither contributes to the other. Lesions are usually radiographically distinct from one another, and other periodontal lesions are usually present in the mouth. Treatment of either lesion will not relieve the other, however, periodontal treatment may be compromised if pulpal disease is not addressed.
2. Pulpal disease may arise from bacteria in a periodontal lesion invading the pulp via lateral or accessory canals. Suspect this scenario when no other likely cause of pulpal disease is present (other than the periodontal lesion). Treatment of the periodontal lesion will not undo the irreversible pulpitis.
3. The most critical combination is that of periodontal lesions arising solely as a result of pulpal pathology. Successful endodontic therapy can result in remission of the periodontal lesion, resolution of osseous defects, and regeneration of the gingival attachment (Fig 6.16). Such

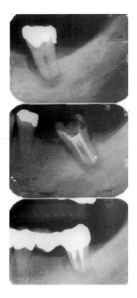

Fig 6.16

Top: severe bone loss, class III mobility, and mesial periodontal defect which could be probed to the apex of the tooth would generally require extraction. Middle: Endodontic treatment was attempted despite difficulty with constricted/obstructed canals, and 6 months later the mobility has decreased and mesial periodontal defect can no longer be probed. Bottom: 5 years after treatment, the tooth remains stable and asymptomatic, and was then employed as a fixed bridge abutment. It remains in function some 20 years later!

lesions tend to be isolated, or unusually severe in relation to other areas of bone loss. When radiographic vertical bone loss or furcation involvements are not clinically detectable with a periodontal probe, it is highly likely that the periodontal lesion is secondary to the pulpal pathology.

It is not understood how periodontal defects and pockets arising from pulpal pathology resolve completely, while 'true' periodontal lesions seldom resolve without surgery and, even with treatment, usually do not regenerate totally.

Unfortunately, the definitive test to determine a pulpally induced periodontal lesion is the performance of endodontic treatment, a costly test if the lesion does not resolve and the tooth is lost! In such cases, overall treat-

ment goals, treatment options, cost-effectiveness, and patient desires have to be weighed before multi-root endodontics are used as a diagnostic procedure.

Dysfunctional teeth

Dysfunctional teeth are those that cannot perform their normal functions as a result of defects in formation or insults suffered after eruption. Malposed teeth are excluded from this category, and will be dealt with later in this chapter when the functional diagnosis is discussed. We will consider four general categories of dysfunction.

Malformation

Poorly formed teeth that are dysfunctional may exhibit:

- Enamel defects, poorly formed or 'chalky,' which do not provide the structural strength required in occlusion or are overly susceptible to caries.
- Abnormal crown morphology, which does not provide function and occlusal support (dwarfing) or which, as a result of severe anatomic anomalies, predisposes to caries and/or makes restoration difficult or impossible (accessory cusps, deep developmental grooves or clefts, 'twinning').
- Abnormal root morphology, which does not provide support for occlusion (short, blunted roots) or which predisposes to caries and/or periodontal lesions (deep axial grooves, furcations close to cemento-enamel junction).

Poorly formed teeth may have minor problems which simply bear watching, or severe problems that so jeopardize the tooth as to rule it out of any long-range plan.

Occlusal wear

Loss of occlusal tooth structure may be dysfunctional if its nature and severity are excessive in relation to the age of the patient.

- Faceting, or circumscribed wear spots in the enamel involving few teeth, may be an accommodation to the overall occlusion and within normal limits, or it may be indicative of occlusal trauma, which can produce mobility, tenderness, and severe localized bony defects in the presence of periodontal inflammation.
- Generalized faceting may also be a normal accommodation to the overall occlusion, especially in elderly patients, or it may result from habits of bruxism and/or clenching, which can lead to more serious damage over time.
- Severe wear resulting in loss of enamel and exposure of dentin is more serious because the exposed dentin is more susceptible to continued attrition as well as caries. The situation is worse when enamel is lost in one arch but not in the other, in which case the arch with enamel may not wear further, but devastate the opposing dentin. Although bruxism is often a factor in severe occlusal wear, other factors should also be considered.

End-to-end occlusion, occupational environments (masons, quarry workers, anyone working with fine abrasives) or poor choice of restorative materials, for example, placement of porcelain crowns or denture teeth against enamel or, worse, against an already worn natural dentition, can lead to abnormal occlusal wear.

Worn teeth may be a normal result of years of use, but unusual or severe wear may suggest functional or psychological problems and can greatly complicate dental treatment planning, because restoration of such severe wear is generally more complicated. It usually involves the extensive use of cast restorations, and such restorations must be designed for greater stresses than normal.

For example, if we are planning restorative dentistry for a middle-aged patient with large masseter muscles and a long history of nocturnal bruxism (Fig 6.17) the severe wear must inform our choice of materials (gold castings over silver amalgam or resins), and our execution (removal of more tooth structure to allow maximum thickness in the restoration).

Once restored, we would have to consider fabrication of a hard acrylic night guard appliance to help preserve and protect the restorative effort.

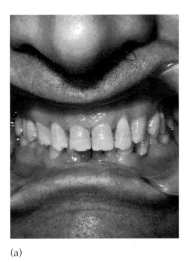 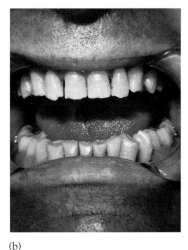 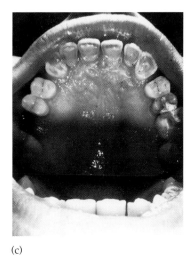

(a)　　　　　　　　　　　(b)　　　　　　　　　　　(c)

Fig 6.17

This 40-year-old man admitted to both nocturnal bruxism and clenching during the day. His masseter muscles were hypertrophic and hypertonic, and, in addition to the tremendous abrasion and loss of enamel shown, he had generalized severe periodontitis with 20–50% bone loss throughout.

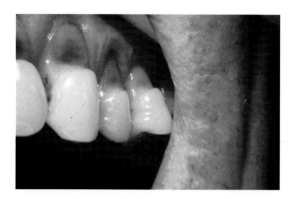

Fig 6.18

Severe gingival abrasion/abfraction, in this case related to 'sawing' motion with hard bristle toothbrush.

Abrasion, erosion, abfraction

Loss of tooth structure at the gingival or cervical region is a complicated problem which can be related to overzealous home care (hard brush, sawing action), chemical action (high acid diet, gastric reflux, bulimia), or traumatic occlusion in which stresses may concentrate at the neck of the tooth (Fig 6.18). These problems become dysfunctional when sensitivity inhibits regular hygiene or limits the dietary choices of the patient, when the pulp is threatened, or when the structural integrity of the tooth is compromised.

Fracture

Fracture of tooth structure creates dysfunction depending on its type and severity. Categorized into two main groups, fractures may be complete, in which case the fractured segment separates, or intact, in which the fractured segment does not separate (typical 'cracked tooth' syndrome).

Some complete fractures may be so minor that, even if dentin is exposed, they can simply be smoothed or at most sealed with bonding agent or conservative bonded restoration. Major fractures involving extensive dentinal exposure, loss of a cusp, or pulpal exposure require definitive treatment for long-term clinical success.

Nevertheless, it is often possible to employ interim restorations of various types, to buy time, assess pulpal status, or contain costs. The patient must be fully apprised of the limitations of such restorations including the risk of early failure, pulpal damage from additional trauma, and axial fractures resulting in loss of the tooth. On the other hand, these risks are often minimal, and countless teeth have been successfully restored with less than definitive restorations which nevertheless served for decades.

In the nonseparation fracture, or 'cracked' tooth, fluids and organisms can penetrate the enamel and enter the dentin, even while the tooth appears intact. The diagnosis can be difficult, as illustrated previously in Fig 6.12, and the prognosis is often guarded.

Defective restoration

A defective restoration is one of the most common dental dysfunctions and can result from normal wear and tear, unusual oral conditions, or failure of the treating dentist to meet the standard of care (Fig. 6.19). Defective restorations may lack marginal seal, proper morphology (over- or undercontoured), occlusion ('high' spots, excessive lateral contacts, or lack of occlusal function and support) or esthetic value. These issues are often matters of clinical judgment, and a pragmatic approach is required, because, at some level, every restora-

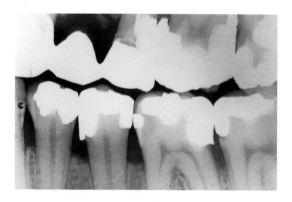

Fig 6.19

In addition to the small problem with overhanging margins, this patient had an incomplete root canal treatment (upper premolar) and the fixed bridge was an eyesore as well.

tion leaks, every contour is less than perfect, and beauty is indeed in the eye of the beholder.

The determination that a restoration is 'defective' should be based on careful assessment, sound clinical judgment, and a balancing of the cost, benefit, and risk of retreatment.

Disfigured teeth

Disfigured teeth are those that present an unnatural and displeasing appearance as a result of stains, developmental defects, or nonesthetic dental restorations. There is certainly some overlap between this category and that of dysfunction, because many dental defects are both dysfunctional and disfiguring, as are many defective restorations.

Disfigurement is considered separately for two reasons: first, quite often a tooth or restoration is reasonably sound and functional, but looks hideous; second, the judgment of what is disfigured, or unesthetic, is as much the purview of the patient as of the dentist. We should refrain from making judgments about the appearance of patients' teeth, eliciting their feelings first.

Disfigured teeth generally fall into three categories: stained, misshapen, and teeth with discolored or nonesthetic restorations.

Stained teeth may be extrinsically or intrinsically stained (Fig 6.20). Misshapen teeth result-

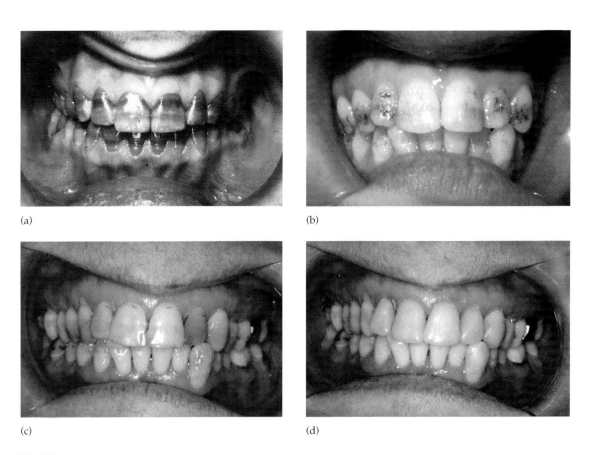

(a)   (b)
(c)   (d)

Fig 6.20

(a) Tetracycline staining, intrinsic. (b) In 1973, severe congenital pitting has accumulated considerable extrinsic stain, which was not removable without mechanical excavation of the pits. (c) Twenty-five years after original bonding (central incisors rebonded 10 years previously), the patient is ready for another complete makeover. (d) In 1998, upper and lower anteriors were stripped back to enamel and dentin, and direct-bonded composite resin reapplied.

ing from fracture or developmental defect may or may not concern the patient, depending on individual taste and tolerance. Current technologies in bonding, whether direct bond composite resin, or laboratory processed partial porcelain veneers, offer many options to restore or enhance esthetics.

Discolored and nonesthetic restorations can affect how patients feel about themselves generally, as well as how they feel about their mouths and teeth. Initially restored with composite resin in 1981, the patient in Fig. 6.21 eventually sought definitive care involving full mouth crown and fixed bridge rehabilitation, carried out 10 years later.

The final dental diagnosis, including etiologic and contributing factors, can be expressed in the same summary statement form, as follows:

- Teeth show severe, generalized occlusal wear, dentin exposed throughout the posterior; low caries rate and few restorations. Missing tooth number 14 (shown in Fig 6.17a).
- Teeth have severe intrinsic stain, probably due to tetracycline therapy. There is abnormal enamel formation on molars (shown in Fig 6.20a).
- Patient has extensive restorations, many defective and unesthetic, with generalized recurrent caries. Missing upper right lateral incisor and lower first molars due to caries-related abscesses in late teens/early twenties (shown in Fig 6.21a).

More commonly, the dental diagnosis is documented either pictorially or written out on a dental chart (Fig. 6.22).

FUNCTIONAL DIAGNOSIS

Based on the findings from the examination of the occlusion and temporomandibular joint, and the myofunctional analysis of tongue, lip, and cheeks, the functional diagnosis can be

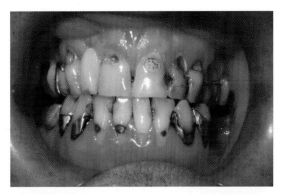

(a)

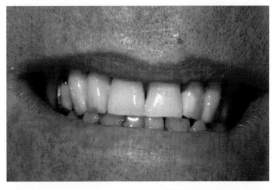

(b)

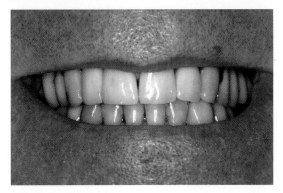

(c)

Fig 6.21

(a) A long history of failed restorations and recurrent caries made for skepticism on the part of this patient, who in 1981 was 'patched' with resins and amalgams. (b) The resulting improvement in esthetics, coupled with the success of a lower fixed bridge over 10 years' time, prompted the patient to seek more care. (c) In 1992 most of the teeth were restored/replaced with crowns and fixed bridges, which are presently doing well at 6 years, with an excellent prognosis for long-term success.

DENTAL AND RADIOGRAPHIC FINDINGS								
			RADIOGRAPHIC					
TOOTH #	EXISTING REST.	CL. CAR.	BW car. oh con	PERIAPICAL bone & root end pathology	VITALITY	MOBILITY	SUMMATION SURFACES	PROCEDURE
1	X							
2	MO/A							
3	MO/A	O	D					
4	MO/A	FRACTURED						
5					4			
6	M/R				5			
7	D/R	DISCOLORED						
8	M/R							
9	M/R		D					
10			M		3			
11					3			
12	MOD/A	O		P.A. LUCENCY	10 (N.V.)			
13	MO/A	D			4			
14	X							
15	MO/A	M(OH)		MESIAL TIPPING		2		
16	—	—	—	IMPACTED				
17	—	—	—	IMPACTED				
18	FCC	B(G)	OH	THICKENED PDL		1		
19	MODB/A	MARGINAL DITCHING						
20	DO/A							
21	DO/R		DO?					
22								
23						1		
24				BONE LOSS		2		
25						2		
26						1		
27								
28			OPEN CONTACT					
29	X							
30	X							
31	MOL/A	B	M	MESIAL TIPPING		1		
32	X							

NAME **JANE DOE** DATE **11-20-98**

Fig 6.22

The dental diagnosis is generally based on and depicted by a pictorial or written tooth chart such as this one.

made. It is a critical piece of the puzzle, because it considers how and whether the entire system, teeth, periodontium, joints, and neuromusculature, is serving the intended purpose. Does the system function effectively in mastication, deglutition, and speech? Do the components of the system function in comfort and harmony with one another? How does the entire system relate to the health and well-being of the patient?

The functional diagnosis is a difficult piece, because we are assessing a system rather than a single tooth or soft tissue lesion. Our knowledge and understanding of these functional relationships have grown, yet there is much that has not been standardized by definitive research. We still work with empirical principles; we rely on the gathered wisdom and experience of respected clinicians and we temper that with our own experience and observations.

We must take a pragmatic approach. Despite apparent deviations from normal, does the patient really have a problem? Does the patient encounter difficulties in mastication, deglutition, or speech? Does an occlusion that deviates from the textbook description of normal (Angle class I), but which serves the patient well, really deserve to be called a 'malocclusion'?

We might postulate that, in the absence of clear pathology, whatever occlusion, temporomandibular joint function, lip, cheek, or tongue function the patient may have is, for that patient, 'normal.' This definition of health should color the entire functional diagnosis. It suggests that not all edentulous spaces demand fixed bridges, not all class II occlusions need to be in class I, and not all clicking temporomandibular joints require orthotic splints and physical therapy.

ILLUSTRATIVE CASE HISTORY 6.23

This is illustrated with the case history shown in Fig. 6.23. These 1981 photos (Fig 6.23a) were made of a 35-year-old physician, who had been followed on periodic recall visits since 1973. Severe occlusal abnormalities were present from the outset, including anterior open bite, CO–CR discrepancy of more than 2 mm, no cusp–fossa relationships in the posterior, and consistent interposition of the tongue between anterior teeth on swallowing. His treatment had been confined to regular preventive counseling and prophylaxis and minor operative dentistry. Incisal wear was seen as a problem, and smoothing/polishing of rough incisal edges was done as needed. A night guard appliance was considered a potential next step.

An appliance was fabricated in 1995 when the patient reported discomfort in the joint during athletic activities, and regular maintenance was continued.

EPILOGUE CASE HISTORY 6.23

Now aged 52 (Fig 6.23b), the patient still exhibits abnormalities in static and functional occlusion, occasionally uses the orthotic appliance at night (Fig 6.23c), and remains free of symptoms. Diagnostic casts (Fig 6.23d) illustrate the probable atypical 'habit' position producing and aggravating incisal wear.

The concept of a 'healthy but abnormal' functional pattern is useful, because many if not most dental patients present findings that deviate from textbook norms, but which do not demand 'treatment.' Care must be taken, however, not to overlook subtle functional problems which may be masked by other conditions, or reflected in other components of the system. A disharmony between the occlusion and the temporomandibular joint (TMJ), for example, may in fact produce myofascial pain or other symptoms of the temporomandibular disorder-type, or it may precipitate a traumatic occlusion leading to severe occlusal wear, pulpal involvement, or aggravated periodontal bone lesions. One cannot rule out functional pathology without assessing the entire system. Symptoms of functional pathology may arise so gradually that the patient may not be aware of them. As with most oral and dental problems, pain is seldom present in the early stages. Finally, many patients possess such high levels of tolerance to insult and injury that they fail to seek timely care. With these concepts in mind, let's look at the functional evaluation of the occlusion, the temporomandibular joint, and the myofunctional analysis.

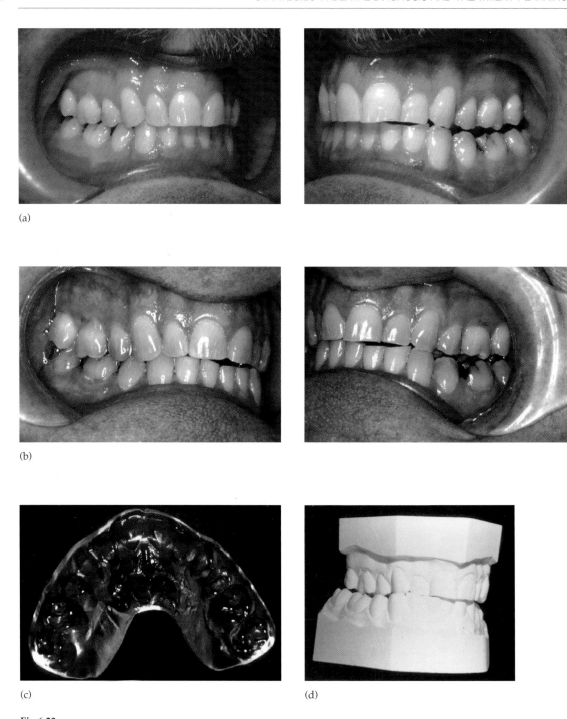

Fig 6.23

(a) Clinical appearance in 1981 of a 'healthy abnormal' occlusion. This 35-year-old physician had already been followed for almost 10 years, with no symptoms or functional complaints. (b) Now aged 52, the pattern continues through 1998. A neutral splint (c) has been available as needed for 2 years. Patient remains fully functional and symptom free. (d) Diagnostic casts illustrate the probable atypical 'habit' position producing and aggravating incisal wear.

Occlusion

The array

The number and distribution of teeth need to be adequate for function, esthetics, and support of the occlusion. The normal complement of 32 teeth is more than sufficient, and seldom accommodated by typical arches. For most people, 28 teeth seem to be the norm, and clinical experience would suggest that adequate function and support are obtained with 'first molar' occlusion, that is, 24 permanent teeth.

Pathology ranges from too many (impacted or crowded third molars, supernumeraries) to too few. Missing teeth within the array may result in tipping and/or drifting of adjacent teeth or the supereruption of opposing teeth. Missing posterior teeth may increase the functional load of remaining teeth, compromising them structurally, periodontally, or orthodontically.

Alignment

Alignment refers to positional relationships of the teeth, the overall arch form in mesiodistal, facial–lingual orientations, the occlusal plane, and axial orientation of the teeth. Normal alignment implies snug contacts between all teeth which preclude food impaction, but allow cleaning with dental floss. A line passing through the center of each tooth should describe a smooth arch form, more or less symmetrical left and right. All teeth should fall approximately into the same occlusal plane vertically, so that marginal ridge height is fairly even from tooth to tooth. Root orientation should allow normal forces to be directed approximately along the long axis of the teeth. It is obvious that most normal healthy occlusions deviate in some degree from the 'dentoform' model just described. The degree to which deviation from the norm constitutes pathology depends on both the severity of the deviation and the individual's tolerance of it. An open contact that shows signs of periodontal inflammation, pocketing, or bleeding is a pathologic finding. A similar open contact that, for whatever reason, shows no sign of periodontal problems may be dismissed as 'healthy abnormal.'

Maxillomandibular relationship

This is the most critical factor in assessing the occlusion, because the patient may have sufficient numbers of teeth in the array, well aligned within the respective arches, yet with such disparity between the maxilla and mandible that the patient is dentally disabled.

ILLUSTRATIVE CASE HISTORY 6.24

Oral Surgeon: Dr Donald Pricco

The case illustrated (in Fig. 6.24) begins with a healthy 42-year-old man, in 1976. His complaint was not cosmetic, as he had been comfortably prognathic all his life (Fig 6.24a,b). Rather, he was growing increasingly frustrated at not being able to chew effectively or, as he put it, 'always being the last one left at the dinner table.' Orthognathic surgery to reposition the mandible, followed by occlusal equilibration and selected crowns and fixed prostheses (Fig. 6.24c,d), created a functional occlusion which remains healthy and stable more than two decades later.

EPILOGUE CASE HISTORY 6.24

Orthognathic surgery was done in 1976. Prosthetic and restorative dentistry followed and continue as needed to the present. Now, in 1998, he is nearing retirement, continues to enjoy comfort and function, and is maintaining teeth and periodontal tissues well. Prognosis remains good for continued oral health (Fig. 6.24e).

It is impossible to isolate occlusion from the temporomandibular joint. The normal inter-arch relationship can be simply described as follows: maxillary and mandibular teeth meshing together comfortably and in harmony with the temporomandibular joint, with freedom in all excursive movements. Both static and dynamic relationships must be considered.

In the static occlusion, or full closure of the teeth, posteriors should interdigitate to provide efficient mastication and occlusal stability.

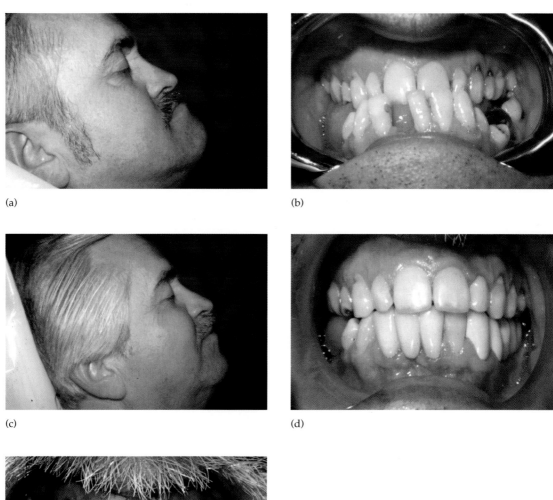

(a)

(b)

(c)

(d)

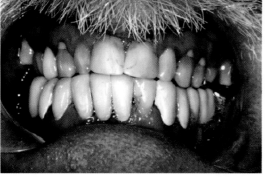

(e)

Fig 6.24

(a) Class III malocclusion, before treatment. (b) Patient's chief complaint was functional, not cosmetic. (c) Profile view after orthognathic surgery. (d) Minor equilibration and some restorative dentistry provided comfort and full function. (e) Twenty years after surgery, the patient continues to enjoy comfort and function, and has maintained teeth and periodontal tissues well.

Anteriors should contact lightly in full closure, preferably with modest vertical and horizontal overlap of upper teeth over the lowers. These simple conditions may be met despite molar relationships other than class I (Angle), and many so-called malocclusions are comfortable, functional, esthetically satisfactory, and free of pathology. In full closure (CO, IP), the condyles should be comfortably seated in the glenoid fossae, neither forcibly retruded nor significantly protruded down the articular eminence. The question of what is significant deserves discussion and requires consideration of the retruded or centric relation position.

Centric relation (CR, RP) is that position of the mandible first created by the prosthodontist only to be hopelessly confused by the periodontist and totally ignored by the orthodontist. This tongue-in-cheek definition serves to illustrate the controversy surrounding the concept. Centric relation has been described as the most retruded position of the mandible from which lateral movements can be made. It has been described as that position in which the condyles of the mandible are in the uppermost, rearmost position in the glenoid fossa. It has been described as the position in which small amplitude opening and closing movements are purely hinge motions, without translation of the condyle.

Clinically, the position is highly significant in that it is fairly stable, readily reproducible, and predictably functional. Although long-term changes such as condylar head remodeling may affect the exact location, the CR/RP position can be consistently located before, during, and after clinical treatment. It remains stable on repeated observations, and is readily reproducible by way of hinge axis location and transfer, allowing dentists to duplicate on an articulator the precise arc of closure of the mandible, and the maxillo/mandibular relationship in the retruded position. Finally, clinical experience has consistently demonstrated that occlusions equilibrated to or restored in the centric relation position will be stable and functional. This predictability of success is the key to the clinical significance of the position.

As CR is stable, reproducible, and functional, it has been inferred that it is a physiologic norm. There is no evidence to support this. Indeed, although some deviations from CR in full closure appear to produce or contribute to temporomandibular joint pathology, we also see many functional individuals with normal health who have gross discrepancies. We also see many severely dysfunctional individuals with very slight or no discrepancies.

The multitude of asymptomatic patients with CO–CR discrepancies suggest that we must view centric relation as a reference point for a range of normal. Indeed, well-accepted studies suggest that most normal individuals reach full intercuspation (CO) within 1–1.5 mm of their retruded (CR) position.[1]

In the dynamic occlusion, movements from full closure are guided by teeth, and the condylar heads functioning in the glenoid fossa. They are influenced by the neuromuscular components and, as the mandible is in effect 'suspended' in space, infinite variety of movement is possible.

Tooth guidance patterns include pure canine guidance (cuspid rise), anterior group function, working side anteroposterior group function (working side only), and balancing side involvements. These last may range from momentary contact in initial movement, to balanced occlusion of a well-worn dentition, to sole guidance on a balancing side tooth with no working side contact (generally considered undesirable).

Temporomandibular joint condylar guidance acts in concert with tooth guidance, but presents much more potential for variation. The osseous anatomy may remain fairly constant, but the influence of muscles, ligaments, and even the articular disk can change, sometimes quite quickly.

The schematic shown in Fig 6.25 illustrates in only two dimensions some of the various combinations of tooth and condylar guidance in straight protrusion. The clinician must consider all excursions and all three dimensions of movement in assessing the dynamic occlusion.

Temporomandibular joint

There is a wide range of normal in the temporomandibular joint and its related musculature. The normal healthy joint is symmetrical upon observation, and pure opening movements are generally free of deviations or noises. Palpation over the condyles during opening/closing and lateral excursive movements should reveal smooth and quiet joint function in the normal range of motion. Palpation of associated musculature primarily addresses the temporalis and masseters. Internal and external pterygoids may also be palpated (not without difficulty), and palpation of the digastric and sternocleidomastoid muscles, the hyoid region, the

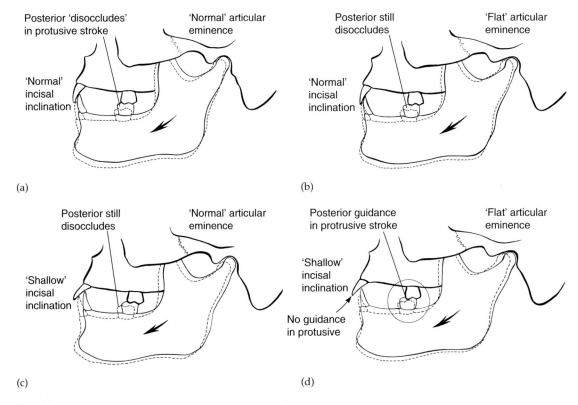

Fig 6.25

Hypothetical combinations of tooth and condylar guidance in protrusive excursions. This schematic depicts the relationship in two dimensions only. Actual mandibular movements entail three dimensions, and any combination of tooth and condylar guidance in any direction! (a) With 'normal' tooth and condylar inclinations, posterior teeth disocclude in protrusive stroke. (b) A 'flat' articular inclination combined with normal anterior guidance still allows posterior disocclusion in protrusive. (c) Conversely, a relatively shallow incisal guidance may be overcome if normal articular inclination disoccludes posteriors. (d) Trouble may come, however, when an anterior open bite or shallow incisal guidance is combined with insufficient condylar inclination, leading to posterior guidance in protrusive (circled). Generally speaking, when excursive movements are determined by posterior teeth alone, the results can be traumatic to teeth, joints, and supporting tissues.

occipital region, and even the shoulder musculature can be instructive. Muscles palpated should be supple, free of spasm or tension, and non-tender to palpation.

Significant abnormalities in the temporomandibular joint, which are potentially pathologic, include the following:

- Pain: any report of pain in or around the temporomandibular joint, especially if associated with functional movements such as chewing or wide opening, should be investigated as an indication of possible pathology.

This includes symptoms such as headache, earache, and stiff neck or shoulder.
- Tenderness to palpation: such tenderness directly over the joint or in the associated musculature is significant.
- Limitation of motion: inability to open normally or move in excursions is suggestive of disorders of the temporomandibular joint.
- Deviation: asymmetric function of the joints, producing large amplitude deviations in opening and/or protrusions, can be a significant finding.

- Noises (crepitus, rustling): many, if not most, joint sounds are benign. In the absence of other signs and symptoms a noisy joint may be assumed to represent simple arthrodial crepitus. However, some joint sounds may be significant. Noises accompanied by other signs and symptoms, noises that come on suddenly (as opposed to a long-standing crepitation) or after a trauma, or noises that are increasing in frequency or amplitude should be investigated.
- Vibration in condylar movement (clicking, popping, or 'clunking'): as differentiated from joint noise, roughness or vibrations such as clicking, popping, or 'clunking' can be readily palpated, and may represent dislocation and reduction of the articular disk, or actual subluxation of the condyles ahead of the articular eminence. As with joint noises, joint vibrations are neither rare nor pathologic in themselves.

Combined with other symptoms, especially pain, or with 'locking' of the joint (either open or closed), vibrations may indicate significant joint pathology or dysfunction. What is clear is that both joint noise and vibration may exist and persist after pain and dysfunction have resolved. What is also clear is that many temporomandibular disorders may resolve through adaptation over time. Knowing this, our diagnosis and treatment must be conservative, lest we create more problems than we solve.

The 'gold standard' for screening and initial diagnosis of the temporomandibular joint and associated musculature consists of three factors:[2,3]

1. A patient history that addresses the issues noted above including jaw joint or facial pain, such as headaches, locking or other functional jaw problems, noises and discomfort in biting/chewing, and history of head/neck or jaw injury, or previous treatment for jaw joint problems.
2. A clinical examination including measurement of range of motion on opening (interincisal) and in lateral excursions; palpations for tenderness over the joint and in the masseter and temporalis muscles; palpation for joint sounds/vibrations including crepitus and clicking; and clinical signs of excessive occlusal wear, mobility, fremitus, and soft tissue alterations suggestive of parafunction and stress. Inspection of symmetry and alignment of face, jaw, and dental arches completes the basic assessment.
3. Temporomandibular joint imaging is used to supplement, when appropriate, the history and examination. Such radiographs include plane transcranial films, tomograms, computed tomography, arthrograms, and magnetic resonance imaging (MRI) studies. A number of these imaging techniques are useful for diagnosing gross disorders, fractures, missing condyles, dislocations, severe arthritic changes, cysts, or tumor masses in the joint region. They are less useful for diagnosing functional problems such as myofascial pain/dysfunction (MPD) or internal derangements of soft tissue. Arthrography is diagnostic of soft tissue derangements, but is somewhat invasive. MRI scans can be definitively diagnostic, but are technique sensitive and can be difficult to interpret.

Many technologies have been proposed and employed in the assessment and diagnosis of the temporomandibular joint. Unfortunately, few of them have demonstrated a degree of scientific validity sufficient to justify their cost.[4]

Myofunctional analysis

The diagnosis of abnormalities in lip, cheek, and tongue function depends greatly on careful observation and the dentist's skill in obtaining patient histories. As with many of the factors in the function diagnosis, deviations from the clinical norm may or may not be harmful to the system, but we must be aware of such deviations whether or not we attempt to correct them. Indeed, the correction of myofunctional abnormalities is more challenging than most of the problems we have discussed so far. A carious lesion can be excavated and restored, a periodontal pocket surgically eliminated, a class II malocclusion corrected. Unconscious habits of a lifetime are tougher to change, and yet we cannot ignore them, because they can drastically affect the course of oral health and disease, and the outcome of dental treatment. Available treatment modalities can be applied to correct or alleviate myofunctional problems; failing that, the clinician must at least be acutely aware of how the problem is likely to affect the prognosis of dental treatment.[5,6]

The standard of clinical normality in the myofunctional environment is that lips, cheek, tongue, and associated musculature should perform comfortably and efficiently in normal function. Muscle tension should be minimal when the system is at rest. Parafunctional movements and habits should not compromise the system. Potential pathologic findings include, but are not limited to, the following:

- Lips with unusual anatomic form, asymmetric, abnormally short, with changes in surface tissue suggestive of sucking or lip-biting habits, with poor muscle tone, flaccidity, or incompetent in rest (open, for example, as with mouth breathing).
- Cheeks with hyperactivity or overdevelopment of masseter, heavy linea alba, or obvious tissue changes indicative of parafunctional activity involving the cheeks.
- Tongue of abnormal size or configuration, with surface features suggesting parafunctional activities (for example, serrations on anterior border mirroring linguals of upper anterior teeth, or on lateral borders mirroring linguals of posteriors), or short lingual frenum, preventing normal speech or swallowing.
- Assuming sufficient numbers of teeth in the array, difficulty in chewing and/or swallowing food must be considered highly significant.
- In the postadolescent patient, a swallow in which the tongue tip does not contact the anterior palate (rugae) area may represent pathology. Common associated signs are pursing of the perioral muscles, contraction of the mentalis muscle in the chin, and interposition of the tongue between teeth during the swallow, either anterior or lateral, on one side or both.

Related findings are mouth breathing and habitual tongue postures between teeth. Mouth breathing, especially in children, can play a significant role in malocclusions and their treatment. In the adult, abnormal tongue function may be involved in mobility and migration of periodontally involved teeth, and in the instability of fixed and removable protheses.

Abnormal speech patterns may be significant in terms of muscle function and tooth positions. Lisping, sibilant or hissing 's' sounds, or other apparent speech defects should be evaluated as potential oral–myofunctional problems.

Existing appliances

Obviously, the functional evaluation must consider the status of any existing appliances. The patient's assessment of comfort and function is of primary importance, as it is that patient's interest we are here to serve. In the absence of pathology, even the loosest, least esthetic, worst-designed partial prosthesis

---

Examples of functional diagnoses associated with previously illustrated cases:

- Normal healthy class I occlusion with slight clicking in right TMJ (asymptomatic) with normal range of motion, and no functional complaints (shown in Figs 4.23 and 4.25).
- Deep class II occlusion, with severe occlusal and incisal attrition. Nocturnal bruxer, with 'type A' personality. Unusually heavy linea albae (shown in Fig 6.17).
- Post-orthodontic (4 bicuspid extraction) adult class I, atypical wear, with unilateral partial posterior open bite. Habitual latero-protrusive posture producing incisal wear. Patient wears an orthotic appliance on an as-needs basis (shown in Fig 6.23).
- Marked class III malocclusion, with notable mandibular prognathism, and difficulty in chewing (takes him longer to finish meals) (shown in Fig 6.24).

may be successful for the patient who likes it and functions well with it. We must be careful, however, not to overlook subtle or chronic pathology involving appliances the patient finds acceptable, so that serious but symptomatic problems with appliances do not go untreated.

DEVELOPING THE MULTIFACTORIAL (PROBLEM LIST) DIAGNOSIS

Once all the pertinent factors in the diagnosis have been considered, the list is finalized and pulled together. A critical last step is the assessment of the extent to which some of the findings are interrelated, that is, impacting on each other. In the boxes are two hypothetical problem list diagnoses that illustrate this:

To illustrate the concept and application of the problem list diagnosis further, please consider the following clinical case history (Fig 6.26).

ILLUSTRATIVE CASE HISTORY 6.26

Concepts illustrated: Development of multifactorial diagnosis, identification of interrelated factors, and treatment planning taking them into account.

This 39-year-old woman in good physical health is seen first on an emergency basis with complaint of pain in the upper right premolar region (Fig 6.26a). Radiographic and clinical

---

Patient no. 1. 22-year-old female college student in good general health
Chief complaint (CC): left central incisor turning dark, was traumatized about 4 years ago.
Dental goal: have front tooth 'fixed', and any other necessary work done.
Marginal gingivitis generalized, home care regular but not highly effective.
Pericoronal inflammation associated with mesioangular, partially impacted lower third molars nos 17 and 32.
Numerous proximal caries (per chart), upper and lower posterior.
Nonvital darkened upper left central incisor no. 9 (source of CC).

Factors are generally unrelated to one another.

Patient no. 2. 52-year-old male postal employee with adult-onset diabetes, non-insulin dependent, and on regular oral medication
Chief complaint: sharp edge on lower right molar – bothering for some time.
Dental goal: 'get teeth in shape – would like to keep teeth.'
Generalized chronic periodontitis; locally severe bone loss (upper right posterior, lower anterior).
Partial edentulism, not replaced, with some tipping and supereruption.
Some caries (per chart), slight but extensive occlusal wear, breakdown of old restorations, several fractured cusps (including chief complaint).
Apparent loss of vertical dimension, CO not same as CR, bilateral clicking in TMJ.

All factors are probably interrelated to some degree.

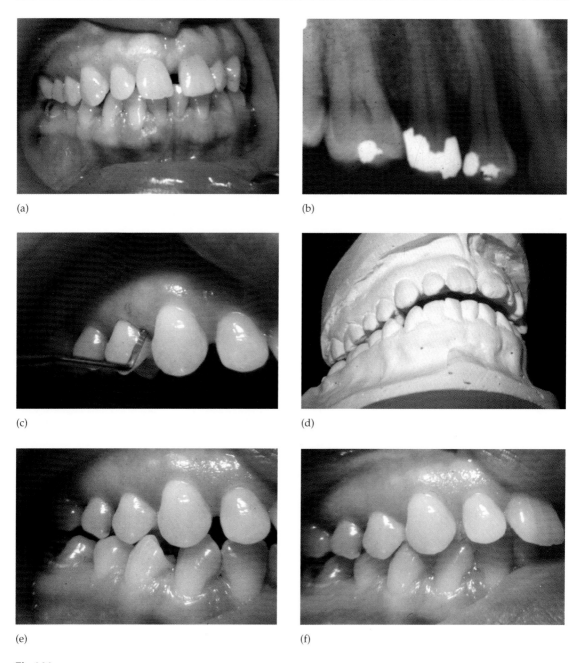

(a)   (b)

(c)   (d)

(e)   (f)

Fig 6.26

(a) In 1976, this 39-year-old woman presented with a complaint of pain in the right premolar. There were no findings of dental origin (caries, periapical involvement), and the overall periodontal picture was excellent. Note, however, the space between upper and lower right canines in full centric closure, and bear it in mind. (b) A closer look (radiograph) reveals a periodontal problem, which was localized to the upper right premolars. (c) Probe depths were significant on tooth number 4 (5–7 mm pockets), and number 5 (8–10 mm pockets). Depths throughout the rest of the mouth were normal. (d) Diagnostic models illustrate anterior open bite, and resultant lack of anterior guidance in excursions. (e) Right lateral excursions are guided by the premolars alone. Canine teeth did not contact in the functional range, despite normal alignment and good vertical overlap. Lack of canine protection was contributing directly to the problem on the premolars. (f) Carrying the investigation further, we observe the tongue during a swallow. Consistently interposing between upper and lower anteriors, the open bite is maintained, with canines precluded from normal contact.

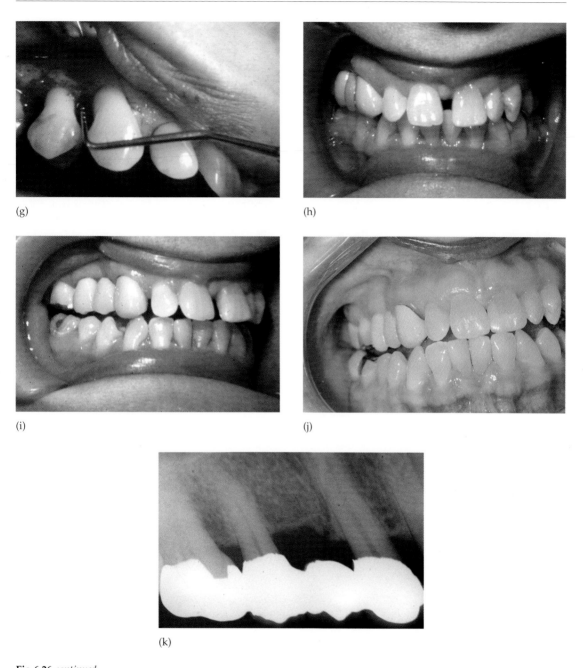

(g)

(h)

(i)

(j)

(k)

Fig 6.26 *continued*

(g) Surgical exploration reveals severe infrabony defects. (h) After extraction of number 5 and osseous surgery on number 4, a fixed prosthesis is placed, double-abutted posteriorly. Centric contact is established on the canine. (i) Canine guidance is established in lateral excursion. (j) The prosthesis remains in service 22 years later, with canine guidance still operative. (k) Radiographically, the prosthesis and its abutments appear sound and healthy in 1998.

examination revealed no findings of dental origin (caries, periapical involvement), and the general periodontal condition was excellent. A closer look at the radiograph (Fig 6.26b) reveals bone loss involving teeth numbers 12 and 13, and probing of those teeth (Fig 6.26c) left no doubt about the diagnosis of 'acute periodontal pain.' If we stop there, we may select an appropriate treatment for the local problem, but miss the big picture! As there were no other pockets over 3 mm throughout the mouth, further investigation of this localized problem is essential.

Note the apparent space between upper and lower canines (Fig 6.26a), and the anterior open bite seen on study casts (Fig 6.26d). In lateral excursion, guidance fell solely on first and second premolars; neither canine teeth nor other anteriors were in contact in the functional range despite normal alignment and good vertical overlap. The lack of canine or anterior protection was contributing directly to the accelerated periodontal breakdown on the premolars (Fig 6.26e). Once again, we must not stop, for there is more happening here. Given normal eruption forces, the canine teeth should be in functional contact, but they are not. If we observe this patient during a swallow (Fig 6.26f), we can see a tongue thrust which, interposed between upper and lower anteriors, has maintained the open bite and, most critically, has led to excessive lateral forces on the premolars aggravating the periodontal condition to the point of tooth loss. The problem list diagnosis for this patient looked like this:

Treatment began with a surgical exploration (Fig 6.26g) which revealed infrabony defects on the first premolar (a furcated root) going almost to the apex, and the tooth was removed as a result. The second premolar was treated with osseous contouring and repositioned flap, and the prosthetic treatment, taking all the problems into account, consisted of a fixed bridge from the canine (which was put into contact in centric closure and lateral excursion) (Fig 6.26h,i), to a double-abutment premolar–molar anchorage. This established maximum stability of the prosthesis in light of the occlusal and myofunctional environment. The case was watched closely for several years for any sign of loss of canine contact as a result of tongue thrust (which was not likely to go away).

EPILOGUE CASE HISTORY 6.26

This case was first diagnosed and treated in 1976. Today one might consider osseous grafting and guided tissue regeneration instead of extraction of the premolar. The functional problems would still have to be dealt with, however, and establishment of anterior guidance would still have to be considered!

The clinical photos and radiographs (Fig 6.26j,k) show the case 22 years later. The prosthesis and its abutments remain healthy and stable, bone level is good, and the canine guidance is still discluding posteriors in

---

Patient DL. 39-year-old woman in good general health

Chief complaint: throbbing pain upper right premolar area – recent onset.

Dental goal: relief of pain, and long-term good care and retention of all her teeth.

Localized severe periodontitis (upper right premolars), otherwise healthy perio.

Traumatic occlusion (lateral guidance) on upper right premolars, with lack of canine or anterior guidance (anterior open bite), with tongue thrust swallow pattern.

All factors are interrelated to some degree.

lateral strokes, with little or no attrition of opposing canine (attributable mostly to good luck).

The natural aging dentition has darkened a bit, so the shade match is no longer great, and 22 years of passive eruption/recession have uncovered the delicate metal collar so cleverly hidden in 1976.

Long-term success can be attributed to excellent maintenance by the patient, technical quality of the prosthesis, and, not least, to the fact that all etiologic and contributing factors were identified and dealt with in the treatment plan.

Given a carefully crafted problem list diagnosis, the dentist can develop an appropriate treatment plan, which addresses all the problems, deals with etiologic and contributing factors, relates well to the individual patient, and is in a logical and effective sequence based first on urgency, then on efficiency. The following chapters offer strategies in the development of such plans.

REFERENCES

1. Reider, CE, The prevalence and magnitude of mandibular displacement in a survey population. *J Pros Dent* 1978; **39**:324–9.
2. McNeill C, Mohl ND, Rugh JD, Tanaka TT, Temporomandibular disorders: diagnosis, management, education, and research. *J Am Dent Assoc* 1990; **120**:253–63.
3. Mohl ND, Temporomandibular disorders: The role of occlusion, TMJ imaging, and electronic disorders. *J Am Coll Dentists* 1991; **583**:4–10.
4. Lund JP, Widmer CG, Feine JS, Validity of diagnostic and monitoring tests used for temporomandibular disorders. *J Dent Res* 1995; **74**:1133–43.
5. Barrett RH, Hanson ML, *Oral myofunctional disorders*. Mosby: St Louis, MO, 1978.
6. Hanson, ML, Barrett RH, *Fundamentals of oral myology*. Thomas: Springfield, IL, 1988.

7

SOME GENERAL PRINCIPLES

The synthesis of a dental treatment plan can be a simple process. Based on the multifactorial diagnosis, one merely matches each problem with an appropriate treatment, puts the treatment into some reasonable sequence, and does it. Given a young adult with mild local gingivitis, a partially impacted and symptomatic lower third molar, and two occlusal pit caries on upper first molars, the case rather plans itself.

Scale/polish and oral hygiene counseling, removal of the offending third molar, and restoration of the caries, followed by establishment of a recall/maintenance schedule, should do the trick. However, some thought may need to be given to sequence. Do we scale first, debriding at once the inflamed third molar area before extraction? Or should we remove the tooth, allow some healing time, and then clean the teeth (assuming the patient's home care will have suffered somewhat after surgery)? Is the patient diffi-

cult to schedule or does he live some distance away? Perhaps the entire treatment plan can be carried out in one visit! In any event, the plan is readily generated from the diagnosis, and you don't need much 'strategy' to construct it.

Many clinical situations are not that simple, however, and even some that seem simple at first may present complications if the plan is not carefully conceived and executed (Fig 7.1). The simple schematics illustrate two seemingly similar treatment situations. In both, a missing lower first molar may be considered for replacement by a three-unit fixed-bridge prosthesis. In Fig 7.1a the abutment teeth appear sound, are relatively parallel to one another, and the curve of occlusion is apparently normal. In Fig 7.1b, however, the second molar is supererupted, tipped, has had deep caries and a large restoration in close proximity to the pulp, and the bone level is close to the furcation. Using the tooth as an abutment

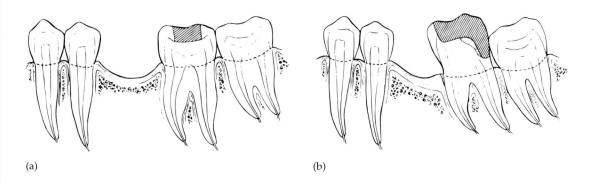

(a)   (b)

Fig 7.1

(a) Simple fixed bridge case; (b) same teeth involved, but situation, and plan, become much more complex.

presents challenges in bridge design and fabrication, including difficulty in preparation (parallelism and path of insertion), occlusion (curve of Spee), pulpal management (previous deep caries, risk of exposing mesial pulp horn), and periodontal maintenance (as a result of the furcation and the margin, which is likely to encroach upon it). It is very likely that additional treatment steps (endodontic therapy, post and core, periodontal therapy) might be required in the course of treatment. Each of these steps has some potential for failure which could result in failure of the entire effort. The cost in time and money is greater, adding to the risk.

It is critical to recognize such complexities, especially when they are subtle in appearance. We will look at a number of clinical case examples to illustrate various strategies that might be applicable in typical general practice situations.

SIMPLER IS BETTER

This is a pretty broad statement, but if nearly 30 years of general practice have taught me anything, it is that the fewer steps in the plan, the less there is to go wrong. Complex approaches, especially where each step is dependent on the preceding step, can be risky. Restoring a broken molar with a full-cast crown is a high percentage procedure, but some crowns will, for a variety of reasons, not succeed long term as we would wish. If we add to this picture a root canal treatment, and post/core before crowning, we increase the failure risk considerably. If we also have a periodontal procedure in the picture the prognosis becomes more and more questionable, because the chance for failure, although minimal for each of the procedures individually, adds up when overall success depends on every component treatment succeeding long term.

A number of strategies that you will see in subsequent chapters aim at simplification of treatment, and this is why. The more things we do to a tooth, a dentition, or a patient, the greater the chance that one of them will fail and compromise the overall treatment as a result.

PATIENT-ORIENTED, GOAL-ORIENTED TREATMENT

Each patient is an individual, with hopes and desires, fears and aspirations, and his or her own idea about what he or she wants and needs when seeking dental treatment. Our treatment plans must be responsive to these individual differences and we must be prepared to offer alternatives or alterations to dental treatment to fit our patients, and serve their needs, not our own. This concept has been discussed at the outset of this text, and I will not dwell on it much further. Suffice it to say that the most sophisticated, creative, state-of-the-art plan is of little use if the patient is not interested or willing to accept it.

This is why it is so important to identify general goals with the patient early in the process. Plans that address the patient's stated goals and felt needs are more likely to be accepted, carried out, and maintained long term.

Finally, we must be prepared to present and discuss treatment in basic terms. Questions such as 'How will it look?,' 'Will it be comfortable?,' 'Will it be healthy?' and 'How long will it last?' deserve answers.

THE KEY TOOTH CONCEPT

In the face of complex dental problems, it is helpful and often essential to identify those teeth that may be utilized effectively in a course of treatment. We call these 'key' teeth, and they must possess or be capable of attaining two attributes: stability and favorable arch position. Such teeth can be depended upon to stand by themselves and provide normal function over time, and to serve, if necessary, as abutment teeth for fixed or removable prostheses, or to reinforce other teeth when splinted together. The 'ideal' key teeth are healthy canines and first molars, which most often fulfill the criteria of stability and arch position. Indeed, it is sometimes possible to restore and rebuild an entire dental arch using just four key teeth – the canines and first molars. Other teeth may meet the 'key' criteria (sometimes canines and molars do not), and distribution (location) of such teeth is also a critical factor.

STABILITY

A key tooth must have sufficient root surface in healthy bone to act as an abutment tooth or, at the least, to ensure its own retention long term. Factors to consider include root morphology and the level of alveolar bone in relation to tooth length (crown : root ratio).

Root morphology includes length, diameter, and configuration – that is, the shape and number of roots. Root length is especially critical when lateral forces are likely to be encountered, usually in the anterior. General bulk (diameter) can be as important as length because the surface area of root in bone is at issue. Cylindrical roots are preferable to conical; dilacerated or clubbed roots are even better, provided root canal therapy is not likely. Multiple roots are more stable than single roots as long as furcations are well below the alveolar crest.

Root length in bone may be compromised by periodontal bone loss and/or supererup-tion. Crown to root ratios should be as small as possible, 1 : 2 being optimal.

Finally, a stable key tooth must either have a healthy pulp or be amenable to endodontic therapy if necessary.

FAVORABLE ARCH POSITION

Both the location and orientation of the tooth are important. The most stable tooth imagin-able is a full bony impacted canine, with large root, infinite crown to root ratio, and a presumably healthy pulp. It is of no clinical use whatsoever, as it is buried! Stable teeth positioned outside the range of functional occlusion, or severely tipped or supererupted teeth, are not key teeth.

Generally, key teeth should be located within the normal dental arch from second molar to second molar and be aligned rela-tively parallel to the forces of occlusion, and approximately perpendicular to the occlusal plane. Small deviations can be overcome.

DISTRIBUTION

The number of key teeth and their spatial relationship to one another are also important. Assume a lower arch with just two key teeth. If those are a lower right first and second molar, their value is limited, no matter how stable they may be. If the two teeth are lower right and left second premolars, there is at least bilateral support, and one might consider using them as overdenture abutments. If the two teeth are lower right and left canines, the range of options widens considerably. Options now include overdenture, overdenture built over a bar splint, crowns and bar with antero-posterior partial denture, or anterior bridge canine-to-canine with partial denture.

CREATING KEY TEETH

Sometimes key teeth can be created by improv-ing stability, arch position, or even distribution. Let's look at some of the strategies to convert a questionable tooth into a key tooth.

ATTAINING STABILITY

Restoring or improving stability can be accomplished with the following.

Periodontal therapy

Procedures that regain bone support, such as successful fill of osseous defects or bone grafts of various types, often combined with guided tissue regeneration using various types of membranes, can greatly enhance the stability of otherwise questionable teeth.

Crown shortening

Although often necessitating endodontic treat-ment, reducing the length of the clinical crown out of the bone improves (reduces) the crown : root ratio, and enhances stability. The most extreme example is the overdenture abutment, which is usually reduced almost flush with the gingiva, improving the stability markedly.

Shortening may be employed after periodontal therapy, offering both esthetic improvement and improved stability.

Splinting

Teaming two adjacent teeth with crowns cast or soldered together can create, in effect, a multirooted tooth, which may be more stable than either of the individual teeth alone. A good example of this is the use of splinted first and second premolars for partial denture abutments. Neither tooth would serve well by itself, but splinted together they create the effect of a molar root system.

ATTAINING FAVORABLE ARCH POSITION

Arch position problems can often be resolved through minor orthodontic procedures. However, if drastic repositioning is required, the orthodontic procedure itself may compromise root length and periodontal support. The role of tooth movement in complex case planning is explored at some length in Chapter 9.

It is technically possible to improve distribution of key teeth by autogenous transplants – surgically removing and reimplanting teeth in new locations. The prognosis of such teeth is questionable, however, because they are subject to possible external resorption or other unpredictable consquences.

The development of dependable dental implants, using Branemark's concepts of 'osseointegration,' now enables us to create key tooth analogs, to solve distribution and location problems. Implants are not a panacea, however. They are substantially more costly, require more time, and are often highly technique sensitive both in their placement and in their involvement in subsequent prostheses. They are sometimes incompatible with natural dentition when employed as abutments, and they

cannot be placed willy-nilly into the mouth expecting the same good predictability everywhere. I address the use of implants as a strategy in treatment planning in Chapter 12. For the present, we should consider them as substitutes for 'key' teeth in some situations, not all, and for some patients, not all.

TOOTH INVENTORY – TO IDENTIFY 'KEY' TEETH

One of the most basic tools in dental treatment planning is the tooth inventory. It can be used to simplify dental treatment, or to assess the degree of complexity that we are are facing in a difficult case. Its main purpose is to identify: 'key' teeth or potential key teeth for use as abutment etc; 'sound' teeth, healthy and retainable teeth which, although capable of standing on their own, are not 'key' tooth material; and those teeth that might be eliminated altogether as a result of their instability, unfavorable arch position, or questionable prognosis.

It is useful to assign appropriate symbols to the teeth evaluated so that upon completion of the inventory a clear picture emerges. The following symbols will be used in the illustrative cases:

+	Indicates a key tooth that is stable and in a favorable position in the arch.
(+)	Indicates a potential key tooth which would require some alteration of position or enhancement of stability.
0	Indicates a sound, retainable tooth, capable of standing by itself.
(0)	Indicates the same as '0', but is in need of some treatment or modification.
—	Indicates a tooth that is to be eliminated from the treatment plan.

The tooth inventory is applied/illustrated in a number of case histories in later chapters. The following case is a good illustration of the use of the inventory and the identification/creation of key teeth.

ILLUSTRATIVE CASE HISTORY 7.2

Concepts illustrated. *Tooth inventory, identification of 'key' teeth, enhancing stability by periodontal therapy, crown shortening and splitting.*

This 48-year-old woman was aware that something was seriously wrong with her teeth as a result of mobility and recurring gum abscesses (Fig 7.2a). She had been told that she might lose her teeth. She wanted desperately to keep all her teeth, with the retention of as many teeth as possible becoming a primary goal. After examination, radiographs (Fig 7.2b) and diagnostic models (Fig 7.2c) were obtained, the problem list in the box was developed.

Given the complexity of the case, a tooth inventory is done, identifying 'key' teeth (and potential 'key' teeth), sound and potentially sound teeth, and teeth with no hope of long-term retention or usefulness (Fig 7.2d). The

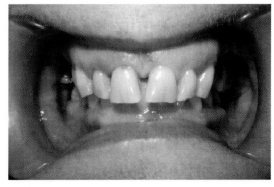

(a)

Fig 7.2

(a) Initial presentation, early in 1976: 'I want to keep my teeth.'

symbols clearly map out the location of sound teeth and key teeth. The upper anteriors might have been considered expendable (–) in favor of an anterior fixed bridge, but the patient's stated desire to keep 'all her teeth' made them candidates for periodontal therapy and splinting, hence they are tentatively labeled as 'potential sound teeth' (0), pending outcome of initial treatment.

Patient DG: 48-year-old female, menopausal but otherwise in good general health
Chief complaint: aware she has 'gum problems,' some teeth are symptomatic
Dental goal: retention of all her teeth if possible
Generalized moderate-to-severe periodontitis, most involved are teeth nos:
 1   (5–7 mm pockets, tipped, supererupted, class III mobile)
 5   (8–10 mm pockets, severe vertical bone loss, class III mobility)
 7–10 (5–7 mm pockets, moderate bone loss, 1 : 1 crown/root ratio, class II mobility)
 12   (5–7 mm pockets, class II mobility)
 14   (8–10 mm pockets, severe bone loss into furcation, class II mobility, suppuration)
 28–29 (5–6 mm pockets, class I mobility)
Generalized caries and broken down restorations, most severe nos 13 and 14
Deep class II, with loss of posterior support, compromised vertical dimension

Many factors are interrelated.

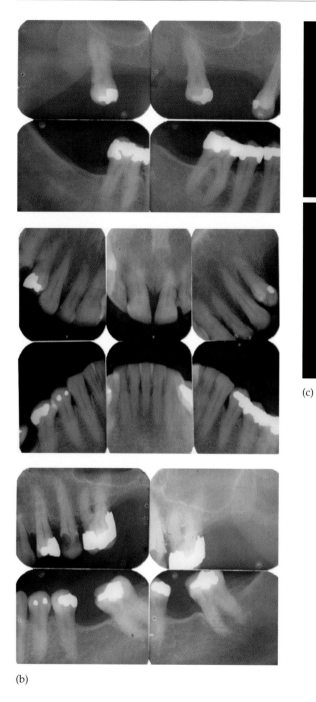

(b)

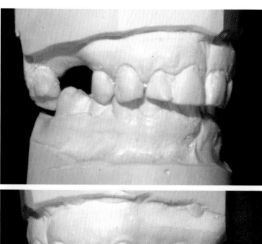

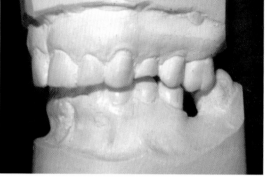

(c)

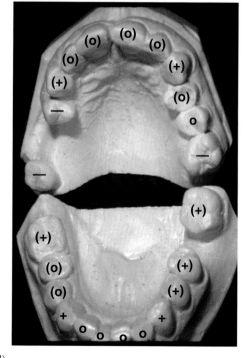

(d)

Fig 7.2 *continued*

(b) Full mouth radiographs, January 1976. Note severe bone loss in maxilla, less advanced in mandible (nos 28 and 29 had 5–6 mm pockets). Generalized pocketing in the maxilla was most notable on teeth nos 1, 5 (note hint of infrabony defect approaching apical third), 7–10 (more infrabony defects), 12, and 14 (furcation involved). (c) Diagnostic casts: note that even though centric stops are present, the loss of posterior support, tipping, mechanical breakdown, and deep class II relationship have all contributed to a loss of vertical dimension. (d) A tooth inventory is performed.

No. 1.   Third molar, supererupted, stubby root, and severe periodontal involvement, extract—"**–**"
No. 5.   First premolar, periodontally condemned—"**–**"
No. 6.   Canine, although requiring periodontal therapy, a potential key tooth—"**(+)**"
No. 7.   Lateral incisor, severely involved periodontally, but if treatable may be potentially sound—"**(0)**"
No. 8.   Same as no. 7—"**(0)**"
No. 9.   Same as no. 7—"**(0)**"
No. 10. Same as no. 7—"**(0)**"
No. 11. Canine, requiring periodontal treatment, a potential key tooth—"**(+)**"
No. 12. First premolar, requiring periodontal treatment, may be potentially sound—"**(0)**"
No. 13. Second premolar, heavily restored, but good root in bone—"**0**"
No. 14. First molar, severe periodontal involvement, with caries and supereruption, a hopeless situation—"**–**"
No. 18. Second molar, excellent root in bone, slight tipping and large restoration, plus minor periodontal involvement make this a potential key tooth—"**(+)**"
No. 20. Second premolar, good root in bone, large restoration and minor periodontal involvement make for potential key tooth—"**(+)**"
No. 21. First premolar, even better root in bone; minor periodontal treatment would produce potential key tooth—"**(+)**"
No. 22. Canine, typical key tooth—"**+**"
No. 23. Lateral incisor, even with slight bone loss a sound tooth—"**0**"
No. 24. Same as no. 23—"**0**"
No. 25. Same as no. 23—"**0**"
No. 26. Same as no. 23—"**0**"
No. 27. Canine, typical key tooth—"**+**"
No. 28. First premolar, class I mobility with lingual periodontal pockets, sound if treated—"**(0)**"
No. 29. Same as no. 28—"**(0)**"
No. 30. First molar, good roots in bone, despite some pocketing and bone loss, furcation is unaffected; with treatment a potential key tooth—"**(+)**".

(e) Healing but disfigured maxillary teeth are seen 6 weeks after periodontal surgery, March 1976. The patient was prepared for it, and provisional crowns were in the plan. Nevertheless, tears were shed when the periodontal pack was removed.

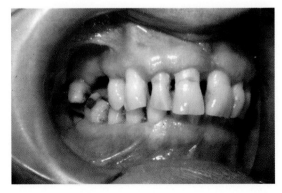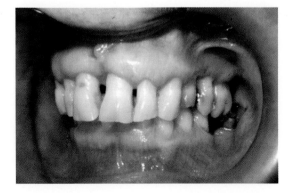

(e)

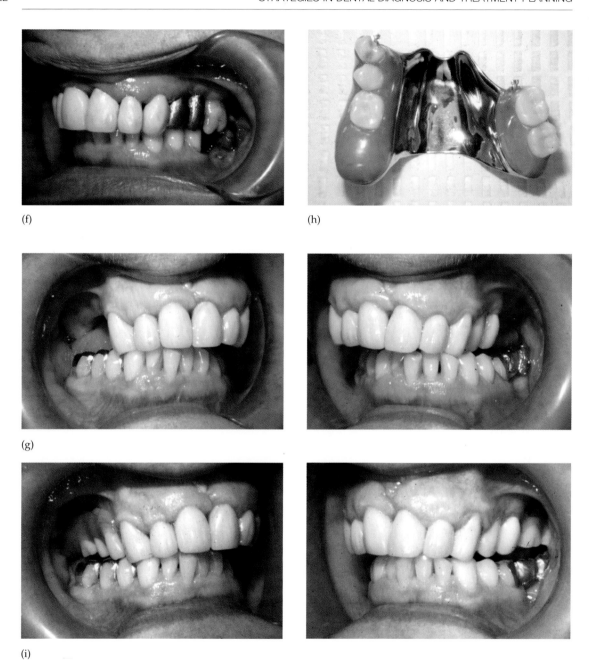

(f)

(h)

(g)

(i)

Fig 7.2 *continued*

(f) Processed acrylic anterior provisional restorations and cast gold provisional splint on nos 12–13 established an enhanced vertical dimension, and provided acceptable esthetics while the tissue matured, July 1976. (g) Splinted crowns (6–8, 9–11, 12–13) with semi-precision keyway attachments set into nos 6 and 13, fixed bridge (18–20) and splinted crowns (28–29–30) shown in lateral excursions (anterior group function). (h) Semi-precision attachments keying into splinted abutments provided sufficient retention and stability even without retentive clasps for this removable partial denture with cast gold base (mucostatic). Wrought wire retentive clasps (lingual only) were later set into the appliance approximately 5 years into its 19-year tenure. (i) Clinical photos (in lateral excursions) at 5 years (1981).

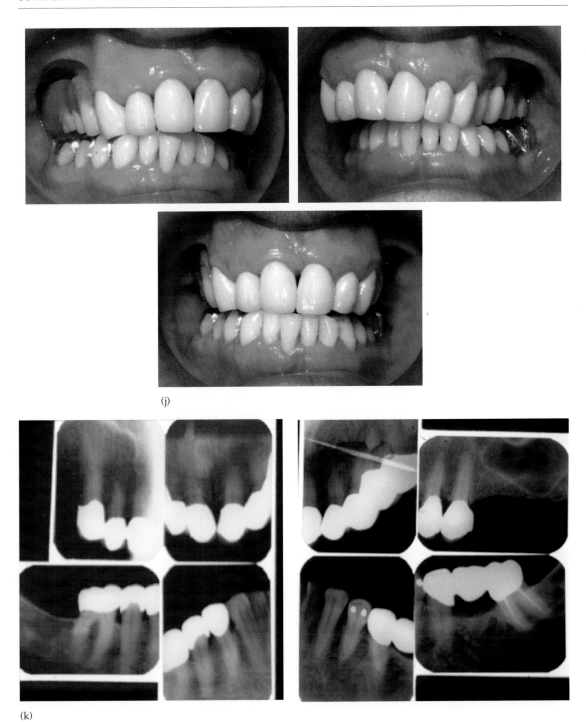

(j)

(k)

Fig 7.2 *continued*

(j) Clinical photos (in excursions) at 12 years (1988). (k) Radiographs at 13 years (1989). The astute reader will notice that root canal treatment has been done on tooth no. 18, which became symptomatic during the 1976 bridge fabrication, and was endodontically treated before cementation.

Periodontal therapy was done, including apically repositioned flaps with osseous recontouring (Fig 7.2e). This case was treated in 1976. Today a less resective surgical approach might be used. Full crown coverage of upper anteriors was planned to shorten clinical crowns, regain lost vertical, and splint weakened teeth. Knowing this, the patient was somewhat less troubled by the esthetic devastation after periodontal surgery. Tears were shed none the less.

Soon after surgery cast gold provisionals were made on numbers 12–13 to gain approximately 3 mm of vertical dimension anteriorly, and the upper six anterior teeth were temporized with processed acrylic provisional crowns. Note that the patient refused extraction of any teeth until absolutely necessary, so number 14 remains in the picture (Fig 7.2f).

After several months tissues were maturing, and the definitive reconstruction was completed, including upper splinted crowns (6–8, 9–11, 12–13) with semi-precision keyway attachments set into numbers 6 and 13 (Fig 7.2g). A cast gold base upper partial denture keyed into the abutments (Fig 7.2h). Lower left fixed bridge (18–20) and lower right splinted three-quarter crowns (28–29–30) completed the effort.

EPILOGUE CASE HISTORY 7.2

This case was first diagnosed and treated in 1976. In addition to using a less resective periodontal surgical approach, consideration might be given to using implants in the upper posterior segments. The cancellous nature of the maxillary bone and the location of the sinuses would complicate such a strategy, however, and the plan as originally conceived is still a viable approach today.

In any event, the patient did exceedingly well with her fixed and removable prostheses, maintaining the periodontal tissues faithfully, and keeping a regular recall schedule for many years. Clinical photos at 5 years (1981) (Fig 7.2i) and at 12 years (1988) (Fig 7.2j) attest to the technical soundness of the plan, and especially the patient's careful home care. Full-mouth radiographs at 13 years (1989) (Fig 7.2k) show no signs of further caries or periodontal disease.

No further treatment other than recall maintenance was needed over 19 years, when we were made aware of the patient's death of natural causes (at age 68). Although a longer lifespan would be desired, she had, at least, reached her goal of keeping her remaining natural teeth all her life.

8

TIMING OF TREATMENT

We must not get further into treatment planning strategies without addressing the issue of timing. The order and pace at which dental treatment is carried out can be as critical to success as the selection of treatment itself. Let's look first at the rational and effective sequencing of dental treatment.

SEQUENCING TREATMENT

The arrangement of procedures into an effective sequence is based on two main criteria: urgency and efficiency in achieving the treatment goal. The initial sequence is often driven by an urgent need felt by the patient, clinical urgency, or practicality; these may or may not coincide. Urgency-based treatment is very much problem oriented, addressing the immediate needs of the patient. Efficiency-based treatment is generally more goal oriented, working toward the long-term goals established by the dentist and patient.

URGENCY-BASED TREATMENT

The patient's most common felt need is relief of pain or discomfort. More often than not, this is what prompts a patient to seek care. Procedures to alleviate or eliminate the patient's pain or discomfort nearly always take precedence in the treatment plan. This is true even when more serious problems are present but asymptomatic. Unless those other problems constitute an immediate threat to the patient's health and well-being, felt needs should be addressed first.

Another common felt need on the part of the patient is loss of esthetics. A chipped anterior tooth, lost restoration, or visible cavity may prompt the patient to seek care. Again, that problem should be addressed first, even at the risk of having the patient fail to return for treatment that is more urgent from our clinical viewpoint. We must certainly inform the patient of such problems, but it is the patient's decision whether or not to deal with them.

The type of procedure selected in meeting the patient's immediate felt need must be based on the overall treatment plan. For example, a patient presenting with pain diagnosed as irreversible pulpitis may be managed in a number of ways. If the patient is new to the dentist, and is being seen after hours on an emergency basis, then opening the tooth to relieve pressure and allow drainage, along with appropriate medication (analgesics, antibiotics if indicated), will address the need without a commitment to a specific, definitive procedure. Indeed, depending on periodontal and overall treatment considerations, such a tooth may be extracted on some subsequent visit. Should other problems need to be addressed in the meantime, vital pulpotomy or pulpectomy as indicated may relieve the symptoms and allow weeks or months to pass before further definitive treatment is necessary.

On the other hand, a patient of record, under control, and well restored, who develops a pulpitis, might be treated immediately with definitive endodontic procedures followed by definitive restoration. Temporary symptomatic relief or palliative treatment should not be considered inferior treatment; it may well be an effective interim measure in the overall plan.

A patient presenting with an esthetic problem as chief complaint may be treated in a variety of ways, depending on circumstances. A lost anterior bridge facing may be treated with some soft white wax if the patient is the mother of the bride en route to the wedding! A broken anterior tooth might be patched with composite resin to solve an immediate esthetic problem, even if the tooth is periodontally condemned and slated for extraction at a later date. Dealing with a patient's felt need doesn't limit us to interim measures. An anterior veneer crown placed to solve an esthetic problem need not wait until posterior periodontal pockets are eliminated and bridges placed. If the patient is made aware of the overall situation, and understands what treatment is necessary to achieve good oral health and function but would like an esthetic improvement right away, that should get precedence.

Effective communication is essential here, both to elicit the patient's felt needs, and to convey the clinical findings to the patient in terms that he or she can understand. Indeed, once the patient understands the big picture, the immediate complaint may be seen as less critical, and be given a more appropriate place in the treatment sequence.

Clinical urgency is based on the following criteria (in order of importance).

Systemic threats

These are conditions that affect or threaten the general systemic health of the patient. A suspected malignancy must be assessed and dealt with immediately. Extreme hypertension may contraindicate any dental treatment until it is evaluated and addressed. Such situations must be handled with care and tact, because the patient's felt need in seeking dental care may be totally unrelated to the systemic problem. Although some patients are grateful that a systemic threat has been discovered, others, out of fear or ignorance, may resist referral to a physician (or specialist) and insist that their dental needs be attended to. Conflict in these cases is nonproductive and generally unnecessary. A gentle and caring explanation of the potential import of the systemic finding is essential.

Occasionally it is necessary to compromise, and one may find oneself smoothing a tooth or replacing a missing filling for a patient with a suspected malignant oral lesion. This need not endanger the patient so long as biopsy and/or referral is also carried out. On the other hand, a patient whose blood pressure is extremely elevated (for example, 205/110) presents the dentist with a real risk of medical emergency. Patients with dental problems who also exhibit signs and symptoms of contagious or infectious disease (mononucleosis, hepatitis, venereal disease) put at risk not only their own health, but that of the dental team as well. Such problems must take precedence over dental treatment.

Immediate dental or oral threats

These are conditions that are currently producing pain or discomfort or that, in the dentist's judgment, threaten the vitality of the pulp or the integrity of the periodontium. This criterion is likely to coincide with the patient's felt need in seeking treatment, for relief of acute symptoms nearly always takes precedence in urgency-based sequencing if systemic threats are not involved.

Secondary to the relief of acute symptoms is the treatment of potentially acute problems, such as excavation of deep carious lesions or removal of gross periodontal insults. Addressing such potential problems often takes precedence over more serious conditions, such as terminally involved periodontally condemned teeth, or nonvital teeth with periapical radiographic lesions. The reason is twofold: first, the likelihood of painful symptoms arising in long-standing chronic periodontal or pulpal infections is less than in the potentially acute situation; second, quick action may save a cariously involved tooth from irreversible pulpal damage, whereas the nonvital apically involved tooth has already lost its battle.

Treatment of these urgent conditions is often palliative or interim in nature. Indeed definitive treatment is often contraindicated.

For example, it may be better to place a sedative temporary restoration in a deep excavation than to subject tooth and pulp to the greater insult of crown preparation, impression, and placement of a metallic restoration. Definitive treatment is also contraindicated if other problems demand immediate attention as well. Excavations and sedative temporaries, pulpotomy/pulpectomy and temporary restoration, relief of traumatic occlusal contacts, local curettage or irrigation of acute periodontal lesions are all examples of priority measures in treatment to relieve acute symptoms or address threats to pulp and periodontium.

Although relieving symptoms and intercepting potential acute problems, these types of urgent treatment may also be investigative in nature, that is, they may assist in developing the overall plan and sequence. A deep carious lesion that, upon excavation, does not encroach on the pulp can be treated with an appropriate definitive restoration at a later date.

If, on the other hand, the excavation reveals a large carious exposure, we have confirmed the need for endodontic therapy, post and core, and crown in the next phase of treatment. Indeed, should pulpectomy be attempted and the root canal system prove impassable, extraction and bridgework may become the definitive plan.

Many procedures, both urgent and definitive, can be investigative or exploratory in nature, and should be done early in the treatment, because their outcome may inform later stages of treatment.

Asymptomatic, potential oral threats

These are dental conditions that, although asymptomatic, have the potential for acute exacerbation. This level of clinical urgency includes treatment of apically involved non-vital teeth, extraction of hopelessly involved teeth (caries, periodontal disease, severe malposition), and, in some cases, the removal of partially erupted but asymptomatic third molars (potential sites for pericoronitis). The degree of urgency here depends on the clinical picture and logistics of the patient's treatment plan. For example, the partially erupted third molar might be left alone if the patient is proceeding with other care and can be monitored, but should probably be removed if the patient is leaving for a year's tour at a research site in the Antarctic! The likelihood of acute flare-up in relation to accessibility of emergency care is of prime importance in determining the degree of clinical urgency.

The clinical picture is also important. Using the same example of a partially erupted third molar, we can envision holding off on treating a situation in which the pericoronal tissues are clean, pink, and firm even though pericoronal pockets are present, but we would assign urgency to a similar third molar with inflamed, spongy tissues, plaque, debris, and a generally unhealthy 'look' to the tissues.

An asymptomatic periapical lesion that is small and well circumscribed may be put off, whereas another lesion, also asymptomatic but encroaching on adjoining teeth, the sinus, or the mandibular canal, may be more urgent.

There are many times when a patient is aware of asymptomatic problems but chooses to wait until symptoms develop before acting on them. Periodontally condemned teeth may serve for many years, impacted third molars may sleep quietly, and patients, having been informed of the risks entailed, have every right to decline or defer treatment. Indeed, when a long-standing asymptomatic problem is finally treated there may be complications that create more and greater problems than we started with. A mandibular paresthesia, or a severe alveolar osteitis arising from removal of an asymptomatic third molar, may make for a very unhappy patient if we 'urged' treatment on him or her.

Another common situation is the discovery of a radiographically insufficient endodontic fill, a 'short' fill, an untreated canal on a molar, or an old pulpotomy. Obviously if such teeth are to play strategic roles in a treatment plan ('key' teeth, abutments etc), then retreatment is probably indicated, albeit risky. One problem is that such teeth may not be amenable to retreatment, and may be compromised or lost in the attempt. Although treatment of such teeth is justifiable if they are integrally involved in overall treatment, they are often better left alone if possible. The patient should be informed of the problem and asked to watch for symptoms or changes. Periodic radiographic reassessment is certainly indicated.

In summary, the treatment of asymptomatic but potentially urgent problems, which do not threaten the patient's systemic health, do not involve strategic teeth or areas in the overall plan, and do not threaten other teeth or structures, can often be postponed indefinitely. The risk versus benefit principle must be applied, and the patient must be actively involved in the decision to treat or postpone treatment of such problems.

Once a sequence of treatment steps has been established to address felt needs and clinical urgencies, the balance of the treatment is generally laid out in sequence based on efficiency. It may, however, be necessary to carry out some or all of the urgent treatment before finalizing the overall plan. This is true when life-threatening conditions are discovered, when the patient requires immediate relief of symptoms, or when the investigative nature of the urgent treatment steps will better inform our plan and sequence for the balance of treatment.

Thus urgency-based sequencing is problem oriented, but not necessarily goal oriented. Indeed, until immediate felt needs (such as relief of acute pain) are met, it is difficult or impossible to consider long-term goals. Today's toothache must be relieved before we can discuss tomorrow's goals. The investigatory nature of urgent care is also key. It makes little sense to establish a goal of keeping teeth only to find, after debridement, full radiographs, and periodontal evaluation, that the prognosis is hopeless and teeth must be extracted! At some point, however, we must progress from urgent care to a plan and sequence based on efficiency in achieving treatment goals.

Sadly, many patients and dentists never make this transition. Instead, they go from crisis to crisis, treating only what hurts, and in the long run fail to reach any goal at all. The dental patient who, having been given the opportunity, rejects goal-oriented treatment must accept responsibility for the outcome. It is usually unproductive to debate with such patients. A genuine concern expressed for the patient's health and well-being, along with an 'open door' policy should the patient change his or her mind, is generally the best approach. I have found that, over time, even the most difficult patients may come around given the opportunity. On the other hand, if the dentist fails to present goal-oriented treatment to a patient, tacitly treating the patient through crisis after crisis without attempting to break the cycle, it may be considered a breach of the standard of care.

EFFICIENCY-BASED, GOAL-ORIENTED TREATMENT

Sequencing of this treatment means that the desired goal is attained in as few steps or appointments as possible, and that treatment is carried out with as little redundancy as possible, with care taken not to perform treatment early in the sequence that might be undone later.

An example of reducing steps in treatment is the situation of a symptomatic, partially erupted, lower third molar, opposing an asymptomatic upper third. Removing the upper along with the lower is more efficient, as the unopposed upper is both nonfunctional and likely to supererupt, requiring later extraction. Performing operative dentistry in quadrants reduces the total number of visits and anesthetic administrations necessary. Indeed, a well-rounded general dentist may carry out multiple procedures in an anesthetized quadrant, doing, for example, root canal procedures as well as operative dentistry at the same visit. Minor periodontal surgery may be performed in a quadrant along with an extraction.

Redundancy can be avoided by not treating small-to-moderate carious lesions on teeth slated as abutments to be crowned, because the caries can be removed and blocked out with light cured resin or glass–ionomers at the preparation appointment. Obviously, this should not be done if deep caries encroach on the pulp, or a core build-up is indicated as a result of lack of sound coronal tooth structure.

Redundancy can also be avoided by postponing restorative or endodontic procedures on periodontally questionable teeth pending outcome of periodontal treatment. Such teeth may be extracted later or, if not, may require a different restorative plan as a result of the altered periodontium or modification in the overall plan.

As it is not always possible to envision the entire treatment plan at the outset, the goal-oriented treatment is often broken into three sequential stages. If treatment is carried out within this general framework, it will generally be in an efficient sequence:

1. Establishment of a healthy oral environment.
2. Restoration of form, function, and esthetics.
3. Maintenance of the environment and the dentistry placed therein.

ESTABLISHMENT OF A HEALTHY ORAL ENVIRONMENT

The concept of the mouth as an ecosystem rather than a complex mechanical device is a key in goal-oriented treatment planning. Both dentists and the public have likened the mouth to a pop-up toaster which, if broken, can be taken to a repairman (the dentist) who putters around a bit, replacing a few springs and wires, making it right again. This mechanistic approach is responsible for much of the failure in dental treatment. The environmental model serves us better, because the mouth is an ecosystem (living organs, teeth, soft tissue, and numerous and diverse microbes) with most of the problems of our own macroenvironment. Pollution, blight, mismanagement, and even 'crime' are problems in the oral environment as well.

Most important, patients present vastly different scenarios, with different sets of 'rules' in their individual oral environments. Some people have tremendous hereditary or acquired resistance to insult, teeth that are resistant to caries, healthy periodontal tissues which seldom see dental floss; they are seemingly 'made of iron.' Others present with a fragile and delicate system, continually susceptible to disease, seemingly made of 'glass.' Sometimes this corresponds to general systemic health, but not always.

The critical issue is that dentistry performed in an unhealthy or unsound oral environment is doomed to failure. Treatment must always begin with the establishment of basic oral health. Assuming that immediate needs (urgencies) have been addressed, the following are typical types of treatment which go to the establishment of a healthy oral environment.

Control of etiology

'Preventive' measures to control etiology remain paramount to long-term oral health and successful dental treatment. Basic plaque control must be taught, encouraged, coached, and continually reinforced. Although research has shown that the role of dental plaque is more complicated than once thought, clinical experience continues to demonstrate that 'clean teeth will not decay,' and that the patient's acquisition and application of effective plaque control can work miracles.

Fluorides continue to play a key role. Fluoridation of water supplies (or daily supplementation) remains one of the most effective public health measures ever conceived. Topical fluorides in a wide variety of applications continue to add to our armamentarium of preventive therapies. Xylitol gum and various selective dietary choices can play a role, and the elimination or control of cariogenic foods and snacks remains critical. Antibacterial rinses such as chlorhexidine and others (usually containing fluoride) can help shift the balance of health and disease.

Direct and early involvement of the patient, as discussed in earlier chapters, is imperative, because most preventive measures depend on patient cooperation and commitment.

Control of periodontal pathology

This is critical to a healthy oral environment. The periodontium is the foundation upon which the dentition (and our dentistry) rests.

Deep pockets and calculus deposits (especially subgingival) may render the most ardent preventive efforts ineffectual. Preliminary periodontal therapy, including thorough root planing and calculus removal, must be done early in the treatment sequence. It may be appropriate to defer some or all definitive periodontal therapy to allow the patient's home care combined with root planing to stimulate as much healing and repair as possible. Therefore, although initiation of periodontal therapy generally takes precedence in establishment of the healthy environment, other procedures may be performed concurrently. Definitive periodontal therapies generally require considerable time, several months or more, to heal fully and mature. Other treatment may often proceed during this time, but care must be given not to do complex restorative and prosthetic procedures until the foundation has been secured.

Surgical procedures (excisional and reparative)

These procedures, including necessary extractions, edentulous ridge reductions or augmentation, removal of cysts, foreign bodies, root tips, or impacted teeth, will generally be performed early in the establishment of a healthy oral environment. Some procedures such as frenectomies, vestibular extensions, and gingival grafts directly enhance the environment.

Efficiency may be enhanced by carrying out several minor surgical procedures at once, as with removal of a hopeless first molar combined with sliding flap or 'free' autogenous graft to establish a keratinized attachment on a second premolar (now the terminal tooth and potential abutment).

A word of caution is in order in sequencing surgical procedures. Having established the importance of daily home care (plaque control), and having painstakingly instructed the patient on how to achieve it, we should not immediately perform surgical procedures which, with their attendant postoperative swelling and tenderness, will prevent the patient from effective home care. Minor local procedures may not create a problem in this regard, but more involved surgeries (multiple third molar removals) should either precede preventive counseling, or be postponed until the patient has had time to develop and practice plaque control. Even then it is usually necessary to review and reinforce those skills after an interruption in the home care routine. This is especially true after periodontal procedures, because they not only interrupt the patient's newly established home care routine, but often change the architecture of the periodontium in the treated areas, calling for modifications in the patient's plaque control technique.

Caries elimination

This is critical to establishment of a healthy environment and, once complete, may result in a measurable improvement (increase) in salivary pH. When carious lesions are many and/or severe, they may well have been addressed with excavations and temporaries in the urgency phase of treatment. The use of temporary or interim sedative restorations can be an appropriate and effective way to eliminate caries without committing to a choice of specific restorative materials. Until a high caries environment has been modified, definitive restorations such as silver amalgam and composite resin should be used with caution, and cast restorations are usually contraindicated.

If, on the other hand, caries are neither severe nor extensive, caries elimination can be accomplished with definitive restorations at this early stage. Efficiency suggests performing such restorations in quadrants or clusters, reducing the number of visits, anesthetic administrations, and total time required.

Finally, there are situations in which caries are incipient, requiring re-evaluation over time rather than immediate restoration, or postponement of restoration until other planned treatment has been done nearby. In such cases full caries elimination may be safely postponed with the patient's knowledge and assent. Postponement of restoration may also be indicated in areas of periodontal surgery, because less bleeding and better access after pocket elimination may facilitate restoration, and preparations (design and margin placement) may be more appropriately planned in a postperiodontal environment.

Elimination of endodontic and apical pathology

If not already addressed as an urgency, this is another critical piece in establishing a healthy environment. It can often wait for the completion of caries control, because that will sometimes result in the discovery of old exposures (or the advent of new ones). Consider three anterior teeth, one with a periapical lesion, one with deep caries, and a third with an old leaking restoration. Endodontic therapy on the apically involved tooth should not precede excavations/restorations on the other two, because they could be candidates for endodontic therapy as well, and efficiency would obviously be enhanced by doing two or three anterior root canals at the same time.

On the other hand, there are cases where endodontic therapy should be instituted early in the game, for example, to establish the viability of a tooth in the overall plan, or in the case of a suspected endoperio lesion (see Chapter 6) in which endodontic therapy is needed before, or in concert with, periodontal treatment.

Correction of functional disorders

Treatment addressing the occlusion, temporomandibular joint, or neuromuscular components that are compromising the health of the oral environment is generally done after preventive, periodontal, surgical, caries elimination, and endodontic procedures have been performed or at least started. This is due to the typically diffuse nature of functional disorders and the occasional difficulty of accurate diagnosis. By eliminating or control-

ling these other problems, we may alleviate symptoms mistaken for functional disorders. At the least, we eliminate other potential causes and ensure more accurate diagnoses. In addition, it is usually more efficient to deal with functional disorders last. Periodontal treatment, caries control, and the like can be done in the presence of orthodontic appliances, but it is not easy. Occlusal adjustments done before excavations and interim restorations may have to be redone after the occlusal anatomy has been altered. Appliance therapy (for example, splints etc) is complicated if periodontal, surgical, or restorative procedures are not performed first. An obvious exception to this is the removal of gross occlusal interferences to relieve acute discomfort.

Taking precedence in the sequence are procedures that address functional disorders which are currently symptomatic or which are clearly contributing to an unhealthy environment. Examples include severe malocclusion, lost vertical dimension resulting from wear, anterior collapse caused by lack of posterior support, myofascial pain/dysfunction, or obviously harmful lip, cheek, tongue, or speech abnormalities.

Less critical are functional disorders which, although not immediately critical to oral health, must be corrected before definitive restoration or prosthetics to ensure good long-term results. Thus a CO–CR discrepancy which is not by itself an immediate problem may require correction before the placement of multiple posterior fixed bridges.

In summary, the establishment of a healthy oral environment should result in the elimination of active disease and potentially pathologic conditions. The patient should be free of major symptoms and in control of oral hygiene. Teeth to be retained should be pulpally and periodontally viable; this is the foundation for all further treatment.

Should financial limitations, systemic problems, or other factors prevent or postpone more definitive treatment, the establishment of a healthy oral environment can often preserve the dentition for many years, allowing for definitive treatment in the future. On the other hand, failure to establish oral health before definitive treatment may doom such treatment to failure.

RESTORATION OF FORM, FUNCTION, AND ESTHETICS

Definitive restorations (whether they are amalgam, composites, glass–ionomers, ceramics, or castings) and prosthetic appliances (either fixed or removable) generally constitute the second stage in the treatment sequence. The sequencing within this stage may itself be based on urgency, and then efficiency. The urgency factor here is not one of relief of an existing problem, but the need to avert potential crises. The prime example is the unrestored, endodontically treated, posterior tooth, which is at risk of fracture down the root or through the furcation. Definitive restoration (or temporization) is called for early in the sequence. The urgency is somewhat less for premolars, depending on the occlusal situation, and endodontically treated anteriors generally present even less risk. Indeed, an endodontically treated incisor with no restoration (other than the sealed access opening) may be left 'as is' indefinitely. Even heavily restored, endodontically treated anteriors are at less risk of catastrophic fracture, because anteriors are more susceptible to incisal angle fracture or horizontal fractures, rather than longitudinal breaks.

Another example of urgency is the restoration of periodontally treated teeth where existing tooth form or faulty restoration predisposes to further periodontal problems. Rough restorations, improper anatomy, or overhanging margins, if not corrected before periodontal treatment, ought to be corrected as soon after as is practicable.

The patient's felt needs must also be considered in sequencing the restorative treatment. Esthetic improvements may not be at the top of the dentist's list, but we must respect the patient's concerns in this regard.

Summarized, sequencing in this stage is based first on potential urgencies attempting to avert crises. Once urgent needs are addressed, efficiency dictates the sequence of restorative/prosthetic treatment.

A good example is the clinical situation in which crowns or fixed bridges are indicated in both anterior and posterior areas of the mouth. The sequence depends on the situation. If loss of posterior support has created excessive wear or shifting of anterior teeth, it may be critical in the restorative stage to reestablish good bilateral posterior support first, so as to allow effective anterior restorations and ensure their survival. Conversely, a similar situation may call for definitive restoration of the anterior segment first, to establish guidance in excursions, thus allowing later placement of posterior restorations with normal anatomy.

When there is no clear-cut clinical indication, patient preference should be taken into account. An esthetic concern may suggest starting with anterior segments, whereas a perceived lack of chewing ability may have us start at the back to establish comfort, function, and security in mastication.

In certain situations, simultaneous anterior/posterior restoration is indicated. This is certainly true when attempting to regain lost vertical dimension, when the establishment of tooth guidance involves both anterior and posterior teeth, or when the restorative or prosthetic plan (long span bridge or removable partial denture) is an anteroposterior restoration.

There is seldom a 'right' way to approach sequencing of the restorative/prosthetic stage of treatment. Alternatives must be considered, and each case judged on its own merits. The critical concept here is that the sequencing of the restorative/prosthetic stage must be based on sound clinical reasoning. There is also seldom a 'right' way to sequence treatment, no hard and fast rule that always applies. Alternatives need to be considered and weighed, and reasoned choices made.

Some sequences are self-evident. If crowns and/or fixed prostheses are to be combined in an arch with a removable partial denture, they will of course be made first, so the removable prostheses can adapt to them. Likewise, supererupted teeth needing to be removed or shortened must be treated before an opposing restoration or prosthesis is made.

Anticipatory restorations are another sequencing alternative, an example being fabrication of an upper posterior bridge without opposing lower teeth. As fixed prostheses generally precede removable, the anatomy and curve of occlusion need to anticipate the later opposing prosthesis. It is often useful to wax the anticipatory restoration against a trial setup of denture teeth representing the future opposing prosthesis. Those very teeth may then be used later, ensuring optimum occlusion in the final result.

The same principle applies when upper and lower crowns are to be placed opposing one another, but when time or financial limitations require that restorations be done one arch or quadrant at a time. The arch restored first does not have to match the opposing teeth (which may be flat, rough, uneven), but should anticipate the future work on the opposing teeth. It may be necessary to grossly recontour those opposing teeth to allow good anatomic form and to establish proper curve of occlusion. The first arch restored must harmonize (that is, make light occlusal contacts free of interference in excursions) with the postponed arch, but it may not fully 'occlude' until the second arch is later restored.

A third example of anticipatory restoration is an edentulous upper arch in need of immediate prosthesis, but where the lower partially edentulous arch requires a much longer course of treatment before definitive restoration. Once again, the upper prosthesis may harmonize with the lower without fully occluding with it, so that the later lower work can match good anatomy and curve of occlusion.

The importance of careful and thorough treatment planning is obvious in anticipatory restorations. With it, a long sequence of steps will fall into place at the end. Lacking it, the end-result can be very disappointing.

The end-point in the restorative/prosthetic stage is a dentition (natural or prosthetic) that provides good form, function, and esthetics: a healthy, well-restored mouth. That is a goal every dentist can appreciate, understand, and strive for, and which, approached carefully, competently, and in logical sequence, is attainable. Once reached, however, the next stage in goal-oriented treatment becomes paramount – namely the maintenance of the healthy oral environment and the restorations placed therein.

MAINTENANCE OF THE ORAL ENVIRONMENT AND ITS RESTORATIONS

An effective maintenance program must be tailored to each patient. No single recall interval, no routine set of procedures is universally appropriate or effective. The long-term success of the maintenance stage depends greatly on patient involvement and commitment, which must be established from the very start of the dentist–patient relationship. Basic oral health theory and practice must be operating throughout the entire treatment sequence, not started at its conclusion. Finally, the maintenance stage of the treatment sequence must address both environmental and mechanical maintenance.

Environmental maintenance

This involves the review, refinement, and reinforcement of the patient's daily preventive regimen. Human nature is such that enthusiasm wanes and skills deteriorate over time. Periodic recall/maintenance sessions must provide a review of motor skills and positive reinforcement of whatever success (mo matter how limited) the patient has had, along with sincere encouragement toward improvement when necessary. A hearty pat on the back coupled with a gentle (figurative) kick in the pants can be an effective combination. The frequency of the recall is critical. Some highly self-motivated patients, having thoroughly mastered oral health maintenance skills, show little loss of enthusiasm or effectiveness when seen on annual recall. Other patients (perhaps most patients) need review and reinforcement more frequently – visits at intervals of 3–4 months are not unrealistic in many cases. The patient should be involved in establishing an appropriate interval between visits that is based on a personal assessment of skills, motivation, and need for review.

Periodic maintenance programs must also be tailored to individual problems. Patients who present with a high caries rate or extreme periodontal breakdown must be maintained more carefully and seen more frequently than those whose presenting dental problems were minimal. Indeed, the greater the adjustment the patient needed to make in lifestyle (diet patterns, oral hygiene, or acceptance of prosthetic appliances), the greater the need for close, careful maintenance to support the changes. Many patients, despite their best efforts (and ours as well), are unable to achieve a consistent level of oral health maintenance and may require more interventions. People with disabilities, whether physical or mental, may not be able to master the basic necessary skills. Many normal healthy people are not endowed with the manual dexterity and fine motor skills necessary for total plaque control. Although the dentist cannot accept total responsibility for his or her patients' oral health maintenance, high-frequency recall visits may be needed.

The specific elements of maintenance sessions are also highly individualized, based on patient need. Review and reinforcement of the daily oral hygiene regimen is a standard, but the amount of time and emphasis placed upon them depends on how well that patient is doing. Mechanical removal of calculus and stain is also a standard maintenance procedure, but may be a major effort in some cases, or simply a 'check scale' in others.

Finally, we must consider where and to what extent our treatment has altered the oral environment and help the patient adjust the regimen originally established to deal with those changes. The most obvious example is the postperiodontal surgery situation, in which much of the gingival topography may have been altered. Gingival position may be different – more root surfaces are exposed. Relearning plaque removal and introducing additional devices may be necessary. Even a localized procedure such as a graft or frenectomy may alter the topography enough to require retraining.

Similar changes occur with extensive restorations, extractions, and prostheses. Each of these represents a change in the oral environment and each requires individual strategies for health maintenance in, under, and around them. Multiple abutments or splinted teeth must allow for access to proximal brushes, threaders, and the like, and techniques must be taught and reinforced regularly. Removable partial dentures present special challenges as a result of anatomic irregularities created for rests and clasps, and the greater tendency for plaque accumulation under and around the removable appliance.

Once again the techniques necessary to maintain oral health and clean the appliance must be taught and reinforced. In many cases completion of the restorative phase simplifies oral hygiene rather than complicating it. Even so, it is necessary to assist the patient in adjusting the daily oral health regimen to the new situation.

Mechanical maintenance

Dentists can be victims of their own terminology. We often hear the term 'permanent' filling or bridge as opposed to 'temporary.' To many people the connotation is that the restoration will last forever. Fabrication of miniature mechanical devices expected to perform comfortably and efficiently 24 hours a day, year after year, in a hostile biomechanical environment is difficult enough. That the device should also last forever with little or no upkeep is unrealistic. Yet we create that expectation if we fail to establish the need for regular mechanical maintenance and an understanding on the part of the patient that mechanical devices wear out or break, just as natural teeth do. If a less durable material is chosen because of financial constraints, the patient must understand the need for maintenance and/or replacement. The dentition is a complex biomechanical system, and it requires maintenance and repairs no matter how carefully it is restored. It is also going to wear out some day. A healthy oral environment is absolutely essential to the survival of mechanical restorations, and makes their replacement with new restorations possible.

MODEL TREATMENT SEQUENCES

A sequential approach to treatment that is based first on urgency, and then on efficiency in achieving treatment goals, has been established in general terms. Priorities within each of those stages have been discussed. Using those general concepts as guides, a model can be developed that places specific treatment steps into the sequence. This model should serve as a guideline, not a set of rules.

SYSTEMIC TREATMENT

This addresses the general health status of the patient and its relationship to the oral cavity and dental treatment. It may include the following elements.

Treatment of systemic disease (referral/consultation)

- Dentist detects significant hypertension; refers patient for medical evaluation and/or treatment.
- Dentist suspects possible diabetic condition and refers patient for medical evaluation and/or treatment.

Treatment of oral disease, or coordination of systemic treatment in progress

- Dentist performs a biopsy of an oral lesion. The results, which suggest a malignancy, are referred to physician for further (head–neck) evaluation and treatment.
- Dentist prescribes penicillin for dental abscess, taking patient off medically prescribed tetracycline acne regimen and informs prescribing dermatologist.

Prevention of systemic disease by premedication

- A prophylactic antibiotic regimen is prescribed for patients with mitral valve prolapse before invasive procedures.
- Presurgical antibiotic coverage is given to susceptible patients – brittle diabetics, immune compromised individuals, or others with history of poor resistance to infection.

EMERGENCY/INVESTIGATIVE TREATMENT

This addresses those dental problems that constitute the patient's chief complaint, are producing symptoms, or are potential sources of acute symptoms. The following are examples:

- Relief of dental pain as a result of pulpitis is accomplished with excavation/sedative temporary restoration, pulpotomy, or pulpectomy.
- Relief of dental pain caused by periodontal abscess is achieved with irrigation, curettage, or incision/drainage.
- Appropriate analgesic/antibiotic agents are prescribed for above.
- Definitive or palliative treatment of soft tissue lesion is accomplished through excision, cautery, or topical medication.
- Any dental treatment procedure that is exploratory in nature – that is, performed in order to determine the feasibility of further treatment – includes excavations of deep carious lesions, initiation of endodontic procedures to assess prognosis, and periodontal flap procedures to assess actual bone levels.
- Any definitive treatment done to relieve immediate symptoms, such as removal of symptomatic, partially impacted third molar. Even a procedure such as cast crown preparation can be an appropriate 'emergency' procedure, with care taken that the entire dental and oral situation is taken into account. Complicated and irreversible procedures should, whenever practical, await a thorough examination and diagnosis before being performed in their proper sequence.

PREPARATORY TREATMENT

This includes those steps aimed at the establishment of a healthy oral environment. Sequencing within this category is flexible, and should be based on efficiency. Examples of preparatory treatment include:

- Preventive counseling and plaque control instructions.
- Dietary analysis and counseling.
- Fluoride therapy, systemic and topical.
- Periodontal therapy, including scaling/polishing, root planing, definitive surgery for pocket elimination, or repair/enhancement of periodontal apparatus.
- Oral surgery, including removal of teeth, cysts, foreign bodies, exostoses, or modification of the soft tissue to facilitate later treatment. Orthognathic surgery in concert with orthodontic correction.
- Endodontic therapy.
- Caries control, either through excavation/temporary or definitive restoration with 'interim' material (such as amalgam or resin). Restoration with castings will generally await completion of all preparatory procedures.
- Modification of the occlusion, including orthodontic treatment – minor tooth movement or comprehensive therapy.
- Occlusal adjustment to harmonize occlusion with temporomandibular joint, relieve symptoms, or facilitate later treatment.
- Restoration of lost vertical dimension to alleviate symptoms and/or facilitate later treatment.

CORRECTIVE TREATMENT

This includes those procedures aimed at the restoration of form, function, and esthetics. Sequencing within this category is flexible but often critical, because in many complex restorative efforts each step must meld properly into the next. For example, a cast post and core on a lower tooth might have to be fabricated not only with the individual tooth in mind, but also establishing parallelism with another tooth, allowing space for intracoronal partial denture attachments, and considering its relationship with opposing teeth. The following are examples of corrective treatment:

- Operative dentistry, including cast restorations and interim materials, especially when further (prosthetic) treatment is not anticipated.
- Fixed prosthetics and individual crown restorations.
- Removable prosthetics, including partial denture prostheses and full dentures.
- Maxillofacial prosthetic devices, including obturators and facial reconstructive appliances.

MAINTENANCE TREATMENT

This is aimed at effectively supporting the healthy environment and restorations placed therein. In establishing a sequence within this category, timing is all important. The need for maintenance starts as soon as that healthy environment is established; therefore, maintenance might be initiated in some areas even before corrective treatment is complete, and perhaps even before it is begun. Although a course of dental treatment may be completed in a short time, complex cases may extend over weeks, months, or even years. An effective maintenance schedule, then, must be instituted independent of preparatory and corrective treatment.

Finally, although frequency and timing are critical in this phase, the actual content of a maintenance program must be tailored to individual patient needs. Examples of this treatment include:

- Review of principles and modification of home care techniques after periodontal, restorative, and prosthetic treatment.
- Periodic review and reinforcement of same.
- Periodic examination and radiographs to monitor status of restorations and prostheses and to detect incipient pathology.

- Periodic scaling/polishing.

- Fluoride therapy.

- Modification, adjustment, repair, and replacement of restorative and prosthetic hardware.

This outline of treatment stages and examples of the types of procedures likely to be done in each should be viewed as a guide. The basic principles apply, but there are no absolute rules. A good example is that of bite-plane therapy. A simple occlusal coverage splint, fabricated over the maxillary teeth and allowing full occlusal contact without lateral interference, is a useful therapeutic dental appliance, yet it cannot be automatically fixed into a treatment sequence. It may be an emergency/investigative device, relieving acute myofascial pain/dysfunction (MPD) symptoms and allowing for a truer assessment of centric relation position. It may be a preparatory procedure relieving occlusal traumatism within the course of periodontal therapy or aiding in the reestablishment of lost vertical dimension. It may be applied in the maintenance phase, should symptoms develop after corrective treatment or recurrent bruxism threaten the mechanical integrity of dental restorations.

Flexibility is also required in responding to patients' felt needs. A definitive anterior restoration when esthetics is a problem may be done before other, more pressing procedures in the preparatory category. Obviously, such a deviation from standard procedure must be done with due care, and with the patient fully informed of the potential risks entailed.

Once the list of necessary procedures has been arranged in the proper sequence, the general treatment categories can be broken into discrete specific procedures, with time and cost estimates attached. We need to know how many visits, over what period of time, and at what cost in order to present the total picture to the patient. At this juncture it is also possible to consider alternative treatment options as a function of time and money. A well-conceived treatment plan requiring 6–8 months to complete is of little value to the patient who is only available for 3 months. Likewise a treatment plan requiring an investment of thousands of dollars may not be appropriate for the patient barely able to keep up with the cost of food, clothing, and accommodation. Possible options in such situations range from selection of alternative treatment approaches requiring less time and money (and providing a lesser service), to phasing the treatment over time.

In any event it is the responsibility of the dentist to present all practical treatment options to the patient, especially the course of treatment the dentist feels can provide the best result over the longest time. The decision of which option to select rests with the patient. We must not prejudge the patient's willingness to accept optimal treatment or his or her ability to pay for it. Even when financial limitations are made known before treatment planning, the patient should be informed of optimal courses of treatment and their cost. Financial situations change, priorities change, people change. The dentist, while tailoring services to the individual needs and desires of each patient, must give each the option of optimal treatment, or at least make the patient aware that such treatment is available. The patient who chooses a lesser alternative approach has made an informed decision. The dentist has provided that patient with the information necessary to make a good choice. The treatment then rendered is, for that patient, an 'ideal' plan, because it serves their needs in a way that they can accept.

The treatment plan in Fig 8.1 illustrates, on the right side, three treatment options for the maxillary arch, all in appropriate sequence. On the left, the dental chart details the plan options 'by the numbers.' The example plan (Fig 8.2) shows a dental tooth chart with a treatment plan, with appointments sequenced and numbered (along with necessary healing time or intervals between preparation and inserts).

PHASING OF TREATMENT

As distinguished from sequencing, phasing treatment connotes spreading treatment over time, and this can be useful in a variety of clinical situations. Let's briefly address a number of those situations.

	SERVICES NECESSARY	FEES I	FEES II	FEES III
~~1~~		I	II	III
~~2~~				
3	ENDO, ROOT AMP, FCC / EXT	1075	85	85
~~4~~	P/G PONTIC	575		
5	ENDO, POST & CORE, P/G / EXT	1025	85	85
6	P/G	600	600	600
~~7~~	P/G PONTIC	600	600	600
8	P/G	600	600	600
9	P/G	600	600	600
~~10~~	P/G PONTIC	600	600	600
11	P/G	600	600	600
~~12~~	P/G PONTIC	600		
~~13~~	P/G PONTIC	600		
~~14~~	GOLD PONTIC	575		
15	FCC / MO/ALLOY	575	575	65
~~16~~	SEMI-PRECISION CAST BASE RPD	1350		
17	CHROME COBALT & ACRYLIC RPD	/	950	
18		—	—	—
19		8625	5695	4785
20				
21				
22				

TREATMENT PLAN OPTIONS: MAXILLA
I KEEP ALL MAXILLARY TEETH–IDEAL, BUT HIGHEST COST & RISK
ENDO AND DB ROOT AMPUTATION #3, ENDO AND POST & CORE #5
FIXED BRIDGES: 3—5–6—8 9—11—15
(DESIGN 5–6 & 11 FOR RPD LATER–IF NECESSARY)
II MAXILLARY PARTIAL–LESS IDEAL, BUT LESS RISK
EXTRACT #3 & 5
FIXED BRIDGE: 6—8–9—11 FULL CAST CROWN #15
MAXILLARY PRECISION OR SEMI-PRECISION CAST METAL
BASE (MUCOSTATIC) RPD
III LEAST COSTLY VIABLE ALTERNATIVE
EXTRACT #3 & 5
FIXED BRIDGE: 6—8–9—11 MO/ALLOY #15
MAXILLARY CHROME COBALT & ACRYLIC RPD (ALTERED CAST)

Fig 8.1

This detailed list of procedures and fees depicts a complex case (maxilla only) with three possible treatment options. Heavy slash marks indicate specific options for treatment on individual teeth. A blueprint like this is essential to calculate and appreciate the cost differential of the various options.

		SERVICES NECESSARY		FEES		
	1					
	2					
⑤	3	MOD/alloy, base, anes.	100			
	4	DO/alloy, base	65			
	5					
④	6	G/composite, base, anes.	65			
	7	M/composite, base	65			
? ◄	8	Cast dowel & core, P/G crn		200	+600	(elective)
	9	M/composite, base	65			
	10					
	11					
	12					
	13					
⑥	14	MOL/alloy, base, anes.	100			
	15					
2 wks ⑧	16	Surgical removal, tissue impactions	125			
	17	ʺ ʺ ʺ ʺ	125			
2 wks ⑨	18	Full cast gold crown				
2 wks ⑩	19	Gold pontic	1650			
	20	Gold 3/4 crown				
	21					
	22					
	23					
	24					
	25					
	26					
	27					
	28					
	29					
⑦	30	MODB/alloy, base, anes.	115			
	31					
2 wks ①	32	Surgical removal, partial tissue impaction	125			
		Preventive visits (2) incl.	120			
1 wk ②		oral health maintenance				
③		instructions, scaling,				
		pumicing, and topical F				
		Appointments numbered in probable sequence.				
		Approximate total time: 3 months, allowing for				
		healing of 3rd molar extractions.				

Fig 8.2

Using a treatment planning form, specific procedures and fees are listed tooth by tooth. Appointments are numbered to indicate the sequence of treatment, and time intervals are estimated where appropriate. For example, appointments 4, 5, and 6 (operative dentistry) can be spaced at any interval (a day, a week, a month), but 2 weeks must be allowed between preparation and insert of the bridge (appointments 9 and 10), and healing time is anticipated after surgical removal of wisdom teeth (appointment 8).

TRADITIONAL VERSUS OPTIMAL TREATMENT MODELS

Traditionally a dentist might offer patients a range of choices based on cost: minimal treatment at one end, optimal treatment at the other. The assumption was that treatment would be done now, and patients would have to choose the level of care that they wanted or could afford. It was the model seen in most dental schools, in which students needing to complete treatment for graduation might hurry to get periodontal treatment and caries control done, so as to proceed to crowns, partial dentures, etc as soon as possible. This approach did not always serve the patient's best interest, in or out of dental school.

The late Dr Robert Barkley proposed a better model a quarter of a century ago.[1] Instead of using the traditional model holding time constant, and making quality a variable (related to cost) (Fig 8.3), we can look at a phased model (Fig 8.4) in which the long-range goal is optimal dental treatment, with phasing over time making such treatment more affordable to the patient.

The time-variable model of planning begins with the assumption that most patients would prefer to have the best available treatment for themselves and their families. No one wants third-rate care. However, real or perceived financial or other limitations may prevent one from accepting an optimal treatment plan. Instead of having to choose mediocre treatment, we can look at the first stage, establishment of a healthy oral environment, as the first step in an extended course of treatment with the long-term goal being the best possible dental care available. Instead of being considered patchwork or substandard care, basic dental disease control is simply the first step toward optimum treatment. There is more than a semantic difference. To the patient, phasing means working toward an optimal goal at a manageable economic pace. Financial commitments are made a step at a time. The patient can 'try out' some dental treatment on a limited basis before committing to a major investment. For the dentist, it means that many more patients will have committed to an optimum course of treatment: some who will have it immediately, others over an agreed upon span of time, and still others over an indefinite period of time. Patients are not categorized as 'optimum care' or 'minimal care' cases. 'Basic' dentistry is more satisfying when it is put in the context of a first step toward a higher goal.

Although it has numerous advantages, this approach to phasing has a few potential drawbacks. The most serious of these is a dentition that is so debilitated that treatment in segments, or over time, is technically impossible. An obvious example is a severe loss of vertical dimension, because, if it is to be regained, treatment must generally be done throughout the mouth at one time.

Another potential problem with time phasing is that caries control may dictate placement of sound interim restorations (such as large silver alloys) which would then be treated again with crowns in the not too distant future, thus requiring treatment of some teeth twice in a period of months or years. This may not be a serious drawback,

Traditional model

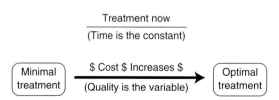

Fig 8.3

Traditional treatment model: treatment is done now, quality is variable.

Time variable model

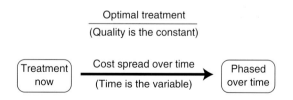

Fig 8.4

Time-variable model: by phasing treatment over time, quality remains the constant.

because excavation of caries and old restorations and placement of 'core' materials are often a prudent step before definitive restoration. In the box is given an example of a hypothetical treatment plan which could be carried out in a fairly short time. The fees are arbitrary, for purposes of illustration.

This plan could be carried out over a longer time period, possibly phased over 3 years, as shown in the second box:

Optimal plan, to be done 'now'

1. Premedicate for invasive procedures – prolapsed mitral valve
2. Remove partially erupted lower right third molar, currently symptomatic — $150
3. Scale/polish and plaque control instructions, emphasis on flossing (two sessions) — $120
4. Endodontic therapy tooth no. 9, asymptomatic, non-vital, with PA radiolucency — $350
5. Operative dentistry: composite resins nos 7 and 8, silver amalgams nos 3, 4, 14, and 29 — $400
6. Cast crown no. 30 — $575
   Fixed bridge replacing no. 19, full crown no. 18, porcelain fused to precious metal no. 20 — $1,750
   Cast dowel and core no. 9 — $200
   Porcelain fused to precious metal no. 9 — $600
7. Recall/maintenance at completion, and every 6 months post-treatment — $60

   Total treatment time approximately 4–6 months, total fee — $4205

Phased plan, to be done over 3 years

Phase 1, first year, establish a healthy oral environment:
1. Premedicate for invasive procedures – prolapsed mitral valve
2. Remove partially erupted lower right third molar, currently symptomatic — $150
3. Scale/polish and plaque control instructions, emphasis on flossing (two sessions) — $120
4. Endodontic therapy tooth no. 9, asymptomatic, nonvital, with PA radiolucency — $350
5. Operative dentistry: as above (composite resins nos. 7 and 8, silver amalgams nos 3, 4, 14, and 29), plus amalgam core no. 30 @ $100 — $500

   Total treatment time approximately 2–3 months, total fee — $1120

Phase 2, second year, replace missing molar tooth:
1. Premedicate for invasive procedures – prolapsed mitral valve
2. Fixed bridge replacing no. 19, full crown no. 18, porcelain fused to precious metal no. 20 — $1750
3. Recall/maintenance every 6 months (2 sessions) — $120

   Total treatment time approximately 3–4 weeks, total fee — $1870

Phase 3, third year, definitive restorations for nos 9 and 30:
1. Premedicate for invasive procedures – prolapsed mitral valve
2. Cast dowel and core no. 9 — $200
   Porcelain fused to precious metal no. 9 — $600
   Cast crown no. 30 — $575
3. Recall/maintenance every 6 months (2 sessions) — $120

   Total treatment time approximately 6–8 weeks, total fee — $1295

With this phased approach, the optimum plan is carried out over a longer time period, at a more comfortable financial pace. Regular payments of $120 per month would allow the entire course of treatment to be paid for as it was completed.

Finally, this plan could be phased over an indefinite period of time (should circumstances require), as shown in the third box.

In this plan, the patient is not labelled 'minimal care' or 'disease control only,' although that is what is being accomplished at the outset. The goal of optimal treatment remains viable, although some years may pass before it is completed. The example shown in Fig 8.5 illustrates such a case in which disease control was accomplished and one quadrant optimally restored, with almost 10 years elapsing before the patient proceeded with the balance of definitive treatment.

PHASING BY QUADRANT

A variation on this theme is to carry out optimal restoration/replacement one quadrant at a time over a number of months or even years. By taking the most urgent areas first and then doing a project each year, full

optimal restoration/rehabilitation can be budgeted over time. This is especially useful in third party relationships (page 151) where there may be an annual benefit limit. Temporary or interim restorations may be necessary to put quadrants 'on hold' for months or years, but this can generally be done safely.

When the goal is optimal dentistry, which may last decades, spreading the care over several years makes good sense.

PHASING BY LEVEL OF ORAL HEALTH

We have already discussed the chronicity of most dental diseases and the futility of dental treatment in the face of uncontrolled caries or periodontal disease. All too often, extensive definitive treatment is carried out without having established the ability or willingness of the patient to achieve and maintain the healthy oral environment so essential to its success. Considerable time, effort, and expense may be wasted, with the result being frustration and discouragement on the part of the patient.

In phasing treatment by level of oral health, we do not deny treatment to patients who do

---

Phased plan, over an indefinite time period:

Phase 1, first year, establish a healthy oral environment:

1. Premedicate for invasive procedures – prolapsed mitral valve
2. Remove partially erupted lower right third molar, currently symptomatic $150
3. Scale/polish and plaque control instructions, emphasis on flossing (two sessions)$120
5. Operative dentistry: as above (composite resins nos 7 and 8, silver amalgams
    nos 3, 4, 14, and 29), plus amalgam core no. 30 @ $100 $500
                                                                                    _____

    Total treatment time approximately 2–3 months, total fee $770

Phase 2, postponed indefinitely, but monitored regularly:

1. Premedicate for invasive procedures – prolapsed mitral valve
2. Recall/maintenance every 6 months (two sessions)
    Monitor clinically and radiographically tooth no. 9, which will need
    endodontic treatment at some point; monitor space for bridge
    (missing no. 19) and consider simple space maintainer if drifting/
    tipping is measurable $120/year

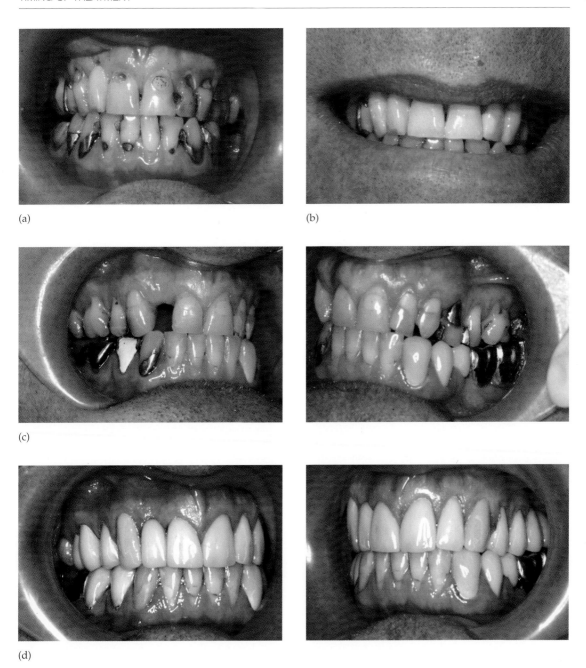

(a)   (b)

(c)

(d)

Fig 8.5

(a) A lifetime of tooth decay, tooth loss, and failed dentistry made this patient skeptical about comprehensive treatment options. He accepted resin and amalgam 'holding' care, and a fixed bridge was placed in the lower left quadrant in 1981. (b) Although not 'definitive' treatment, significant esthetic improvement was a positive factor in the patient's attitude about his dentition. (c) It was nearly 10 years later, in 1990, that the patient sought definitive care. Although some of the holding treatment was wearing out, the patient had maintained his home care, and was pleased that the lower left bridge was still going strong. (d) 8 years later (1998) the phased treatment continues to serve the patient functionally and esthetically.

not perform up to 'our' standards of oral health maintenance. This would be arbitrary and foolish, because we are dealing with human beings, not robots. To accept our patients as human beings is to accept both success and failure, enthusiasm and apathy. The patient must be met more than half-way. We must accept the level of understanding, ability, and motivation the patient presents, and work toward the next level. The type of treatment we render, however, and the timing of that treatment must consider the patient's current level of oral health or be doomed to failure.

PHASING BY CARIES CONTROL

The patient exhibiting a high caries rate must have four treatment approaches applied simultaneously: personal plaque control, dietary control, fluoride therapy, and elimination of carious lesions.

Plaque control and dietary modification

These are clearly under the control of the patient. In many cases they require a significant change in lifestyle and daily routine. Such changes do not come easily, and we must allow for assimilation, relapse, and occasional failure, in the hope of achieving success in the long term. We must be prepared to accept less than total plaque and dietary control, given human nature. The patient who has the self-discipline to exercise total plaque and dietary control is not likely to have excessive caries in the first place. The content and timing of our treatment plan must be sensitive to the patient's ability and willingness to control caries, and not create a situation in which failure is inevitable.

Fluoride therapy

This is effective in the control of caries and involves the patient's use of fluoridated denti-frice, rinses, and/or home-use topical gels, as prescribed or recommended, as well as the professional application of fluorides in a variety of delivery vehicles.

Eliminating all carious lesions

This prevents further loss of tooth structure, eliminates plaque formation/retention areas (the lesions themselves), and will shift the pH and general oral environment toward health and away from disease. The critical question is not whether to remove all caries as soon as practical, but the choice of materials to fill the spaces thus created. Few would advocate multiple porcelain fused to metal crowns as an immediate treatment in the presence of rampant caries, and such treatment would be at grave risk of failure. 'Intermediate' materials, including resin-reinforced zinc oxide–eugenol (IRM), or fluoridated materials, including a wide range of glass ionomers, can be very useful in this area owing to their economy, ease of placement, caries inhibition, sedative properties, and relatively good longevity (6 months to a year or more). When greater strength, retention, or longevity is required, silver amalgam, composite resin, or even temporary metal or resin crowns can be employed, and can often serve for long periods of time.

If we are phasing by caries control, we must assess whether that control has been established. If the patient tells us he is doing daily plaque removal, has eliminated, substituted, or controlled a cariogenic diet, and is using appropriate fluorides, we must take that at face value. We can easily observe whether or not plaque control has been established by direct examination. The other issues depend on the patient's honesty.

A safer assessment of caries control is by direct observation of the extent and rate of caries activity. Careful clinical and radiographic examination at 4- to 6-month intervals, carried out over 1–2 years, allows for a realistic assessment. The benefits are worth the wait. If effective caries control has been established over that time, both patient and dentist can proceed with more definitive treatment with confidence. On the other hand, should there be continuing new and recurrent caries, reinforcement or additional caries control methods are appropriate, and we have not added the complication of failed definitive restorations. The following treatment plan is for a 14-year-old girl who presented with 18 carious surfaces on 12 teeth, and a class II malocclusion, crowding and anterior overbite, with bilateral posterior crossbite.

The second plan is for a 45-year-old man presenting with extensive existing restorations, and 22 carious surfaces (predominately gingival and root caries) on 19 teeth.

Fourteen-year-old female

Phase 1, caries control:

1. Plaque control instructions/counseling
2. Analysis of diet, and modification/counseling
3. Topical fluoride application and home-use gel prescription
4. Excavation/temporization of three deep carious lesions – potential pulpal involvement
5. Removal of all caries: restoration with silver amalgam and composite resin when practical, stainless steel crowns or pin-amalgam cores if necessary
6. Recall/maintenance at intervals of 3–4 months to review/reinforce plaque and diet control, apply fluorides, reexamine for new caries, continue for 1–2 years

Phase 2, orthodontic/restorative, assuming no new caries and patient maintenance:
1. Fixed (straight wire) orthodontic treatment to improve health, function, and esthetics; intensive caries control continued throughout treatment
2. Porcelain fused to gold crowns as needed, replacing interim restorations after orthodontic treatment

Unless caries control has been established, phase 2 is not recommended: The potential benefits of orthodontic and definitive restorative treatment are offset by the risks of placing appliances and then crowns into a high caries environment.

Forty-five-year-old male

Phase 1, caries control:

1. Plaque control instructions/counseling
2. Analysis of diet, and modification/counseling
3. Topical fluoride application and home-use gel prescription
4. Removal of all carious lesions including excavation under and around existing crowns

Phase 2, reconstruction:
Assuming effective caries control has been established, restoration of the dentition will require multiple crowns and fixed bridges, and considerable investment of time and money.
OR... if caries continue to develop or recur, an alternative treatment approach may be indicated.

Phase 2 alternative, transition to prostheses:
Continued minimal restoration/patchwork may be done where possible, leading to eventual extraction of non-restorable teeth, and placement of partial or full removable prostheses.

This last alternative constitutes some of the most difficult and least rewarding of dental treatments that we are called upon to perform. It is preferable, however, to seeing collapse and failure of extensive reconstructive efforts and, for some patients, it is an appropriate and rational treatment choice.

PHASING BY PERIODONTAL MAINTENANCE

Periodontal disease is so strongly behavior related that control and maintenance must precede almost any dental treatment, including definitive periodontal therapy. If the patient is unwilling or unable to carry out effective daily plaque control, treatment efforts are doomed to failure. On the other hand, environmental factors may be present that contribute to the disease (occlusal traumatism) or prevent effective plaque control (rough, overhanging margins, impassable or open contacts). Severe malocclusions may also contribute to the disease and/or inhibit plaque control, and present a special challenge in phasing treatment.

Fortunately, periodontal maintenance efforts can be evaluated readily. Disclosants reveal plaque accumulations, which can be qualitatively classified (slight, moderate, heavy) or quantified with plaque index (PI) or other tools. Steady progress in the patient's plaque control bodes well, and is likely to be accompanied by other observable improvements in tissue color and tone. Reduction in bleeding on probing is another key observable sign of improving periodontal health. Definitive periodontal therapy is generally deferred until such positive changes are observed. It is possible, through frequent sessions of scaling/polishing, to achieve similar improvements without effective home care, but over time the patient's own efforts are paramount.

Antimicrobial rinses, including chlorhexidine and fluoride preparations, can be effective adjuncts to plaque control, and short-duration, broad-spectrum, systemic antibiotics administered during acute periodontal episodes have added another tool in the management of the disease. A hypothetical phased plan based on periodontal mainte-nance might look like the one in the box shown on page 147.

PHASING BY SUCCESS OR FAILURE OF PRECEDING STEPS

This applies the preceding concepts on a wider scale. There are many situations in which a given dental treatment has an inherent risk of failure. That failure may become apparent immediately (longitudinal root fracture when cementing a post), or may be a latent problem. When subsequent treatment is carried out based on the anticipation of success of preceding treatment, the risk is magnified; more is now at stake. For that reason, it is often prudent to allow some time to pass after an initial treatment to enhance confidence in its success. Examples of this application of phased treatment include the following:

Deep excavations of carious lesions

Placement of bases or liners or 'conditioning' with etchant, followed by denting bonding agents, may help maintain pulpal health and encourage or allow secondary dentin formation. Failure is inevitable if the caries have already invaded the pulp or if the operative procedures stress the pulpal tissue beyond its limit. Should irreversible pulpitis develop subsequently, endodontic therapy will be required to retain the tooth, and there is no guarantee that such treatment can be successfully carried out, or that it will itself succeed long term.

Treatment involving such deeply excavated teeth should be phased, if possible, so that definitive treatment (castings, or the use of the tooth as an abutment) is postponed pending evaluation of pulpal status (Fig. 8.6). If no signs or symptoms are seen over 6–12 months, subsequent steps can be carried out, although some risk remains, which must be discussed with the patient. On the other hand, if deeply excavated teeth remain sensitive, become symptomatic, or exhibit apical radiolucencies, they are not good candidates for further definitive restoration or prostheses unless endodontic therapy is successfully performed.

Phase 1, periodontal control:
1. Plaque control counseling, with intense emphasis on sulcular brushing and flossing
2. Prescription or recommendation of antimicrobial rinses
3. Complete calculus removal, that is, root planing (with curettage where appropriate)
4. Relief of gross occlusal disharmonies to control primary and secondary trauma
5. Close maintenance with follow-up scaling/polishing and reinforcement of home care
    Total treatment time approximately 3–12 months.

Goal of phase 1: the establishment of an effective plaque control regimen, and control of acute periodontal lesions as determined by improved tissue color and texture, and reduction or elimination of bleeding.

Phase 2, definitive periodontal therapy:
    Note: this phase should not be implemented unless the phase 1 goal has been attained.
1. Surgical procedures, as appropriate, to eliminate pockets, eliminate and recontour bony defects, osseous grafting to fill same, guided tissue regeneration, autogenous gingival or connective tissue grafts, etc. Supportive topical antimicrobials and systemic antibiotics as indicated.
2. Complete review and modification of plaque control regimens after alterations to the gingival topography.
3. Periodic review of same, with post-surgical scaling/polishing every 3–4 months.
    Treatment time will vary, but maturation of tissues can take many months.

Goal of phase 2: a healthy periodontium, free of significant pockets and/or bleeding, which can be and is being effectively maintained on a daily basis.

Phase 3, restorative/prosthetic:
    Note: extent of restorations/prostheses and choice of materials will depend on success of phase 2 treatment.
1. Restorative and prosthetic dentistry as needed.
2. Periodic recall, with re-evaluation of periodontium and scaling/polishing every 3–4 months.
    Treatment time will vary, depending on patient need.

Goal of phase 3: to establish a functional, esthetic, and atraumatic occlusion, readily maintainable by the patient. Timing and treatment choices will depend greatly on the degree to which of phase 2 goals have been met.

OR... if the patient is unable to gain at least a reasonable degree of control, an alternative treatment approach may be indicated involving removal of teeth and leading toward full removable prostheses.

Endodontic therapy

This is another example of a highly predictable dental procedure which, nevertheless, has some potential for failure. Consider that a 95% success rate still implies that one root canal in 20 will almost certainly fail! As endodontic failure can result in loss of the tooth, treatment should be phased after endodontic treatment to allow some assessment of the result before building further upon such teeth. An asymptomatic tooth is essential, and radiographic evidence of resolving bone lesions is a most welcome sign. In an ideal case, a month to 6 weeks is a reasonable minimum waiting period before proceeding with further treatment. Where unusually large osseous defects were found (especially if resulting in mobility), or where the endodontic procedure was complicated by

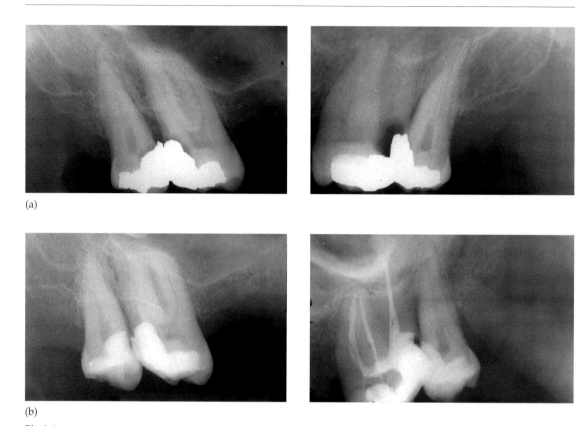

(a)

(b)

Fig 8.6

(a) This patient presented in mid-1990 with six sound upper anterior teeth, missing premolars and first molars, and second and third molars severely affected with recurrent caries. Tooth number 15 was pulpally involved and question-able as to its restorability. The other maxillary molars were potential endodontic candidates as well. (b) Excavations and sedative (IRM) temporaries were placed, and endodontic treatment carried out on number 15. A full 6 months was allowed to pass, while other treatment was done. All the teeth remained asymptomatic and radiographically within normal limits on these late 1990 films.

root morphology, canal size, or other unusual conditions, a longer wait (6–12 months) may be more prudent (Fig 8.7a–f).

Periodontal surgery

This has already been addressed as a reason to delay subsequent procedures. This is especially true when very deep pockets, severe osseous defects, furcation involvements, and the like are encountered. Valiant efforts may be made periodontally to preserve such teeth, but we must then be cautious about the extent to which we involve or depend upon them in further treatment steps. A successful bone graft and guided tissue regeneration may save a second molar, which may then be used as a bridge abutment. However, failure of the periodontal effort would also cost the patient the bridge, and necessitate construction of a partial denture. It would be prudent if some time were allowed to pass after periodontal therapy, to build confidence in the result (Fig 8.8a–d,g). If the surgical procedure proves unsuccessful, or even if the result is less than optimal, further treatment that depends on that tooth can be avoided, or 'escape routes' established. This concept will be explored in later chapters.

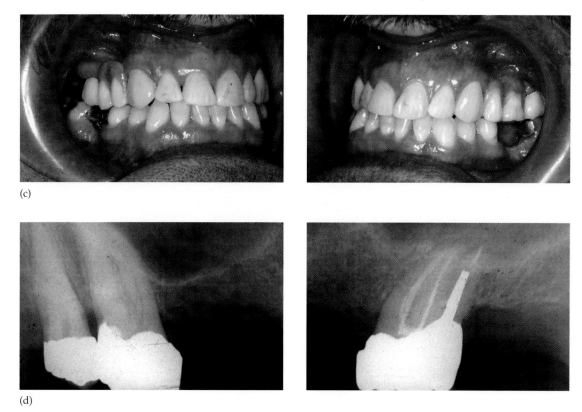

(c)

(d)

Fig 8.6 *continued*

(c) Crowns were placed on numbers 1, 2, and 15. (No. 16 was removed to allow ready access to clean behind no. 15, and because it was of no strategic value.) Attachments placed in the molars and in canine crowns receive a semi-precision, gold base, tooth-borne, partial denture, completed in mid-1992. (d) On the most recent recall, early 1998, both the endodontically treated tooth and the vital molars nos 1 and 2 were asymptomatic, stable, and radiographically within normal limits. Lower fixed bridges, placed in 1993 and 1994, completed the case.

Finally, it is the duty of the general dentist overseeing the total case to identify teeth that are deemed hopeless or nonrestorable before periodontal therapy, and either remove them at the outset, or at least ensure that they are not heroically treated only to be removed after periodontal treatment.

Orthodontic treatment

Whether minor tooth movement, comprehensive treatment, or orthognathic surgery, this treatment creates the need for phasing based on the orthodontic result. A period of retention is generally required after tooth movement, and relapse during or after active retention is a risk (Fig 8.9).

In summary, the number and complexity of treatment steps dictate the degree of caution required in phasing treatment. An anterior tooth that has been endodontically treated, but which requires only a composite to seal the access opening, can be 'finished' as soon as it is practicable. On the other hand, a molar tooth that has undergone periodontal therapy to fill an osseous defect and multiple canal endodontic treatment, and will require a cast

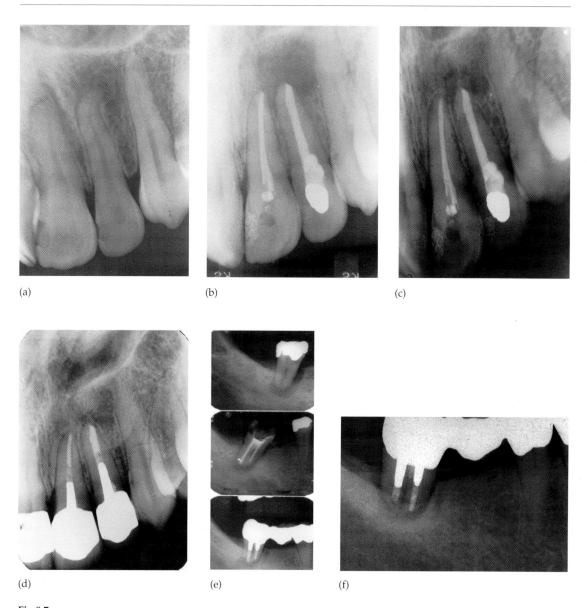

(a)   (b)   (c)

(d)   (e)   (f)

Fig 8.7

(a) Both central and lateral incisor were pulpally involved, probably as a result of trauma some years previously. Severe dilaceration at the apex of the lateral was a complicating factor. (b) A large periapical lesion developed, involving both teeth. Both were mobile, especially the lateral. Surgical access was gained to enucleate the lesion, and apicoectomy was done on the lateral incisor, with gutta percha fills on both. (c) Definitive restoration was deferred, and this 6-month follow-up shows that the apical lesion was clearly resolving. Mobility was back to normal. (d) Post cores and crowns were placed 2 years after endodontic therapy, by which time confidence in the long-term endodontic result was high, with almost complete resolution of the apical lucency. (e) This endo/perio involved lower third molar (top) was so mobile that it had to be stabilized by hand in order to perform endodontic therapy. The tooth was temporized and left out of occlusion, and at 6 months much of the lesion had resolved (middle). An amalgam core was placed and the tooth was left on its own for another 5 years, over which time it stabilized, with no apical lucency. With a reasonably high degree of confidence established, it was then engaged as a distal abutment in a fixed bridge (bottom). (f) The tooth and bridge are still present and functioning well 23 years after the original endodontic treatment.

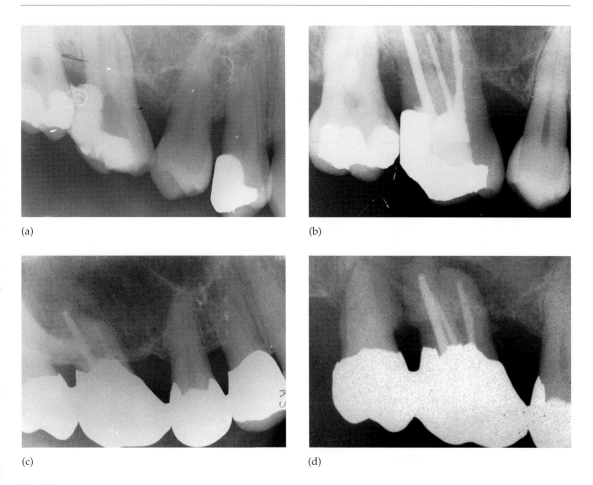

(a)

(b)

(c)

(d)

Fig 8.8

(a) Although this patient came in 1975 seeking endodontic treatment, she had bone loss, mobility, and pockets throughout the mouth. The upper molar (probably no. 2) had to be stabilized by hand while being instrumented. (b) After endodontic therapy, full-thickness flaps and osseous recontouring were done in an attempt to preserve the tooth. (c) Only when the periodontal situation had stabilized (about one year after surgery) was a definitive restoration placed. In this case, all four teeth were splinted, with ample access for proximal cleaning. This quadrant remained stable and functional for more than 20 years. (d) Recently recurrent periodontal breakdown has compromised the molars, and they were removed in 1998. It was a good run, none the less.

post and core, presents multiple additive failure risks. If, after all this, we hope to use it as terminal abutment for a long span fixed bridge, we are putting a large bet on a potentially lame horse. Both dentist and patient must understand and appreciate the risks entailed. Phasing such treatment to allow time to assess success builds confidence in the result, and may prevent disaster.

PHASING IN THIRD PARTY RELATIONSHIPS

The advent of third party involvement in dental care has had a tremendous impact on dental treatment and treatment planning. On the positive side, many patients who could not or did not seek comprehensive dental care before a third party involvement have availed themselves of dental care and treatment, to

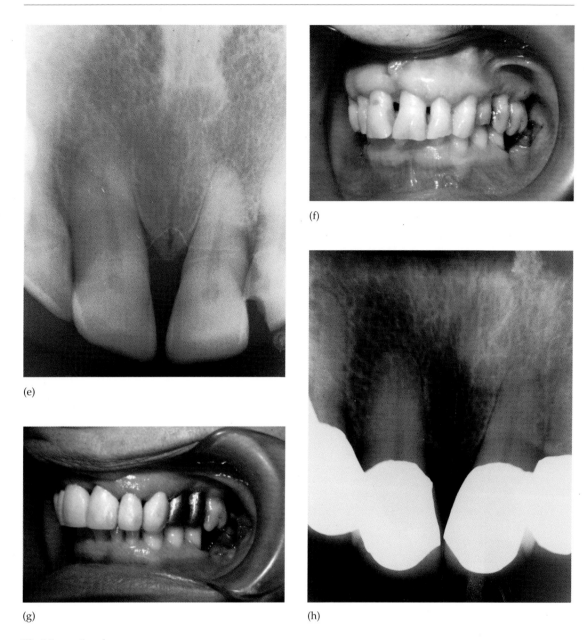

(e)

(f)

(g)

(h)

Fig 8.8 *continued*

(e) Moderate-to-severe periodontitis (5–7 mm pockets, vertical bone loss, class II mobility) made for a guarded prognosis for these incisors. (f) Full-thickness flaps and osseous recontouring (resective surgery) eliminated pockets, but did not ensure long-term retention. (g) Processed acrylic provisionals, with improved crown/root ratio, were followed for a full 3 months before definitive treatment (splinted crowns) was carried out. (h) Radiographic follow-up at 13 years shows stable bone level.

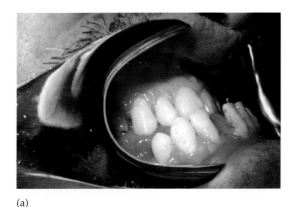

(a)

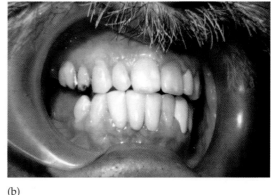

(b)

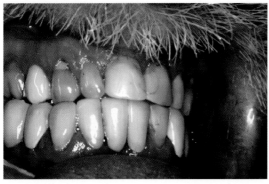

(c)

Fig 8.9

(a) Orthognathic surgery was used to correct a severe class III with functional deficit (inability to chew efficiently). (b) Definitive restorations (crowns, fixed bridges) were deferred for nearly a year, to allow for stabilization of the bite after surgery. (c) This follow-up, at 22 years after surgery, demonstrates ongoing function of the restorations (a cantilever bridge was added 5 years after surgery), but there has indeed been some relapse toward a class III relationship.

the mutual benefit of both patients and dentists. On the down side, third party relationships can complicate the dentist–patient relationship because restrictions, limitations, and paperwork intrude on what was once a simple contract between dentist and patient. These complications can be dealt with in most cases; sound and effective dental care can be rendered, but careful planning and some adjustments may be required. Phasing in third party relationships can be considered in three general situations. In the first, the third party limits the type of treatment and the level of reimbursement, and furthermore prohibits the dentist from performing a higher level of services and charging the patient for the difference. (In the USA, welfare programs such as Title XIX and Veteran's Administration programs fall into this category.) In this situation, planning is difficult if the program will not allow or cover an appropriate course of treatment. Phasing may mean performing palliative or preliminary procedures only, pending the patient's ability at some future time to proceed without the third party assistance. In some cases these types of programs can and do permit reasonable care to be rendered and reasonable remuneration to be made. However, if the limitations of a program appear to dictate irrational or substandard care, the dentist is faced with a dilemma: to provide optimal treatment free of charge is impractical in most cases, yet to perform the 'approved' treatment could constitute substandard care. There is often no solution, and the problem should be discussed frankly with the patient. The dentist may decide not to accept the patient for treatment under the third party restriction, and this is his or her choice. Often, however, at least minimal disease control can be carried out within the framework of a third party program, and it may serve as the first step in a phased treatment plan.

A second situation is that in which the third party, while limiting reimbursement for certain types of treatment, does not prohibit more comprehensive and costly approaches, providing the patient pays the difference. Most fee-for-service dental insurance plans operate on this basis. Benefits are provided under the terms of a contract, but no restrictions are placed on the actual treatment chosen by the patient. Phasing in this situation can be based on annual benefit limitations or on certain waiting periods.

Annual benefit limitations are common to many dental insurance plans. When a proposed course of treatment will significantly exceed the limitation it may be feasible to spread the treatment over 2 or more years, just as in the time-variable model previously discussed. This allows the patient the maximum financial benefit from the plan, while pursuing optimal treatment. Indeed, it is sometimes possible to spread such treatment over 3, 4, or even 5 years. If this is to be done effectively, two factors must be considered.

First, can the treatment be spread over time safely, without jeopardizing the result? Obviously active disease cannot be ignored. Interim restorations may have to be placed where definitive treatment is being postponed. Anterior restorations or prostheses may be subject to excessive stress or breakage if posterior support is not established. In our desire to assist patients financially we must take care not to compromise them dentally.

Sometimes treatment can be timed at year's end so as to encompass the end of one benefit year and the beginning of another. Provided that treatment can be, and is actually divided between the 2 years, then within a 2-month course of treatment, 2 years of insurance benefits may be tapped. Dates of service and fees charged must be recorded and reported

accurately and truthfully; to do otherwise can be construed as fraud and result in serious consequences for the dentist. Careful appointment scheduling is essential, requiring equally careful treatment planning.

Some situations preclude this strategy altogether. A long span bridge may exceed an annual allowance. Do not be tempted to submit a claim for the service as two separate procedures. In rare cases, a prosthesis could legitimately be made as two separate bridges, inserted with temporary cement in two separate appointments, billed accordingly, and later splinted together if indicated. Such machinations can lead to many complications and should be avoided if possible. We must strive to treat patients and their dental conditions, not their insurance contracts.

There must also be sufficient stability in the dentist–patient–third party arrangement to permit long-term planning. Will the present insurance plan remain in effect? Will the patient remain employed so as to be eligible? Might the patient move or be transferred during the course of treatment? If any of these scenarios are likely, long-term phasing may be a bad idea. At the very least, phased treatment to accommodate third party involvement must adhere to all general principles of rational treatment planning so that, should the extended course be disrupted, the patient will be stable and under good control, permitting the balance of treatment to be done at a later time or another place if need be.

Waiting periods associated with third party plans take various forms. The most common situation involves a patient in need of dental care who is not under a dental plan, but who anticipates having insurance in the foreseeable future. It is certainly reasonable to initiate disease-control procedures and postpone definitive treatment until coverage is obtained. Many dental plans limit coverage on replacement of existing prostheses until they have been in the mouth for some period of time (often 5 years). Phasing treatment to postpone needed replacement until coverage is available is possible if the existing prosthesis can be repaired, patched, or otherwise made to serve in the meantime. This will not do if the defect is too severe or the time too long to postpone replacement safely.

Although treatment planning under these conditions is often challenging and frustrating, third party plans can be of benefit to patient and dentist. The principle of quality as a constant and time as the variable applies nicely, and can help bring about excellent results in dental treatment.

A third situation is the capitation or HMO model, in which the dentist provides care and treatment at a fixed rate per patient per month. Ethically and legally this situation demands much of the dentist, because he or she determines what care will be given. Obviously, immediate performance of every possible maximal procedure for every patient would be economically disastrous for the dentist, and it would not necessarily be good patient care, as has been discussed previously. However, postponing costly procedures indefinitely, or simply not disclosing the available options to the patient, may constitute a breach in the standard of care.

In these arrangements, it would be prudent to develop a written phased treatment plan with the patient based on any or all of the strategies discussed here, or on any other good rationale. The plan and the rationale become part of the patient record. This protects the dentist, in justifying what treatment has been done and at what pace, and the patient, in ensuring that treatment will be based on sound principles and serve his or her individual needs. It also facilitates peer review and quality assurance protocols.

PLANNING PHASED TREATMENT

Phased treatment can be an effective approach to optimal patient care, but it requires more of the patient and dentist than an immediate approach. First, complex plans that are phased over long time periods are not easy to draw, and they demand greater care, skill, and judgment than simpler, immediate plans. Care must be taken to ensure that postponing a given treatment will not create greater problems. Judgment is required in making some predictive diagnoses – that is, in foreseeing possible developments in the clinical picture and preparing alternative treatment approaches to meet them.

Phased treatment planning requires a greater commitment of time and effort by the dentist, for which there is neither financial reward nor patient appreciation. The intellectual challenge can be stimulating, however, and the process is generally educational.

Phased treatment planning also requires the patient to be involved in the planning, and committed to the plan and the dental health goals established. Phasing is ineffective without this commitment, because the patient may lose interest and not return, or experience a lapse in the personal oral health efforts essential to success.

As the human body and the mouth are dynamic environments, continual reassessment is necessary in a phased approach, considering the following factors:

- Changes (for better or worse) in the oral clinical picture, in the patient's general systemic health, or in the patient's lifestyle, job, marriage, outlook on life, or attitude toward dental health.

- Changes in costs of rendering care and, subsequently, changes in fees; introduction of third party involvement subsequent to the original treatment plan and phasing.

- Advances in available techniques and/or materials that might allow or dictate different approaches from the original long-term plan.

Alterations made in the phased treatment plan for these or any other reason should be recorded, and the plan redrawn if necessary to reflect the circumstances necessitating the change.

REFERENCE

1. Barkley RF, Must third party dentistry be mediocre? *J South Cal Dent Assoc* 1973; **41**:307–10.

9

ORTHODONTIC INTERVENTIONS

One of the most effective strategies the dentist can employ to simplify treatment and enhance overall results is orthodontic intervention. Obviously, many patients present with malocclusion as their chief complaint, and comprehensive orthodontic treatment is indicated. Many more patients can benefit from orthodontic treatment, whether it is single tooth crossbite correction, uprighting of tipped abutments, or even fairly comprehensive treatment, and whether performed by a specialist or a general practitioner in the course of overall dental care.

The case histories below illustrate the integration of orthodontic treatment into an overall comprehensive plan. Each case presents more complex problems, but in each case the orthodontic treatment itself is fairly simple. Figures 9.1–9.4 show corrections of anterior crossbites. Figure 9.5 illustrates a simple orthodontic approach used to prepare an extensive and complicated restorative/

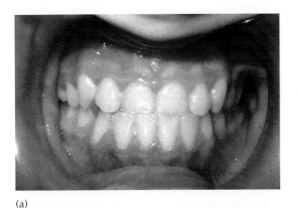

(a)

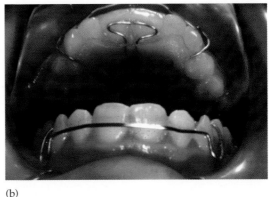

(b)

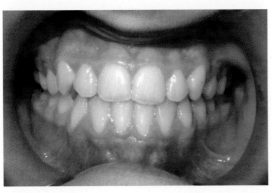

(c)

Fig 9.1

(a) An 11 year old, with central incisors locked in cross-bite. (b) Simple Hawley appliance, with lingual recurves (note stand-off of labial bow over numbers 8 and 9 to allow movement to facial). (c) Less than 2 months of active treatment, retained at night for 6 months.

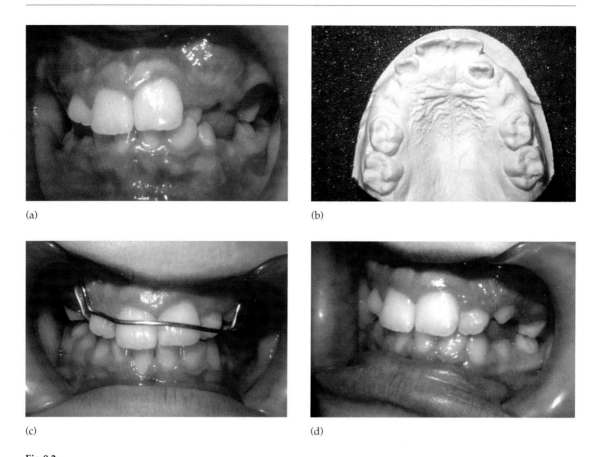

Fig 9.2

(a) Deeply locked lateral incisor crossbite. (b) Study cast. (c) Simple Hawley, with lingual spring moving no. 10 labially. (Labial bow again stands off no. 10 to allow repositioning.) (d) 3 months of active treatment was retained at night for 6 months.

prosthetic case. Figure 9.6 illustrates a rehabilitation case set up orthodontically. The general idea is the same in each of these examples.

ILLUSTRATIVE CASE HISTORIES 9.1–9.4

Concepts illustrated: *simple orthodontic interventions.*

CASE 9.1

This 11-year-old girl's central incisors were locked behind her lower anteriors (Fig 9.1).

Earlier intervention would have been preferable, but a simple Hawley appliance with recurved lingual wires corrected the problem in less than 2 months, and served as a night-time retainer for about 6 months afterward.

CASE 9.2

Potentially more severe, this single tooth crossbite was intercepted at age 8, again with a simple Hawley appliance (Fig 9.2). 3 months of treatment, followed by 6 months of night-time retention corrected the problem and the rest of the teeth erupted normally and in good

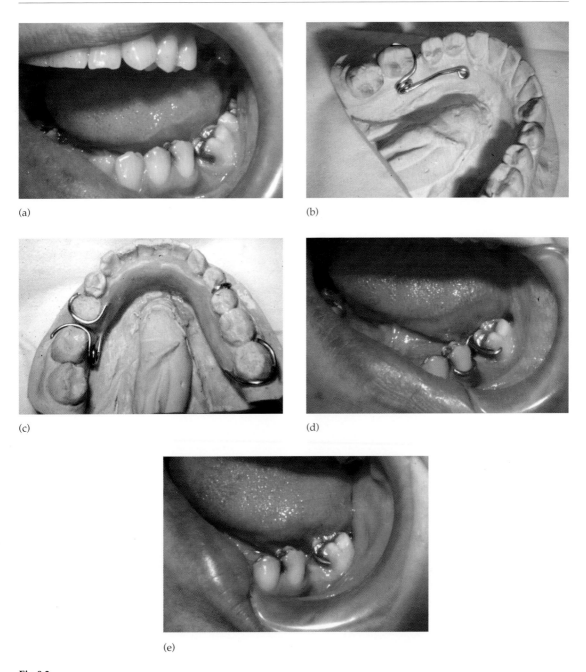

Fig 9.3

(a) Not an uncommon sight, this lower second molar has tipped into the missing lower first molar space. The third molar has erupted and tipped mesially also. (b) Simple coiled wire clasp/activator wire will drive and tip second molar back into extraction site of third molar. No. 17 was extracted the same day the appliance was inserted. (c) Simple clasp wires embedded in self-curing acrylic provide more than ample anchorage to move no. 18. (d) After 2 months, space is being gained and treatment is nearly complete. (e) At 4 months, pontic space is adequate and alignment is favorable for placement of a fixed bridge, which will, of course, retain the orthodontic result. Note the horizontal slot cut into the amalgam mesial of no. 18. The coiled activating wire engaged this slot.

occlusion, averting a potentially serious malocclusion.

CASE 9.3

Early loss of a 6-year molar produced tipping and space loss in the lower left quadrant (Fig 9.3). A difficult bridge situation is simplified with 4 months of orthodontic treatment. Removal of the third molar just before initiation of treatment not only made the mechanics

simpler, but the second molar was then rotated back into newly forming bone (the third molar extraction site). Retention was achieved with the placement of the fixed bridge.

CASE 9.4

This 22-year-old man had prematurely lost upper right posterior teeth and lower left molars, resulting in this pseudo-class III collapsed dentition (Fig 9.4). In centric relation

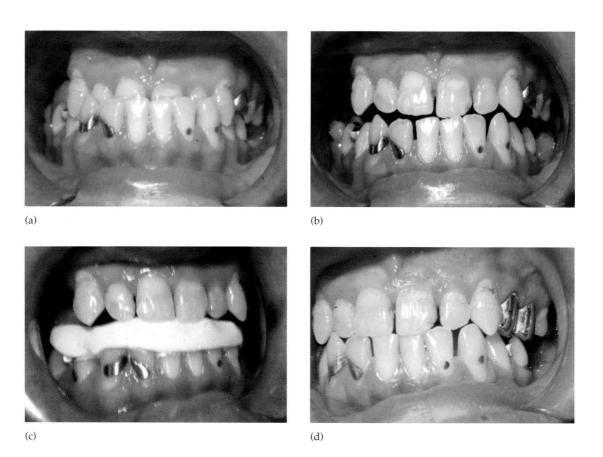

(a)

(b)

(c)

(d)

Fig 9.4

(a) Complex problem, pseudo-class III, anterior crossbite. (b) In centric relation (RP), anteriors are almost end to end. (c) Lacking posterior anchorage, a simple cemented splint/ramp was placed. (d) Within 2 weeks, anterior crossbite was corrected, canines were 'engaged,' and metal provisionals were placed on upper left premolars to hold the regained vertical dimension.

(RP), however, he was almost end-to-end, and a cemented acrylic ramp advanced maxillary incisors in about 2 weeks' time. Once that was accomplished, metal temporaries were placed on the upper left to hold the regained vertical, and straightforward restorative and prosthetic treatment was then carried out. Although the orthodontic treatment was 'simple,' it made a huge difference in this case, converting a very complex clinical picture into a much more manageable situation.

ILLUSTRATIVE CASE HISTORY 9.5

Concepts illustrated: *simplification of a complex clinical scenario through orthodontic intervention, general tooth inventory, strategic extraction of unsalvageable tooth (no. 12), and noncontributing teeth (left mandibular deciduous canine, upper third molars). Phased treatment, short-term success, long-term failure.*

This 38-year-old male engineer realized that his dentition was in dreadful condition and expressed a desire to keep his teeth (Fig 9.5a).

Periodontal support was good, with little or no bone loss (Fig 9.5b), although marginal gingivitis was present. Scattered carious lesions and extensive previous restorative dentistry (along with early loss of 6-year molars and other teeth) pointed to a high caries rate. Tooth no. 12 (already extracted on the clinical photos) had no attached gingiva and the buccal root was denuded of tissue and carious. The problem list in the box was developed.

A tooth inventory was carried out (see Chapter 7) to identify key teeth, potential key teeth, sound teeth, and potential candidates for extraction (Fig 9.5c). Looking at the upper cast (Fig 9.5d) one can envision a simple orthodontic intervention to 'undo' the posterior tipping and drifting, moving upper second molars (nos 2 and 15) distal and buccal, while advancing the upper central incisors. A simple palatal appliance with clasps and recurved springs (Fig 9.5e) was used over a period of 8 months. Anterior teeth were unlocked, second molars were out of crossbite, and a pontic space was developed between nos 2 and 4 (Fig 9.5f).

The result (Fig 9.5g) is a clinical situation which, although still requiring extensive treatment, is no longer complex, that is,

Patient AU:	38-year-old male, in good general health
	Chief complaint: doesn't want to lose teeth, but feels that they are in terrible shape
	Dental goal: long-term retention of teeth, improvement of function and esthetics
	Generalized slight gingivitis, ineffective home care
	Caries and broken down restorations
	Unrestored endodontically treated number 5 with broken file in buccal canal, and successful (5-year) surgical retrofill
	Missing teeth nos 3, 14, 17, 19, 20, 30
	Multi-rooted/bifurcated premolars – problematic if root canal should become necessary
	Tipped and rotated teeth nos 2, 15, and, to a lesser degree, 18 and 31
	Buccally locked upper third molars, and retained lower deciduous canines
	Class III, with molar crossbites and anteriors crowded and locked in alternating crossbite
	Finances somewhat limited; insurance available, with annual limits

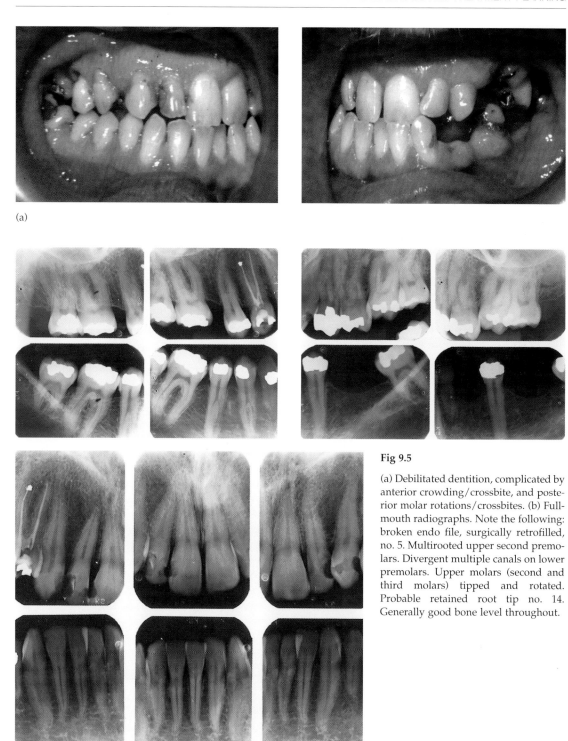

Fig 9.5

(a) Debilitated dentition, complicated by anterior crowding/crossbite, and posterior molar rotations/crossbites. (b) Full-mouth radiographs. Note the following: broken endo file, surgically retrofilled, no. 5. Multirooted upper second premolars. Divergent multiple canals on lower premolars. Upper molars (second and third molars) tipped and rotated. Probable retained root tip no. 14. Generally good bone level throughout.

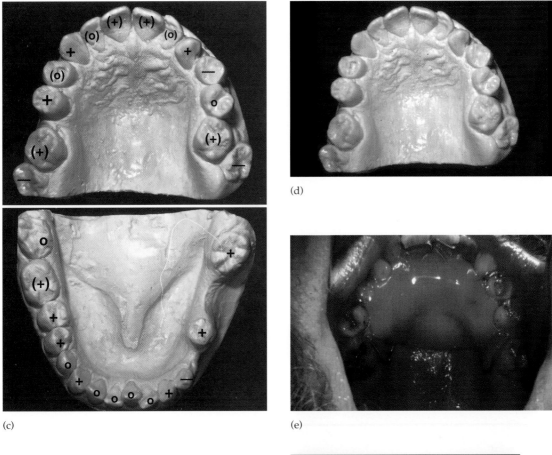

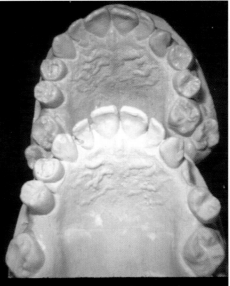

Fig 9.5 *continued*

(c) Tooth inventory: symbols: + = key tooth, 0 = sound tooth, — = potential extraction, (+) = needs treatment to become key or sound. (d) Upper diagnostic cast: we can easily envision advancing incisors while rotating second molars out and back, after removing third molars. (e) Simple palatal appliance (mirror view), with recurved springs acting on incisors and molars, was self-retaining, and had reciprocal anchorage. (f) In 8 months (bottom) anteriors were advanced and aligned, molars rotated and tipped back to allow reconstruction in quadrants.

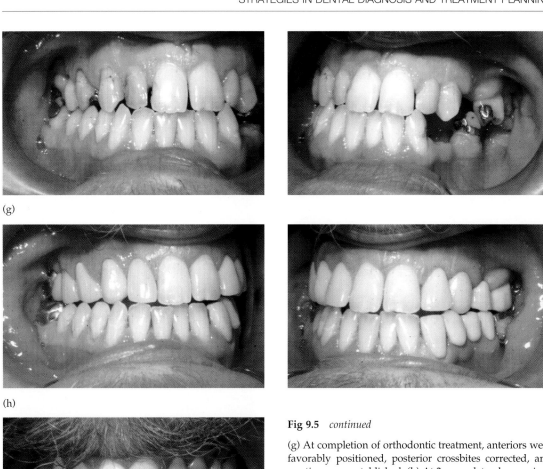

(g)

(h)

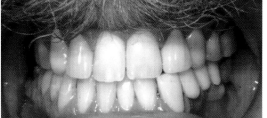

(i)

Fig 9.5 *continued*

(g) At completion of orthodontic treatment, anteriors were favorably positioned, posterior crossbites corrected, and pontic spaces established. (h) At 2 years, lateral excursions demonstrate working side group function, and excellent maintenance of tissue and restorations. (i) At 5 years, the case was stable and prognosis was good. (j) Twenty-one years after completion of treatment, the prognosis is no longer positive. The case has become a 'holding' action, with occasional acute periodontal flare-ups palliated, or teeth extracted if necessary. In the future full dentures may become necessary, but it may take years to reach that point.

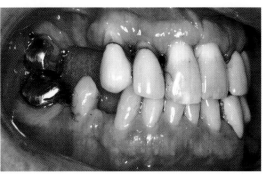

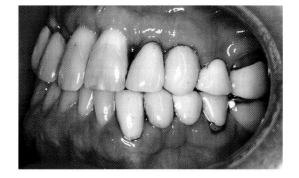

(j)

restorative and prosthetic treatment can be, and in this case was, carried out in sections over time. Insurance benefits were tapped for 3 calendar years (1974–76) and the prognosis after 2 years (Fig 9.5h) was very good. Note the working side group function shown here, and the lower left canine reshaped to mimic an incisor for esthetics. Note also the good tissue color and oral hygiene. The patient continued on regular maintenance, and at 5 years had no mechanical or biologic breakdowns (Fig 9.5i).

EPILOGUE CASE HISTORY 9.5

First treated in 1974–76, this patient was followed and maintained for approximately 8 years, at which time he moved away. He was seen again in 1997, some 21 years after completion of treatment, and the picture was not good (Fig 9.5j).

The patient had lost his job in the late 1980s, suffered psychological and emotional setbacks, and was living alone in a rural area, almost like a hermit. He had moderate-to-advanced periodontal disease, and had lost a number of teeth; his maintenance was poor. The clinical photographs are deceptive, taken after he had been cleaned up and coached back into better home care. His desires now are for maintenance and palliative treatment only, and he returns on a sporadic basis. He is not interested in (nor can he afford) prosthetic treatment, but seems to get along just fine as he is. You cannot win them all.

ILLUSTRATIVE CASE HISTORY 9.6

Concepts illustrated: *simplification of complex clinical scenario through orthodontic intervention, tooth inventory, use of direction-changing coping (telescope), use of orthodontic appliances as temporary partial prostheses.*

This 17-year-old student (Fig 9.6a,b) suffered from congenital partial anodontia, the following teeth never having developed: upper lateral incisors, premolars, and left canine, lower incisors (all four) and premolars (all four). Furthermore, upper central incisors were tipped 12–15 mm apart, right canine was only partially erupted and its root inclined 45° back into the palate. Lower canines were misshapen, and tipped labially at nearly 90° to one another. Finally, many of the deciduous molars were retained, but ankylosed and buried in the tissues (Fig 9.6c). The problem list in the box was developed.

After surgical removal of retained deciduous teeth, study casts (Fig 9.6d) make identification of potential 'key' teeth very simple. Except for their inclination, all extant permanent teeth are 'key'. The plan was to upright upper incisors and lower canines orthodontically, using removable appliances doubling as treatment partials, that is, with prosthetic teeth attached. The appliances were fabricated, placed, and activated, and treatment carried out over 10 months, followed by 3 months of passive retention with the removable appliances (Fig 9.6e–h).

Patient RM: 17-year-old male, in good general health
Chief complaint: missing many permanent teeth, extreme esthetic deficit
Dental goal: improvement of appearance and function
Generalized slight gingivitis, ineffective home care
Molar pit caries, ankylosed and broken down deciduous molars
Missing teeth nos 4, 5, 7, 10, 11, 12, 13, 20, 21, 23, 24, 25, 26, 28 and 29
Tipped and rotated teeth nos 6, 8, 9, 17 and 22
Deep class II anterior overbite with retroclined upper incisors

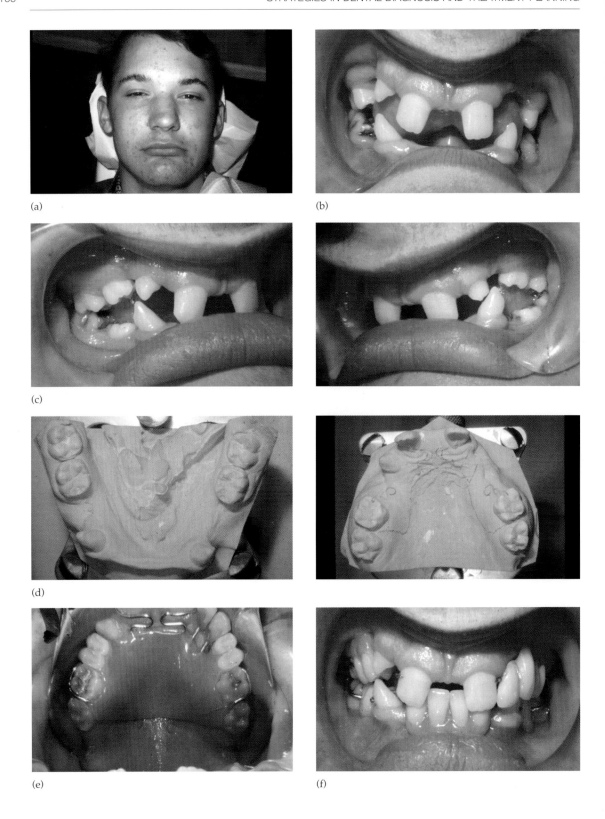

(a)

(b)

(c)

(d)

(e)

(f)

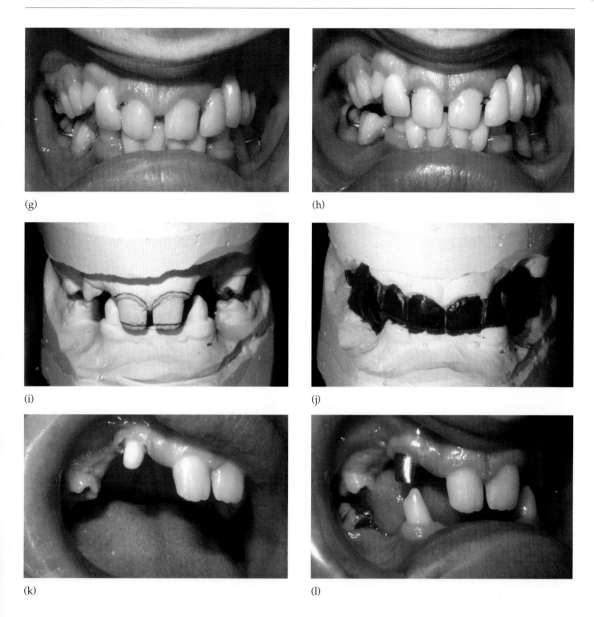

(g)

(h)

(i)

(j)

(k)

(l)

Fig 9.6

(a,b) 17-year-old male with congenital partial anodontia. (c) Retained deciduous teeth were ankylosed, and some were buried beneath the tissue. The patient did not smile much. (d) Mounted models (after removal of deciduous teeth) demonstrate good molar dentition, and potential key teeth (upper centrals and right canine, lower canines). (e) Orthodontic appliances double as temporary partial dentures. (f) Immediate esthetic improvement is seen at the outset of orthodontic treatment. (g) At 8 months, another lateral incisor (no. 7) is added to the appliance. (h) At 10 months, uprighting is almost complete, to be followed by 3 months of passive retentive wear. There was no problem getting this patient to wear 'retainers.' (i) Anterior deep bite was anticipated, with gingivoplasty and elective endodontics on nos 8 and 9 planned. (j) The final reconstructed occlusion was prewaxed on the study casts, then duplicated in stone, upon which thin plastic pull-down 'shims' were made. (k) Tipped canine prepared for telescope coping. (l) Telescope coping inserted, creating parallelism for upper fixed prosthesis.

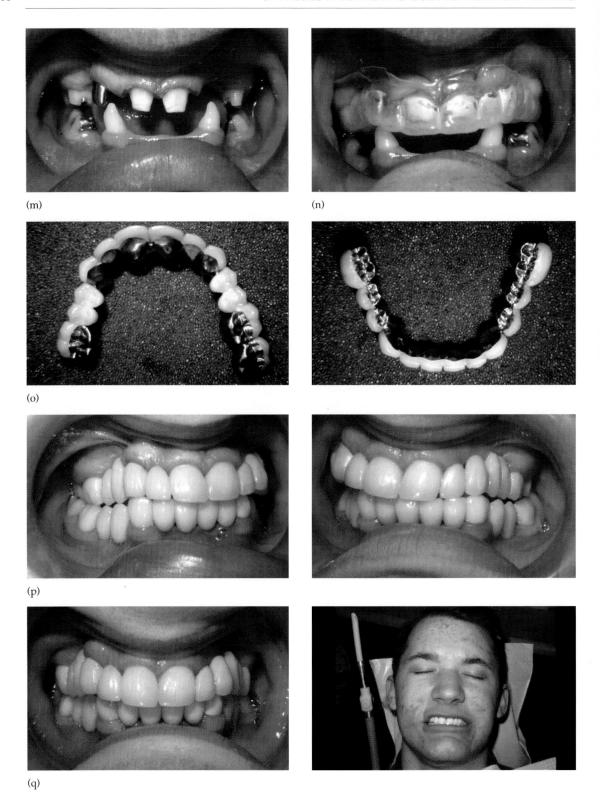

(m)

(n)

(o)

(p)

(q)

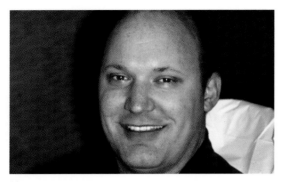
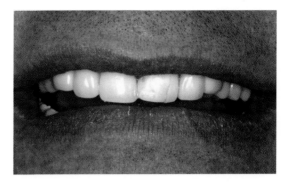

(r)

Fig 9.6 *continued*

(m) Upper arch prepared, with canine coping, and endodontically treated incisors with gingiva reduced. Note the reasonably flat plane established. (n) Preformed shim placed over prepared teeth to verify adequate reduction, and as shell for full arch provisional bridge. (o) Upper and lower long span fixed bridges; upper right uses both molars as distal abutments, reflecting the long span from central incisors. (p) Shown in left and right lateral excursions, with anterior group function guidance. (q) Permanent cementation was done after 6 weeks of comfortable use. (r) At 19 years, the upper bridge has been repaired, and the lower replaced (at about 10 years). The patient was still doing well.

Mounted models subsequent to treatment (Fig 9.6i) illustrate the anterior deep bite problem, and marks on the upper incisors predict the incisal reduction and concomitant gingival repositioning intended. Both central incisors were to be devitalized to accomplish this. The entire occlusion was pre-waxed on the articulated models (Fig 9.6j), then duplicated in stone to make preformed shells for later use in preparation and temporization.

It was decided to leave the upper right canine undisturbed, due in no small part to lack of anchorage to move it. To compensate for its incorrect inclination, number 6 was prepared, and a cast gold coping placed, which was parallel with the molars and incisors (Fig 9.6k and l).

At the time of preparation, the curve of occlusion was improved, by devitalizing the incisors and repositioning the gingiva. Note the nearly flat plane of the five upper abutment teeth, molars, incisors, and canine coping (Fig 9.6m).

The preformed shell fabricated from the pre-waxed occlusion is useful both to assess tooth reduction and then to form the temporary bridge (Fig 9.6n).

Complex, long span, fixed bridges were fabricated to complete the treatment, the upper involving numbers 3—6—8–9—14–15, the lower involving 19—22—27—30 (Fig 9.6o). Working side anterior group function was established (Fig 9.6p), and the bridges were cemented provisionally for 4–6 weeks, using a non-setting temporary cement. Throughout the provisional cementation period the patient was comfortable and functional, and careful occlusal assessment at its end confirmed full intercuspation and freedom of movement in excursions, all in harmony with the temporomandibular joint.

At that point, the prostheses were cemented permanently, and the patient placed on frequent recall (Fig 9.6q).

EPILOGUE CASE HISTORY 9.6

First started in 1977, orthodontic treatment was completed in the fall of 1978. Preparatory procedures, coping on no. 6, endodontics and posts for nos 8 and 9, preparation, and provisional bridges took about 3 months, and the final bridgework was completed in early 1979.

The patient was followed briefly, then left for military service and spent quite some time abroad.

We reacquired contact with him nearly 20 years later, in 1998 (Fig 9.6r). His lower bridge had broken after about 10 years of service, and had been replaced in Germany. His upper bridge had been repaired when he chipped the porcelain on number 9. Both were stable and functioning well (Fig 9.6s). The gingival tissues were in great need of professional attention and reinforced home care, but the foundation remains sound, with good bone around solid roots (Fig 9.6t). The bridgework was now in need of replacement, and plans were made to do so over a 2-year period. The patient is highly motivated to avoid removable prostheses, and with a return to regular maintenance and effective home care, the prognosis looks favorable.

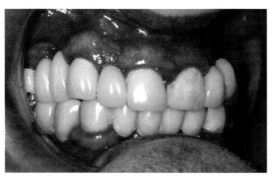 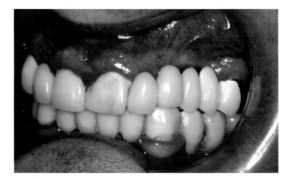

(s)

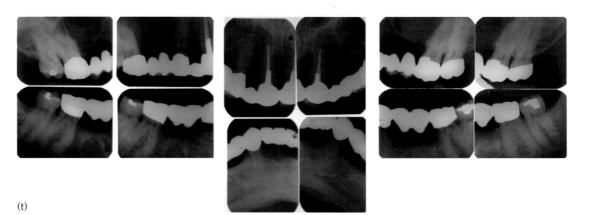

(t)

Fig 9.6 *continued*

(s) Before renewal of soft tissue maintenance, the dentition is a bit the worse for wear. (t) Radiographs are more encouraging, suggesting a sound foundation of roots in bone, encouraging retreatment of this 20-year case, which, with a reinvigorated maintenance program, still has a favorable long-term prognosis.

10

STRATEGIC EXTRACTIONS AND NONREPLACEMENT

There are a number of instances in which the best interest of the patient is served by removing one or more teeth that could possibly be retained, but which do not 'fit' in the patient's overall long-range plan. These are called strategic extractions, and this chapter illustrates the use of this strategy, and discusses instances in which removal and nonreplacement is appropriate.

Nonsalvageable teeth may be truly non-treatable (longitudinal fractures, caries through a furcation, substantially denuded roots), or they may require such extensive and complex treatment (endodontics, crown lengthening, bone graft, post and core, cast crown) that removal and prosthetic replacement are less costly and more likely to succeed long term. Strategic extraction of such teeth becomes the treatment of choice when other sound teeth in the vicinity offer ready alternatives. In some cases the situation may call for heroic measures (see Chapter 11), but the dentist must be prepared to present extraction as the most reasonable option in many cases.

Nonfunctional teeth such as unopposed third molars may often be left alone, provided they present no immediate threat to the patient. It is often good practice to remove such teeth, however, because they may become problematic at a later date, and the patient's ability to withstand extraction later in life may be compromised. No one wants to be removing third molars in a geriatric setting. Extractions become more difficult, more complicated, and present greater risks, both operative and postoperative, with advancing age.

Noncontributory teeth, such as retained deciduous teeth or teeth with unusually small or short roots, are often removed strategically when doing comprehensive restorative and prosthetic treatment, because they do not enhance the clinical scenario, and may make for more complicated treatment than otherwise necessary.

The case history illustrated in Fig 10.1 depicts strategic extractions of several otherwise healthy and sound teeth, in attempting to simplify a complex clinical situation.

ILLUSTRATIVE CASE HISTORY 10.1

Orthodontic treatment: *Dr John Cheek*

Concepts illustrated: *Strategic extractions, orthodontic intervention, reliance on 'key' teeth.*

This 18-year-old woman presented with a chief complaint of poor dental esthetics. Exhibiting a class III relationship with an underdeveloped premaxilla (Fig 10.1a–c), her central incisors had been removed as a result of ectopic eruption in early childhood, and she was left with lateral incisors and a transposed premolar as front teeth. A problem list was developed (see box on page 172).

Some initial discussions were held with the patient and her parents proposing comprehensive orthodontic treatment, including orthognathic surgery to advance and expand the premaxilla. Concomitant rhinoplasty was included in this proposed plan, the surgical and orthodontic phase to be followed by fixed prosthetics in the maxillary anterior. Both the time factor (several years) and the uninsured surgical costs negated this approach.

Given the complexity of the case, a tooth inventory was done, identifying 'key' teeth

Patient SP: 18-year-old female, in good general health
                 Chief complaint: doesn't like the way her teeth look
                 Dental goal: improvement of esthetics, long-term retention of teeth
                 Generalized slight gingivitis
                 Caries and broken down restorations, mostly involving 6-year molars
                 Class III, with crossbite right posterior and anterior, generalized crowding,
                     loss of upper central incisors and transposition of nos 11 and 12
                 Time and finances somewhat limited

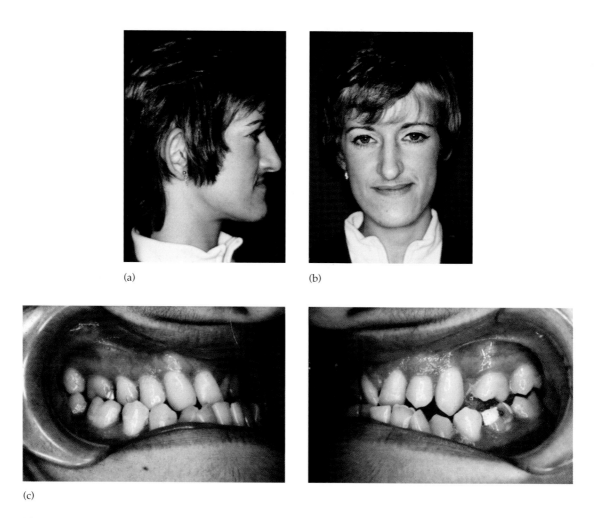

(a)   (b)

(c)

Fig 10.1

(a,b) A skeletal class III relationship: this young woman was reluctant to smile. (c) Lateral incisors (instead of centrals), and the left first premolar presented a very unesthetic picture.

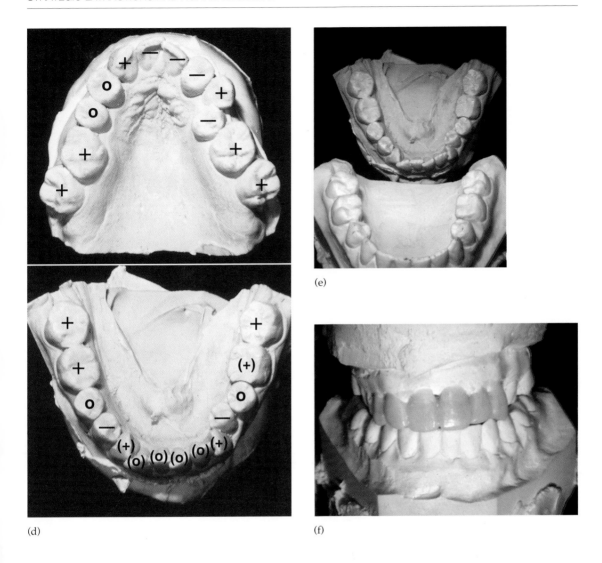

(d)

(e)

(f)

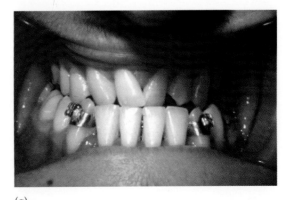

Fig 10.1 *continued*

(d) Tooth inventory identifies stable teeth, 'key' teeth, and potential candidates for extraction. Specifically, upper lateral incisors; and the transposed and malposed left premolars were slated for removal and replacement with fixed bridge using key abutment teeth nos 6, 11, and 14. Lower first premolars were planned for extraction to allow 'uncrowding' of anterior segment, and some retraction to gain a normal anterior overbite. (e) Diagnostic cast (top) and lower diagnostic wax-up with prospective lower orthodontic result. (f) Diagnostic wax-up of upper plan, articulated with lower prospective cast. (g) Completion of lower orthodontic treatment, anteriors now nearly end to end, with band and lingual wire retention in place.

(g)

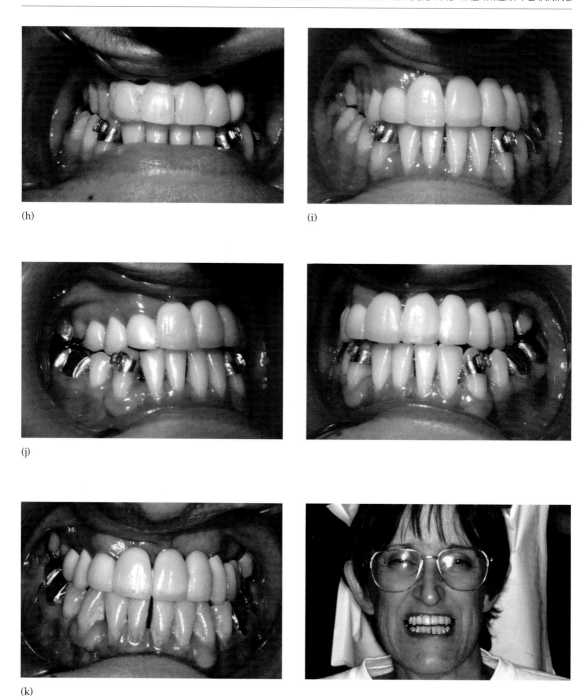

(h)   (i)

(j)

(k)

Fig 10.1 *continued*

(h) Upper strategic extractions were carried out, abutments were prepared, and a provisional was placed, all at the same appointment. (i) Upper bridge placed temporarily, until extraction sites healed. (j) Showing left and right lateral excursions, this 2-year follow-up shows posterior crowns placed to optimize occlusion, grafts done on lower canines, and the retainer about to be removed. (k) Follow-up at 24 years.

(and potential 'strategic extractions') (Fig 10.1d), designed to simplify treatment and reduce total time and costs, was conceived and carried out on the diagnostic casts first.

Lower

Fixed orthodontic treatment would be carried out in the lower arch only, extracting first premolars to uncrowd, align, and retract lower six anteriors. This treatment was performed on a plaster model, which could then be rearticulated with a plaster model of the maxilla (Fig. 10.1e).

Upper

Strategic extractions of the lateral incisors numbers 7 and 10, and the transposed and palatally locked premolars (nos 12 and 13, respectively) would be followed by placement of a fixed bridge anchoring on numbers 6, 11, and 14. This approach was prewaxed on a plaster model, articulated with the projected orthodontically treated lower (Fig 10.1f).

Mandibular orthodontic treatment was completed in 11 months, and canine-to-canine retention established (Fig 10.1g). Caries were all restored and good periodontal health established during that time. Upper extractions were done, and a temporary fixed bridge placed at the same time (Fig. 10.1h). A porcelain-fused-to-gold bridge was placed temporarily, and then cemented to place once extraction sites had healed (Fig. 10.1i).

Over the next 2 years, cast crowns were placed on upper and lower molars which had been heavily restored with silver amalgam. Optimal posterior occlusion was thereby established long term. Free gingival grafts (palatal autografts) were performed on lower canines which, having little keratinized gingiva at the outset, had none after orthodontic movement (Fig 10.1j).

Epilogue case history 10.1

The patient has been seen for regular maintenance for almost 25 years. Home care has been

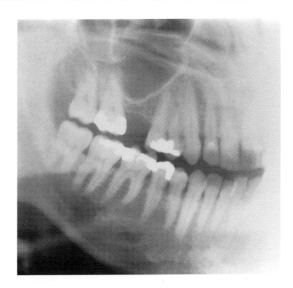

Fig 10.2

Tooth no. 3 has been missing and unreplaced for 22 years.

acceptable, and no further restorative or prosthetic treatment has been required in that time. Now in her forties and a mother of two, she continues to function well with the crowns and fixed bridge (Fig 10.1k).

You will see more examples of strategic extractions in other case histories in this text. It is a useful tool in comprehensive treatment planning.

Another strategy is nonreplacement of missing or extracted teeth. There are many situations in which patients can function quite well without certain teeth, and prosthetic replacement is simply not necessary.

The upper first molar shown absent (Fig 10.2) had been missing for over 20 years. Slight rotation/tipping of the second molar is noted, but no change in the width of the edentulous space could be measured over a 5-year period. The patient doesn't miss the tooth, and the expense and trouble of placing a fixed prosthesis are not justified on the basis of clinical or perceived need.

The 34-year-old man depicted in Fig 10.3a had been missing numerous posterior teeth for some time. His strong gag reflex made impressions difficult, and the very idea of

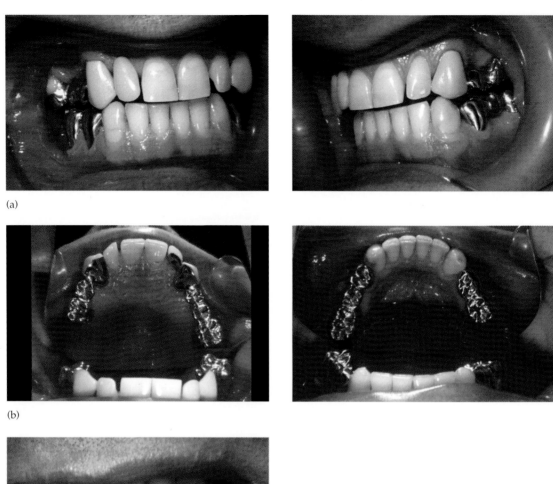

(a)

(b)

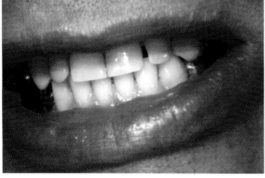

(c)

Fig 10.3

(a) Porcelain veneer was used on canines and upper right cantilever lateral, posteriors are cast gold. Canine guidance is established in excursions. (b) Occlusal scheme was waxed with cone technique (see Chapter 12) to ensure maximum chewing efficiency with relatively few teeth in the array. (c) The patient was very pleased with the result, both functional and esthetic.

wearing removable partial prostheses made him gag. He was in need of restorations on the posterior teeth, and was interested in improving function without necessarily replacing the missing teeth. Simple hygienic cast crowns and bridges, designed for maximum masticatory efficiency, were fabricated (Fig 10.3b), replacing missing premolars and upper lateral incisor, and the patient was very satisfied with the result (Fig 10.3c).

ILLUSTRATIVE CASE HISTORY 10.4

Concepts illustrated: *minimal replacement using cantilever bridges, use of 'key' teeth.*

This pleasant 51-year-old woman had worn upper and lower removable partial dentures for many years. The partials did not fill the anterior spaces resulting from congenitally missing lateral teeth, and she had always been self-conscious about her 'gap toothed' smile (Fig 10.4a). With the exception of no. 24, all teeth were sound and periodontally stable (Fig. 10.4b). The following problem list was developed:

Patient BK: 51-year-old female, menopausal but in good general health
Chief complaint: loose partial dentures, self-conscious about the way her teeth look
Dental goals: better comfort and function, long-term retention of teeth, improvement of esthetics
Good periodontal health, with advanced recession of no. 24 (adjacent to edentulous space)
Caries under and around three-quarter crown restorations
Upper/lower removable partial dentures old and ill-fitting
Some apprehension about dental treatment

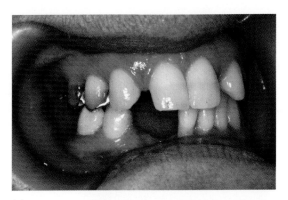 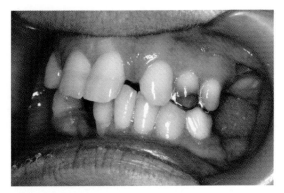

(a)

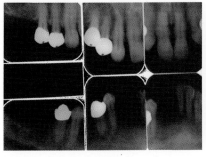 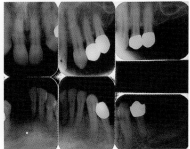

(b)

Fig 10.4

(a) Removable partial dentures replaced upper posterior, and lower anterior and posterior missing teeth, but the lack of space had precluded a solution to the congenitally missing upper laterals. (b) Radiographs confirm a solid foundation (except no. 24, which was removed).

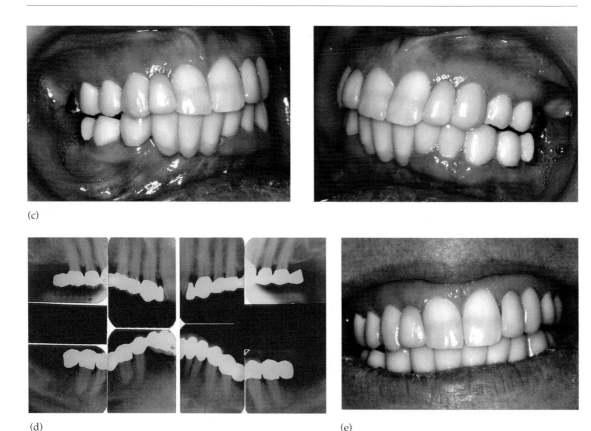

(c)

(d)   (e)

Fig 10.4 *continued*

(c) Lower AP fixed bridge with cantilever posterior pontic, and upper triple abutment bridges with cantilevers both anteriorly (lapped laterals) and posteriorly ('mini-molars'), provided both an esthetic and functional solution. (d) Radiographs at 10 years. (e) Clinical appearance at 10 years. The patient's home care is impeccable.

Some initial discussions were held regarding implant options. The patient was very hesitant about multiple surgeries, and the availability of simpler options led to the following plan.

Upper

Bilateral bridges using triple abutments (canine, first, and second premolars), with cantilevered pontics at both ends. Lateral incisor pontics to 'lap' centrals in a class II, division 2 configuration, premolar-size pontics extending distally. Patient's natural unrestored central incisors are left untouched.

Lower

Strategic extraction of no. 24. Bilateral bridges, cantilevering one premolar distal from no. 20 to 21, and a long span bridge from nos 22–23 to 27–28, cantilevering one premolar distal from no. 28 (Fig 10.4c).

EPILOGUE CASE HISTORY 10.4

The patient has been seen for regular maintenance for 10 years. Home care continues to be excellent, and no further restorative or prosthetic treatment has been required. Radiographs at 10 years demonstrate sound periodontal support (Fig 10.4d).

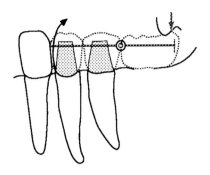

Fig 10.5

Failure of cantilever is ensured when the cantilevered distal abutment is too long, creating a lever arm that tends to lift the anterior abutment crown off the tooth. Note that the moment of force is congruent with the path of insertion/removal of that abutment (mesial of first premolar).

Her only regret is that she waited so long to improve her 'gap toothed' smile (Fig. 10.4e).

CANTILEVERED BRIDGES

Conservative replacement of missing teeth using cantilevered bridges has been an effective treatment strategy for a long, long time. Unfortunately, cantilever bridges have acquired a bad reputation because of their tendency to come 'undone.' It is obvious that extending a cantilevered pontic creates a lever arm which can introduce lateral torque forces to the abutments, and tends to loosen or remove the abutment casting furthest from the cantilever (Fig 10.5).

As they can be such an elegant yet simple solution to so many treatment planning problems, it is appropriate to offer some keys to success in their application. The first two keys are common knowledge, and fairly intuitive; the second two are less obvious, but are often critical to long-term success. The schematics illustrate a common situation, using two premolar abutments to replace (partially) a missing first molar, but the keys apply as well to most other cantilever situations.

Keys to successful cantilevers include the following:

- Never have less than a 2 : 1 ratio of abutment span to cantilevered span (Fig 10.6a,b). Greater abutments spans and multiple abutment teeth may allow for longer cantilever pontic units, but we should never cantilever further than absolutely necessary, regardless of anchorage.

- Occlusal tables must be kept narrow buccolingually, especially the cantilevered pontic, to reduce forces exerted in function.

- Abutment teeth must have average or better clinical crown length; preparations must be full coverage with minimal taper, and incorporate longitudinal grooves if practical. Castings must fit perfectly; and be cemented with a durable cement, preferably one with adhesive properties.

- Path of insertion should be altered where possible, so that it is not parallel with the natural arc of rotation of the cantilever (Fig 10.6c,d). If the preparations are 'canted' slightly (to the mesial, in this case) then the natural arc of rotation does not act to remove the bridge on its path of insertion/removal, but instead tries to move the abutment casting 'through' the prepared tooth. Resistance form is created. It is sometimes necessary to 'shave' the adjoining tooth (in this case the distal of the canine in the incisal one-third) slightly to allow the bridge to seat on insertion.

- Finally, cantilever abutment roots must not be in close proximity, such as illustrated in Fig 10.6e). Solder joints or multiple castings tend to strangle the papillae, and make effective interproximal plaque removal difficult if not impossible. The thin alveolar bone between close roots is at particular risk, there being so little of it. Splinting such teeth together is not a good idea, unless minor orthodontic movement is employed to gain space between roots.

In situations where root proximity is a problem, the use of interproximally chamfered preparations (Fig 10.6f) can allow for an undercontouring of proximal castings, opening the joint for healthy tissue contours, and ready access to threaders and interproximal brushes for daily plaque removal.

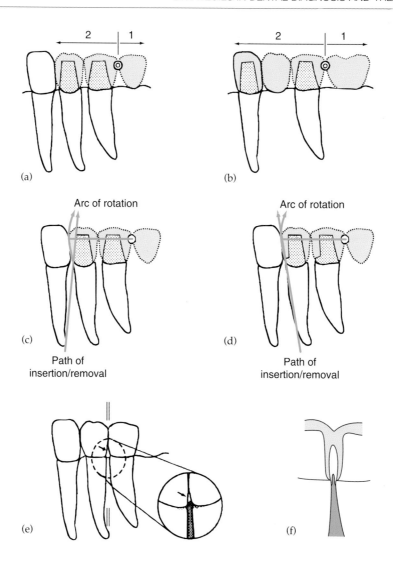

Fig 10.6

(a,b) Maintain an abutment-to-cantilever ratio of not less than 2:1. (c) 'Normal' path of insertion/removal is congruent with arc of rotation. (d) Creating a mesial 'cant' in the preparation provides resistance to displacement when rotational forces occur. (e) Close proximity of roots may preclude splinting of cantilever abutments, or the interdental papilla may be strangled, and access for plaque removal made difficult or impossible. Minor orthodontic treatment may be indicated in such cases. (f) Where inter-root space is adequate but not generous, chamfering the preparations interproximally and undercontouring in the joint area can preserve tissue health and accessibility for cleaning.

Later chapters of this book illustrate the use of 'convertible' fixed bridges, using questionable distal abutments with the option of converting to cantilever should the distal abutment fail. When using this strategy, it is critical to employ these 'keys' in the planning and preparation stage, to ensure success of the converted prosthesis.

Strategic extraction, and nonreplacement of missing teeth or partial replacement using cantilevered bridges are useful strategies, and can often simplify complex and difficult treatment situations.

11

HOPELESS TEETH

There are times when extraction may be the most rational and appropriate option, but circumstances demand at least one good effort, in order to retain a critical tooth or teeth. These situations often arise when traumatic injuries threaten the loss of permanent teeth in young people, or when retention of a questionable tooth is crucial to an overall plan of treatment to which the patient is strongly committed.

When attempting heroic treatment to save 'hopeless' teeth, it is essential that all parties understand the risk, indeed the likelihood, of failure. If dentist, patient, and/or parents are willing to attempt the save, and everyone understands the odds, then one or more of the creative strategies illustrated below may be employed. The cases shown are somewhat unusual, in that all of them have been successful in salvaging the hopeless teeth, at least as of this writing.

ILLUSTRATIVE CASE HISTORIES: 'HOPELESS' TEETH

Concepts illustrated: *techniques in salvaging and preserving severely damaged or debilitated teeth including apexification, electrosurgical management of tissue, use of natural teeth in temporary post-crown restorations, single sitting endodontics, orthodontic extrusion, fabrication, and use of direct/indirect post-copings.*

HOPELESS CASE 11.1

Figure 11.1a shows a successful apexification procedure on the central incisor (no. 8) of an 8-year-old girl (1988). Devitalized by a traumatic blow, successive applications of calcium hydroxide had stimulated sufficient closure of the immature apex (note the difference in root length between central incisors) to permit endodontic fill with 'hand-rolled' gutta percha. The tooth was doing well until a year later (1989), when another trauma resulted in a complete horizontal fracture (Fig 11.1b).

The fractured crown was removed, and the tissue was managed with electrosurgery to clear the fracture margin and obtain hemostasis (Fig 11.1c). This was especially critical on the palatal aspect, where the fracture extended deeply subgingival.

Meanwhile, the crown was cleaned, hollowed out, and a brass dowel post loosely fitted into it (Fig 11.1d). This was carried to the mouth, and passive adaptation of the crown, root, and brass post was confirmed. Light-cured composite resin was then used to affix the post to the crown segment, and the result-

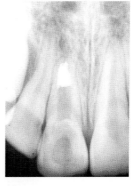

(a)

Fig 11.1

Successful apexification procedure, patient age 8.

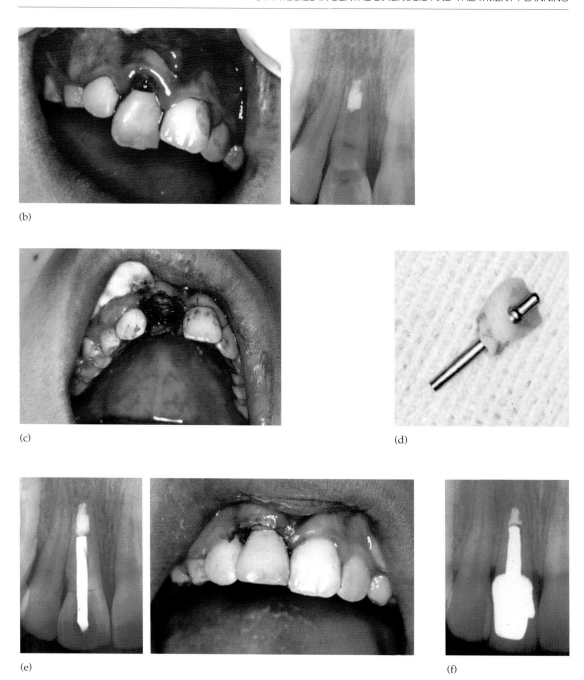

(b)

(c)

(d)

(e)

(f)

Fig 11.1 *continued*

(b) A year later, at age 9, traumatic horizontal fracture. (c) Electrosurgery was employed to access subgingival fracture margins, and to obtain hemostasis. (d) Brass dowel pin (Pindex) was loosely fitted to the crown on the bench. (e) Once fitted passively in the mouth, light-cured composite resin was used to fill the crown portion, and initial curing was done in the mouth. The post crown was removed to complete the light cure, and then cemented with a temporary cement. (f) Six years later, at age 14, a custom-cast post and core was fabricated and cemented permanently.

ing post-crown was cemented into and onto the root with a temporary cement (Fig 11.1e).

EPILOGUE CASE HISTORY 11.1

Six years later (1995) the temporary post and crown came loose, and a custom cast gold post and core was fabricated and cemented permanently (Fig 11.1f). A temporary was made over this post and served until a porcelain-fused-to-gold crown could be placed.

HOPELESS CASE 11.2

This patient, referred from another office in 1986, had a severe vertical fracture of tooth no. 8 (Fig 11.2a).

This 16-year-old girl had no dental restorations of any kind. After exposing pulp the fracture exited the root 5 mm below the alveolar crest, and easily made this tooth a candidate for extraction. She and her parents were desperate to save the tooth.

Electrosurgical debridement and hemostasis were employed to clear the field for a one-

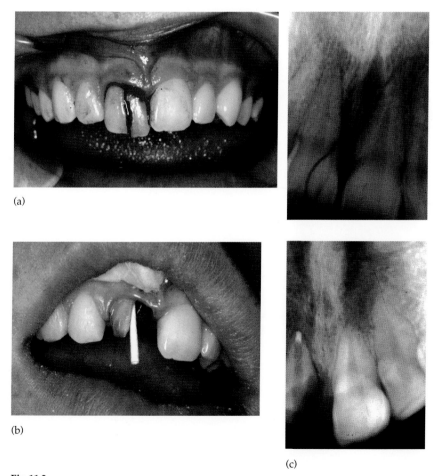

(a)

(b)

(c)

Fig 11.2

(a) Both clinical and radiographic appearance suggest a 'hopeless' situation. (b) After controlling the field with electrosurgery, a one-sitting endodontic treatment was carried out. (c) The apical seal is just barely adequate, as maximum post length was needed in view of the anticipated orthodontic extrusion.

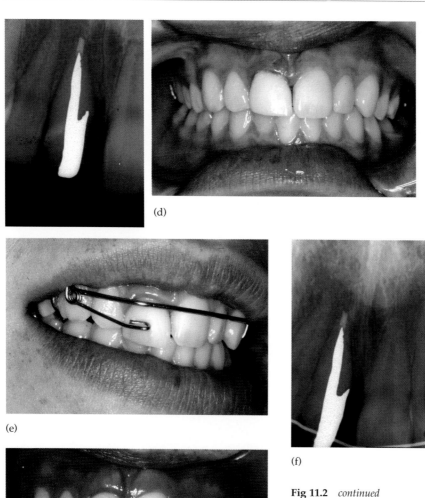

(d)

(e)

(f)

Fig 11.2 *continued*

(d) Having a tooth in place within a day of the trauma was much appreciated by patient and parents, who understood that we were not yet 'out of the woods.' (e) Orthodontic extrusion was used to clear the fracture margin above the alveolar bone. (f) With an acceptable physiologic width for attachment established, definitive restoration could proceed. (g) Eight-year follow-up, demonstrating successful retention of this 'hopeless' tooth.

(g)

sitting root canal (Fig 11.2b). After sealing the apex with gutta percha, as much post space as possible was created, and a direct pattern for cast gold post was made (Fig 11.2c). The post was inserted the following day, and a light cured composite resin provisional crown was 'permanently' cemented to the post (Fig 11.2d).

The tooth was then extruded orthodontically, using a Hawley retainer with a coiled finger spring off the anterior bow (Fig 11.2e). The finger spring engaged a facial 'notch' created in the provisional. The extrusion was monitored weekly, and the provisional was reduced incisally and lingually as necessary. A bonded wire retainer stabilized the tooth after 6 weeks, with the fracture margin ending about 2 mm clear of the alveolar crest (Fig 11.2f).

EPILOGUE CASE HISTORY **11.2**

Eight years later (1994), the patient was kind enough to return for follow-up and photograph (Fig 11.2g). As might be expected following orthodontic extrusion, the gingiva had crept down somewhat, and minor electrosurgical gingivoplasty was performed to 'even up' the crown length of nos 8 and 9. The tooth remains comfortable and functional.

HOPELESS CASE **11.3**

Another variation on the theme, this 11-year-old boy was a sports enthusiast, and a series of sports-related traumas made him a regular in the office for several years. In early 1992 he presented with a full horizontal fracture of tooth no. 8 (Fig 11.3a). One-sitting root canal therapy was indicated, but electrosurgery

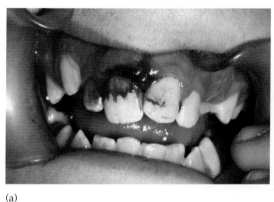

(a)

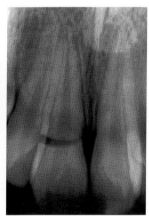

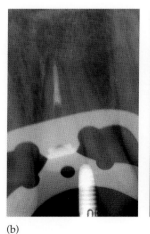

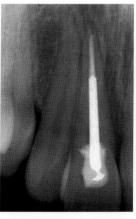

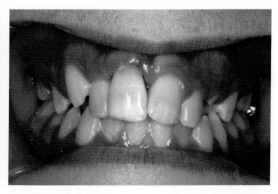

(b)

Fig 11.3

(a) Full horizontal fracture, subgingival no. 8, of an 11-year-old patient. (b) Endodontics done in one sitting, post crown made using patient's own clinical crown and brass dowel pin, 3 weeks after initial trauma.

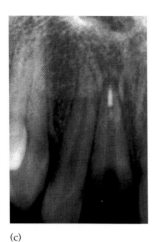

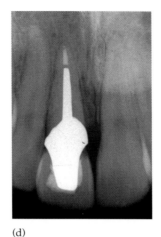

Fig 11.3 *continued*

(c) 6 weeks later another traumatic blow dislodged the temporary post crown. (d) Custom cast post coping was cemented permanently, with the crown fragment still serving as temporary. (e) Orthodontic treatment added to the normal daily stresses on this hybrid restoration. (f) 8 years after the initial trauma, a definitive crown was placed over the post coping, and the crown fragment was finally retired.

(c)   (d)

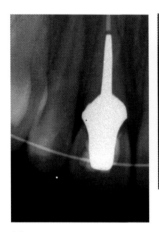

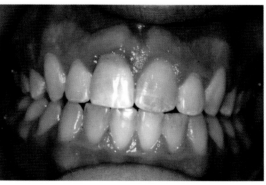

(e)

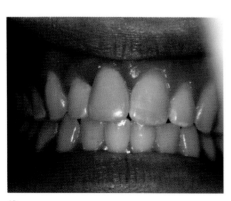

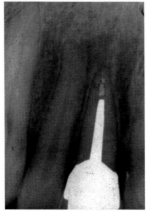

(f)

was ruled out as a result of the severe contusion to the gingival tissues. Instead, a flap was carefully reflected to clear the root for a rubber dam clamp. Endodontic and temporary post-crown procedures were performed, and the flap sutured back to place. The tissue was healing well, and the tooth was comfortable, although still slightly mobile, just 3 weeks after the initial trauma (Fig 11.3b).

Less than 6 weeks later, another sports-related injury caused the temporary post and crown to be knocked loose (Fig 11.3c). Fortunately the root was not fractured, and it was decided to fabricate a post-coping for better retention and to 'bind' the root, creating a ferrule effect. This was done, and the patient's own clinical crown, relieved and filled in with light cured composite, was cemented 'permanently' to the post-coping (Fig 11.3d).

This arrangement held up through 2 years of orthodontic treatment (1993–94) (Fig 11.3e) and continued to serve until late in 1997 when, at age 17, a porcelain fused to gold crown was placed in its stead. The original post-coping remains as the foundation (Fig 11.3f).

HOPELESS CASE 11.4

To illustrate the fabrication of a custom-cast post-coping, we may consider this fragile but critical distal bridge abutment, the hemisected distal root of lower right second molar number 31 (Fig 11.4a). Given all it has gone through, such a tooth (or root) could well be considered 'hopeless.' Nevertheless, the desire to maintain an intact dentition drives

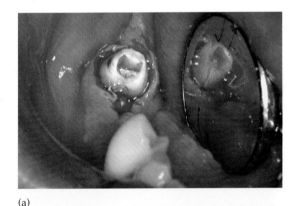

(a)

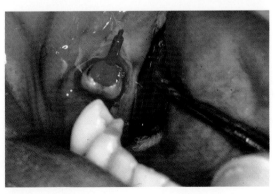

(b)

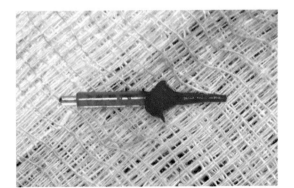

Fig 11.4

(a) Hemi-section of lower molars can often preserve a sound root for many additional years of service. (b) Formed in the mouth, using a plastic core or dowel pin with additional self-curing acrylic resin (Duralay), the intracoronal post pattern should draw easily, and seat positively on the prepared tooth.

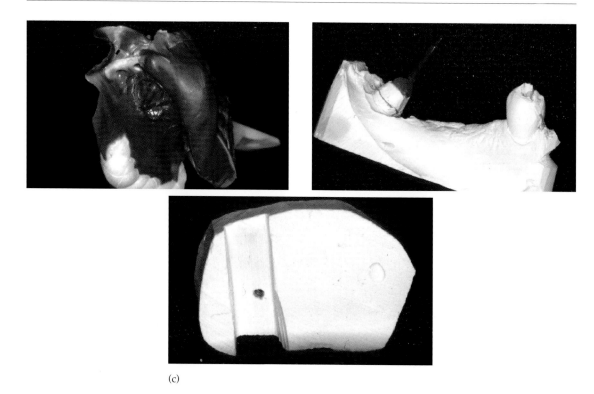

(c)

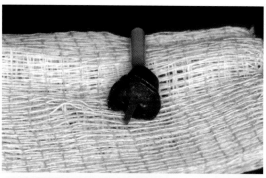

Fig 11.4 *continued*

(c) Demonstrating the steps in the fabrication of direct/indirect post coping. The intraoral pattern must sit cleanly on the indirect die. (d) The coping is waxed directly to and over the post pattern, creating a finished margin and collar of gold, and permitting directional changes for proper parallelism. (e) Bridge preparations, with double premolar abutments in the anterior, hemisected molar root at posterior. As a subgingival gold margin and collar have been established, it is easy to impress the distal abutment.

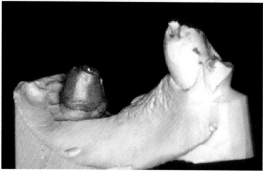

(d)

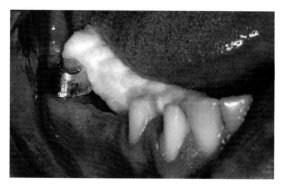

(e)

us to seek strategies to preserve and utilize this delicate little 'hemi-tooth.' A cast post and core would generally be the next step, but we must take great care with such teeth, because intracoronal stresses can easily fracture the root longitudinally. A post-coping is indicated to provide intracoronal retention while at the same time 'binding' the root circumferentially, creating a ferrule effect.

In fabrication of the post-coping, fit is critical. Intracoronal cast posts must fit passively, because 'tight' fits can introduce stresses resulting in subsequent root fractures. Care must be taken in fabrication to limit expansion of the pattern, to keep the casting 'small.' Extracoronal crowns and copings must also fit passively, to allow complete seating, with room for cement. In order to accomplish this, we try to maximize expansion of pattern and casting, keeping the casting 'large.' How do we make a combination casting of post and coping that meets both needs?

One approach is to use a direct/indirect technique. After post space and extracoronal preparation is complete, an acrylic pattern is made directly in the mouth. This one is using a plastic sprue pattern with Duralay resin, making an accurate pattern that seats cleanly onto the top of the prepared tooth (Fig 11.4b). As resin tends to shrink in setting, and as the sprue pattern core has somewhat less capacity for thermal expansion than wax does, the resulting intracoronal casting should fit passively.

An impression is made of the prepared tooth subgingivally, and as far into the post space as practical. The end of the post impression is augmented with wax, which, when the stone model is set, can be located and removed from below, allowing the direct post pattern to be seated accurately on the die (Fig 11.4c).

The extracoronal coping is then waxed over the direct pattern, which will allow the normal expansion of lost wax for a 'generous' fit when cast in gold. The coping also allows a directional change, so that proper parallelism with anterior abutments can be achieved (Fig 11.4d).

Given the multiple procedures (root canal, hemisection, post-coping) performed on the distal root of no. 31, the fixed bridge is double

abutted in the anterior, and designed to be converted to a cantilever arrangement should the 'hopeless' distal anchor root give out in the future (Fig 11.4e). This approach is discussed at length in Chapter 13. The

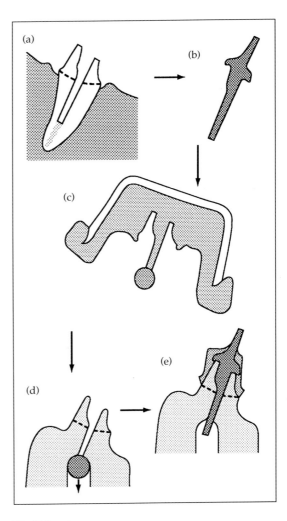

Fig 11.5

Schematic diagrams review the steps in creating the direct/indirect post coping. (a) Post space and chamfer margins prepared. (b) Intracoronal direct post pattern. (c) Impression of tooth and prepared margin, and post space (not necessarily complete). Wax ball added at end of post impression before pouring stone model. (d) Stone die, hollow-ground from below to locate and remove wax ball. (e) Post pattern fitted cleanly onto die, with coping waxed over it. Gold finish margin and collar create finish margin for later overcasting.

schematic diagrams review the steps in creating a direct/indirect pattern for the post-coping (Fig 11.5).

All such heroic efforts are at risk of failure, owing to the number and complexity of procedures necessary, and to the compromised situation at the outset. If all parties understand the risks, and agree that they are worth taking, then applying creative strategies to 'hopeless' teeth can be a rewarding, albeit challenging, part of dental practice. Some of the approaches illustrated here are put to use in the next chapter, dealing with management of complex problems.

12

MANAGING COMPLEX DENTAL TREATMENT SITUATIONS

There are times when we are presented with complex problems that defy our attempts to simplify them. This chapter considers a number of tools, techniques, and tactics that may be applied to some challenging clinical cases.

MANAGEMENT OF VERTICAL DIMENSION

Managing and maintaining vertical dimension is often critical in complex cases. The patient shown in Fig 12.1a was a retired teacher in her early seventies. Other than the normal maladies of advancing age such as arthritis, she was spry, in reasonably good physical health, and mentally sharp. Her upper and lower removable partial dentures had become loose and ill-fitting; abutment teeth were broken down and carious. She had five upper anterior teeth (missing no. 10) and no posteriors. She had two lower canines (missing incisors) and two lower premolars nos 28 and 29, missing all the rest. Periodontal support was excellent for her age, but decades of patchwork had all come due.

She accepted a plan of full reconstruction, involving crowns on all remaining teeth. Upper crowns on nos 6, 7, and 8, and a fixed bridge from no. 9 to 11, would have keyways for a semiprecision, cast gold base partial denture. A lower fixed bridge from no. 22 to 27, and splinted crowns nos 28–29 would have similar attachments. As her only centric stops were on canines, the technical challenge was to maintain her vertical dimension, while preparing all the lower teeth at once. This was accomplished as follows: before preparation, a solid centric stop is marked indelibly on no. 27 (Fig 12.1b). The lower canines are prepared, except that incisal reduction is not done on the centric stop mark. Temporary acrylic is moulded over the prepared teeth, and the patient closed to contact (Fig 12.1c). As the material starts to firm, we can see indentations of the linguals of the uppers, and the original centric stop 'burned through' the material (Fig 12.1d). The temporary material is removed, trimmed and shaped, and returned to the mouth for reline. The centric stop is still visible (Fig 12.1e). The process was repeated to produce a second acrylic appliance, which was used to replicate the vertical dimension in the laboratory, seating it on the stone dies. The second acrylic moulding was not shaped as a temporary, but simply trimmed for easy seating on the dies. The light imprint of the upper teeth was retained, and used to help articulate upper and lower working models.

At that point, the final reduction of no. 27 was done, and acrylic used to fill the void. The patient's vertical dimension was thus maintained in the provisional bridge.

The completed case, with crowns and fixed bridges in the anterior, with claspless semi-precision gold base partial attachments (Fig 12.1f), was very pleasing to the patient, providing comfort, function, and improved esthetics as well. She continued on maintenance for about 10 years, and required no further periodontal, restorative, or prosthetic

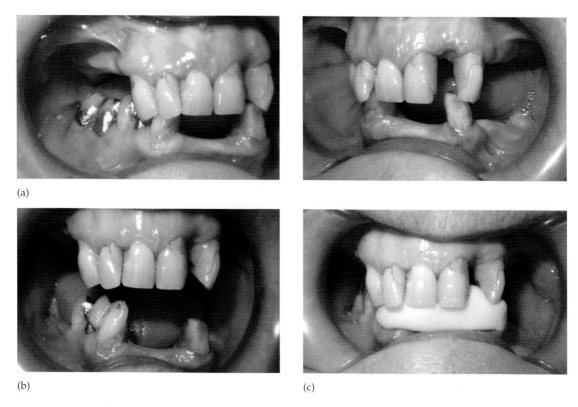

(a)

(b)   (c)

Fig 12.1

(a) Years of maintenance and patchwork were coming due, and sound periodontal structures made reconstruction both possible and desirable. Vertical dimension was acceptable, but was being maintained by two canine contacts, which would be wiped out in the lower anterior bridge preparation process. (b) Blue mark notes and preserves a centric stop on tooth no. 27. This was overmarked with indelible marker. (c) Canines were prepared, except for reduction of the stop on no. 27, temporary acrylic was molded over the teeth, and the patient closed into contact.

treatment. She passed away at age 90, having had 17 years of carefree and comfortable service from her reconstruction.

Regaining lost vertical dimension as a result of loss of teeth, loss of tooth structure, or a combination of both is a complex and challenging process. When significant tooth structure has been lost, it is necessary to establish patient comfort and tolerance while restoring teeth and regaining vertical dimension. We must consider that the functional and habitual forces that caused the damage initially are likely to continue acting at some level. In other words, our restored occlusion must be prepared to take on the stresses that destroyed that natural dentition.

ILLUSTRATIVE CASE HISTORIES 12.2–12.4

Treated by Wm L. Nequette, DDS, FICD, FACD

Concepts illustrated: *techniques in planning and executing reconstructions of severely debilitated occlusions including prewaxing, use of shims, bite-opening splints, gnathologically developed metal occlusals.*

Nequette case 12.2

Figure 12.2a illustrates a combination of tooth loss and attrition resulting in collapse

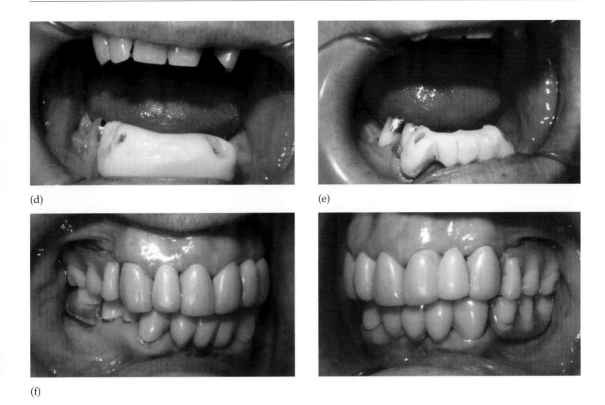

Fig 12.1 *continued*

(d) The contact spot 'burned through' the acrylic. (e) The temporary bridge is shaped, with the contact still in place. Once finished, the stop is reduced and the temporary 'filled in' with more acrylic. (f) The reconstructed case, with upper and lower crowns and fixed bridges, providing abutments for upper and lower partial dentures (cast gold base).

of the bite, into a pseudo-class III relationship. Maxillary anteriors were too short to support restoration, and endodontics, posts, and cores were considered. With pulps barely discernible radiographically, both the practicality and the need for multiple endodontic treatments came into question. A creative solution was found involving pin-retained gold cores. Cast gold, lower premolar temporaries established a workable vertical dimension (Fig 12.2b). Using a fully adjustable articulator and gnathological principles, the upper anterior dies and working model were mounted at the new vertical dimension. Upper six anteriors were fabri-

cated against a prewaxed lower model (Fig 12.2c). The upper anteriors were inserted, impressed, and provided the opposing model for fabrication of the lower anterior segment (Fig 12.2d).

Once anterior guidance was established, upper and lower posterior sextants were restored, using gnathological wax-ups to create optimum cusp–fossa relationships which disoccluded in lateral excursions (Fig 12.2e).

Note that the occlusals are in metal, respecting the environmental forces that had decimated the natural dentition (Fig 12.2f). Anterior group function that disoccludes

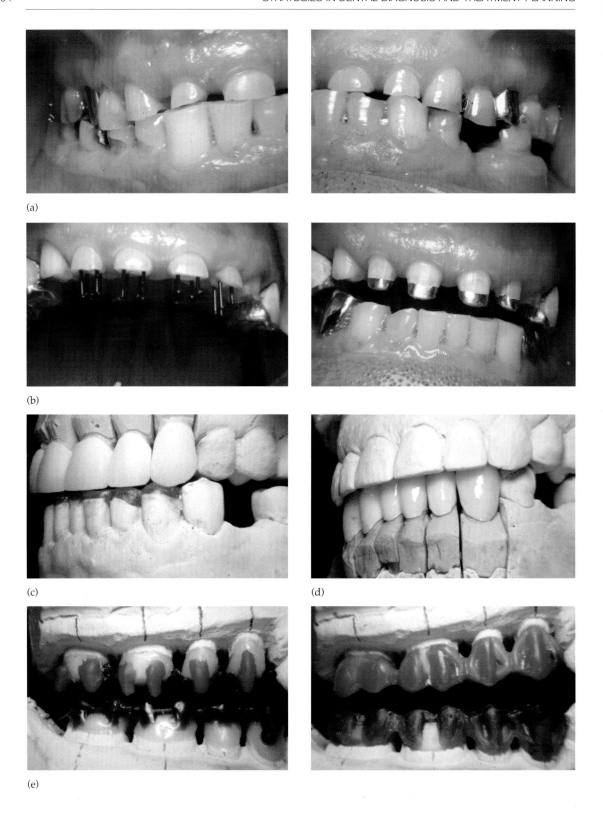

(a)

(b)

(c)

(d)

(e)

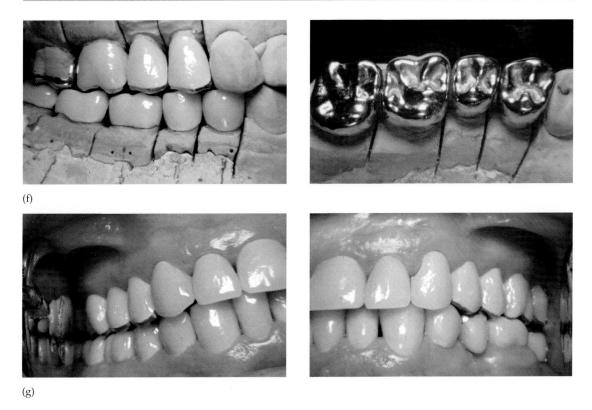

(f)

(g)

Fig 12.2

(a) Severe attrition and loss of vertical dimension, a 'collapsed' bite. (b) Parallel pins (four per tooth) were made to create pin copings, thus obtaining adequate crown length without devitalizing the teeth. Note the cast gold premolar temporaries establishing and holding an enhanced vertical dimension. (c) Upper six anteriors (biscuit porcelain bake) fabricated against prewaxed lower anteriors, to establish anterior group function disclusion. (d) Lower anteriors now being made opposing the newly inserted upper sextant. (e) With anterior guidance established, wax-to-wax development of posterior occlusion is carried out. (f) Posterior occlusals are in metal, in view of the original devastation of the natural dentition. (g) The completed reconstruction.

posteriors in excursions will often reduce parafunctional activity such as bruxing, but there is no guarantee.

The completed reconstruction (Fig 12.2g) provided comfort and function, was esthetically pleasing (Fig 12.2h) and compatible with the periodontium (Fig 12.2i).

Follow-up at 8 years (Fig 12.2j) shows good durability (other than a lost pontic facing on the lower left bridge, which was replaced with composite resin). The patient had suffered a severe heart attack and lengthy recuperation, and periodontal tissues reflected his fragile condition.

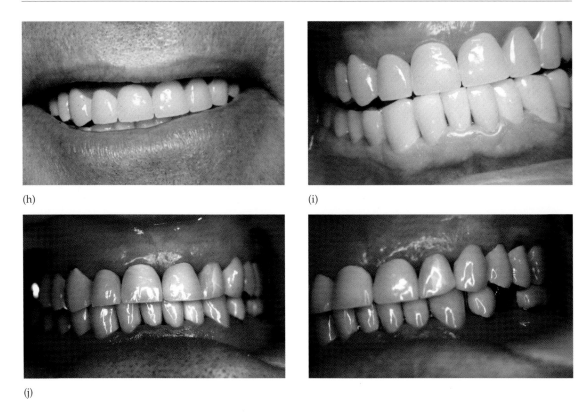

(h)

(i)

(j)

Fig 12.2 *continued*

(h) The patient was pleased with his new smile. (i) Periodontal health and maintenance were excellent. (j) At an 8-year follow-up we see the aftermath of a severe heart attack and lengthy recuperation. Periodontal tissues have lost their good color and tone. A bridge facing has become debonded (no. 20). Functionally, the reconstruction was doing well.

Nequette case 12.3

Figure 12.3a illustrates severe attrition resulting in collapse of the bite, this time in a strong class II relationship. A centric relation mounting on a fully adjustable instrument is used arbitrarily to select a workable vertical dimension (Fig 12.3b). An overlay splint is fabricated at that dimension, and delivered to the patient for a trial run (Fig 12.3c). The patient found the splint and the regained vertical dimension to be very comfortable, and the reconstruction was started, with prewaxing on the same mounted models (Fig 12.3d). The wax-up was duplicated (Fig 12.3e), and thin 'pull-down' shims were made over it. These shims serve

many useful purposes. Placed over the teeth before preparation, they are used to gauge the amount of tooth reduction necessary (Fig 12.3f). They are, of course, used as formers for the acrylic provisionals, giving the patient and dentist a 'preview' of the reconstruction. In the laboratory, they can be used over the mounted upper dies to begin waxing the lowers, replicating the original prewaxed occlusion (Fig 12.3g).

Control of the entire case is maintained as the reconstruction is completed on the instrument (Fig 12.3h). Anterior group function provides guidance in all excursions (Fig 12.3i), teeth fully interdigitate (again using all gold occlusals) (Fig 12.3j), and there is no contact

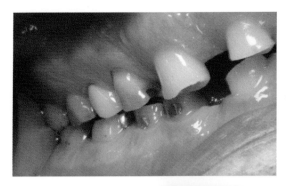
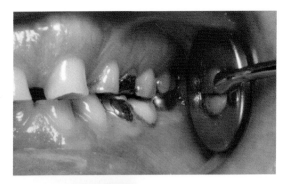
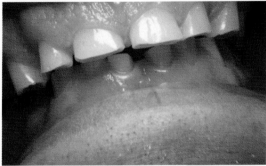

(a)

Fig 12.3

(a) Despite a full complement of teeth, bruxism and resulting attrition have collapsed this class II occlusion. (b) Casts mounted in centric relation on fully adjustable articulator (TMJ), with prospective 'new' vertical dimension. (c) An overlay splint, to be worn by the patient until everyone is comfortable with the prospective vertical dimension.

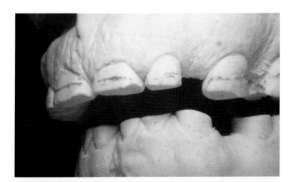

(b)

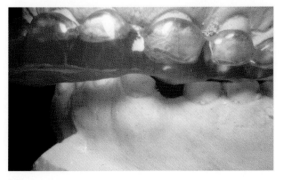
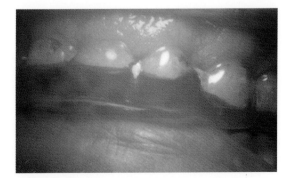

(c)

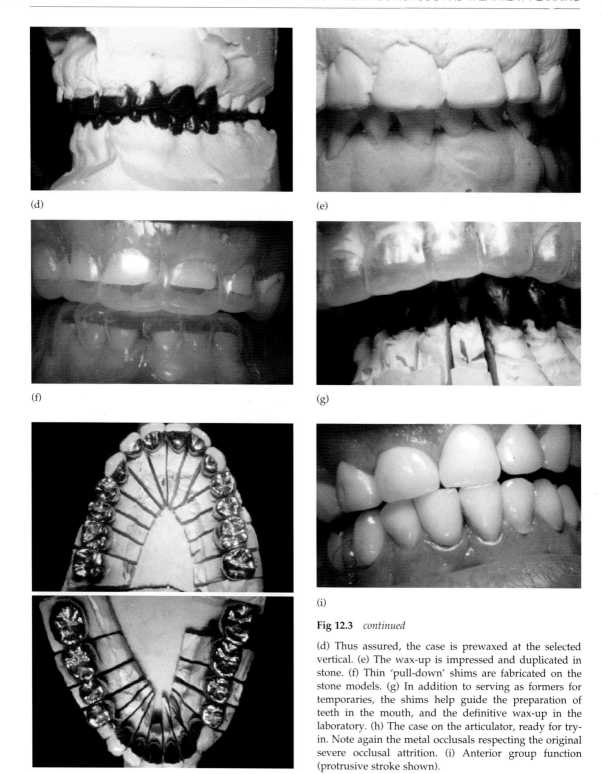

(d)

(e)

(f)

(g)

(h)

(i)

Fig 12.3 *continued*

(d) Thus assured, the case is prewaxed at the selected vertical. (e) The wax-up is impressed and duplicated in stone. (f) Thin 'pull-down' shims are fabricated on the stone models. (g) In addition to serving as formers for temporaries, the shims help guide the preparation of teeth in the mouth, and the definitive wax-up in the laboratory. (h) The case on the articulator, ready for try-in. Note again the metal occlusals respecting the original severe occlusal attrition. (i) Anterior group function (protrusive stroke shown).

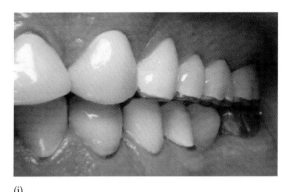

(j)

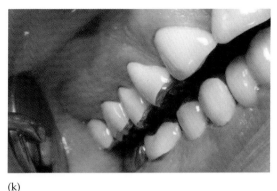

(k)

Fig 12.3 *continued*

(j) Full and functional occlusion. (k) No contact on the balancing (right) side in the left lateral.

on the balancing sides in lateral strokes (Fig 12.3k). Scrupulous attention to detail and carefully planned and executed clinical and laboratory procedures are critical to the management of such complex cases.

Nequette case 12.4

Figure 12.4a recapitulates the approach. Note the attrition of teeth and the habitual laterotrusive wear in the left canine/premolar

area. The prewaxed occlusal scheme (Fig 12.4b) leads to the production of the shims (Fig 12.4c), and to the eventual gnathologically reconstructed occlusion (Fig 12.4d). The completed reconstruction is shown in centric and left lateral excursion (Fig 12.4e).

Systemic factors can further complicate an already complex technical treatment plan. The last two cases again involve significant vertical dimension problems, but with other factors influencing the plan.

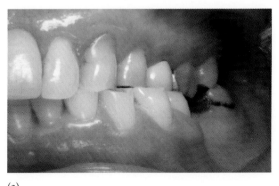

(a)

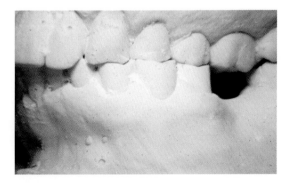

Fig 12.4

(a) More occlusal attrition, note the 'habitual' laterotrusive wear.

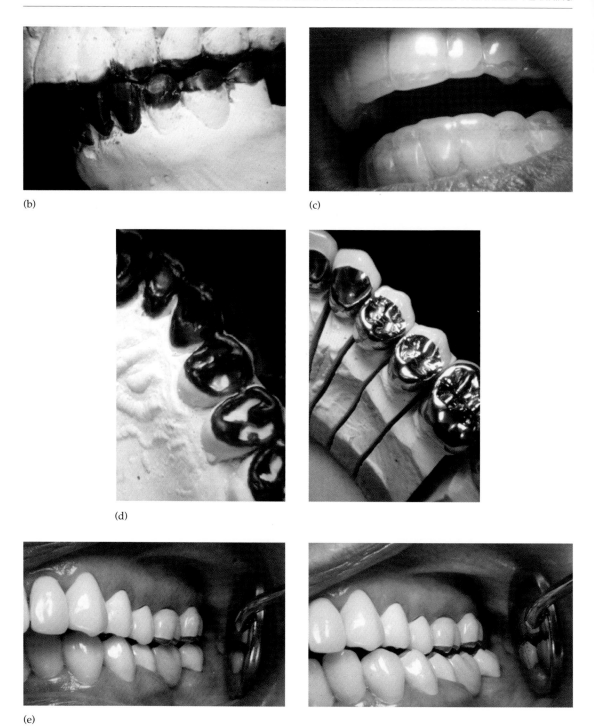

(b)

(c)

(d)

(e)

Fig 12.4 *continued*

(b) Prewaxing the occlusal scheme. (c) Shims in place before preparation. (d) Development of optimal cusp–fossa relationships. (e) Reconstructed occlusion in centric and in lateral excursion.

ILLUSTRATIVE CASE HISTORY 12.5

Concepts illustrated: _vertical dimension issues, non-replacement of missing teeth, complicating systemic factors._

This 68-year-old woman presented with a chief complaint of continual breakdown of her teeth (Fig 12.5a). Lacking molar support on the left, her deep class II bite has deepened as attrition has compromised vertical dimension (Fig 12.5b). She has long suffered from rheumatoid arthritis, and deals with chronic pain every day. Nevertheless, she was warm and pleasant, bearing up well to both her arthritis and to the extensive dental work she was undergoing. Of note is the asymmetry of jaw motions, with a right lateral excursion that involves a shallow disclusion on the working side going from the central incisor all the way back to the second molar, whereas the left lateral had a steep cuspid rise (canine guidance) (Fig 12.5c). The following problem list was developed:

Patient SP:	68-year-old retired kindergarten teacher, rheumatoid arthritic
	Chief complaint: general dental breakdown
	Dental goal: would like to keep teeth
	Many broken down restorations, several nonvital, periapically involved teeth
	Deep class II, with generalized attrition and loss of vertical dimension

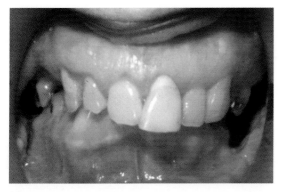

(a)

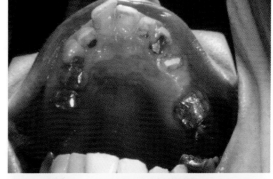

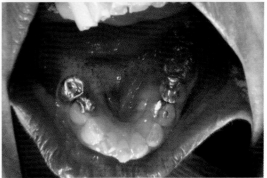

Fig 12.5

(a) Class II, collapsed vertical dimension. (b) Occlusal attrition evidences high stress in the environment.

(b)

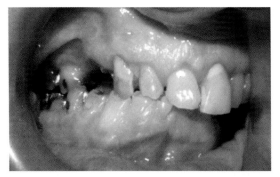

(c)

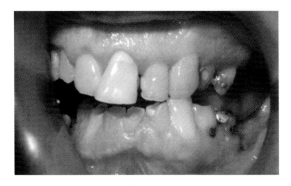

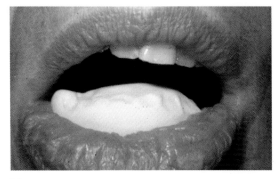

(d)

Fig 12.5 *continued*

(c) Lateral excursions are asymmetric, shallow group function on the right, steep cuspid rise on the left. (d) Lower anterior temporary molded in the mouth captures the asymmetry, at an enhanced vertical dimension. (e) Finished lower anterior provisional mimics the patient's presenting guidance pattern, at an increased vertical dimension. (f) Full provisional crowns and bridges functioning comfortably for 6 months. (g) Finished reconstruction, maintaining the established occlusal relationships. (h) 5-year follow-up.

As the teeth were so debilitated, it was decided to prepare and temporize throughout the mouth, increasing the vertical dimension as each arch was temporized. Lower anterior teeth were prepared first, and a moulded acrylic temporary was fabricated (Fig 12.5d), maintaining the shallow right lateral disclusion, and the steep left side cuspid rise, but at an increased vertical dimension (Fig 12.5e). Preparation and temporization were continued, and the patient functioned comfortably for 6 months, during which time several endodontic procedures were completed (Fig 12.5f).

As she had not had molar occlusion on the left side for at least 30 years, it was decided for the sake of simplicity not to replace the teeth in that area, but to preserve and maintain her preferred functional right side.

Crowns and fixed bridges were fabricated at the established vertical dimension, preserving the asymmetric disclusion but limiting it to the anterior only, to allow posterior disclusion in both directions (Fig 12.5g). Throughout the lengthy multiple procedures the patient was tolerant and in good spirits, and I will never forget the Saturday morning when I found my 5-year-old daughter (who had come to the office with me and was supposed to be watching cartoons in my office) sitting instead on my patient's lap, delighted at being read to by this gracious and gentle lady.

EPILOGUE CASE HISTORY 12.5

At 5-year follow-up, the patient continued to function effectively (Fig 12.5h). It is interesting to note that at about this time a single lower crown came debonded as a result of failure of its core amalgam, and the tooth was built up again, and recrowned. In the 5 years since the reconstruction, the patient had aged considerably. Her arthritis limited her ability to tolerate the dental procedures, she was depressed and irritable, and it was all we could do to get one crown made. Had the reconstruction not been done when it was, there would have been no way to restore her dentition. As it was, regular maintenance was done for about 12 years, and the patient passed away 15 years after the reconstruction, her dentition intact.

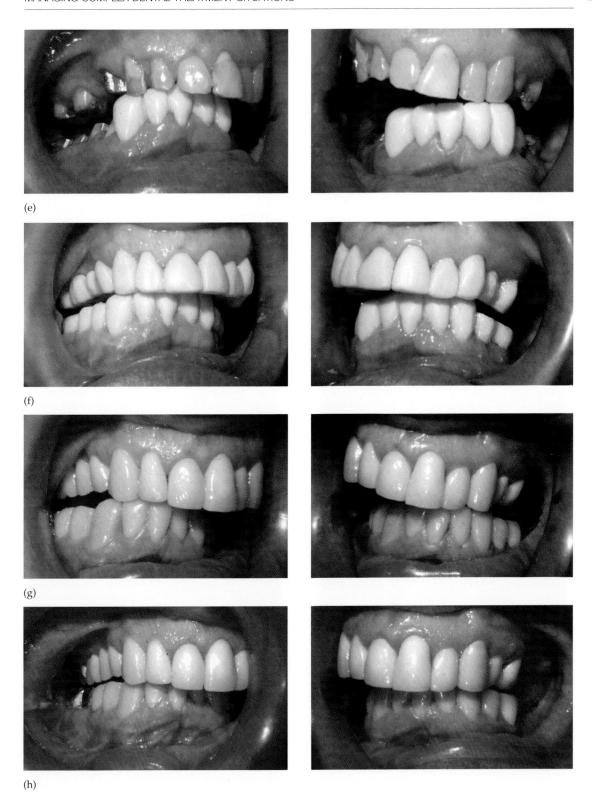

(e)

(f)

(g)

(h)

ILLUSTRATIVE CASE HISTORY 12.6

Concepts illustrated: *vertical dimension issues, phasing based on systemic factors, nonreplacement of teeth.*

This 57-year-old man presented for dental evaluation subsequent to a heart attack, having been advised by his cardiologist to have his dental problems attended to before cardiac catheterization, angiogram, and possible open heart surgery. It was immediately apparent that attending to his teeth was going be a rather large undertaking, and that a phased plan of treatment would be necessary (Fig 12.6a). The following problem list was developed:

Patient SP:	57-year-old engineer, recent myocardial infarction, anticipated angiogram and open heart surgery. Prognosis unclear at this time
	Chief complaint: general dental breakdown, with direction from cardiologist to 'have dental problems attended to' before further heart treatment
	Dental goal: take care of immediate needs
	Local moderate-to-severe periodontitis, some teeth badly involved, others less so, others not at all
	Class II, with severe attrition and breakdown throughout, with significant loss of vertical dimension, along with some supereruption. Anteriors have eroded into each other over the years. Deep carious lesion no. 12

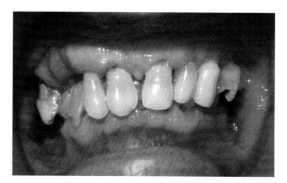 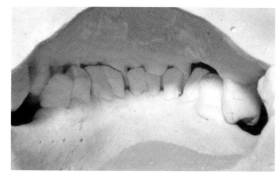

(a)

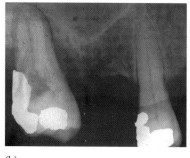 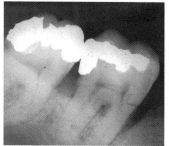 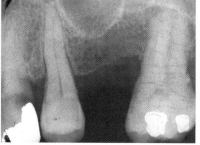

(b)

Fig 12.6

(a) Presenting occlusion, clinical, and diagnostic cast lingual view. (b) Teeth nos 2 (may be 1?), 12, and 30 presented immediate problems.

Phase 1 disease control

A thorough scaling/root planing was carried out under local anesthetic. Teeth numbers 2 and 30 were extracted as a result of advanced periodontitis with bone loss. Tooth no. 12 was excavated, and a vital pulpotomy performed when it was determined that caries had encroached on the pulp (Fig 12.6b).

Intensive oral hygiene instructions were given, and the patient went to hospital.

His angiogram revealed multiple blockages in coronary arteries, and a multiple bypass operation was performed. Happily the patient survived and, as soon as he was cleared for dental treatment, he returned seeking more definitive care. His dental goal now included the hope of keeping the rest of his teeth, and we then planned the second phase of treat-

ment. Study casts reflect the status after extractions and disease control (Fig 12.6c).

Phase 2 definitive treatment

As the teeth were so debilitated, it was decided to prepare and temporize everything. Upper and lower anteriors were prepared, and temporaries placed at the desired vertical dimension, such that restorative and periodontal treatment could be carried out (Fig 12.6d). Cast gold temporaries on lower left premolars were made to help hold that vertical, and guidance in excursions was established (Fig 12.6e). Full-flap periodontal surgery was done on upper anterior teeth; the rest of the periodontium was doing well after root

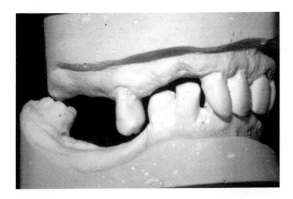
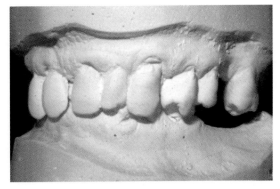

(c)

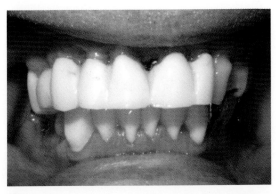

(d)

Fig 12.6 *continued*

(c) Study casts after extractions and disease control.
(d) Acrylic provisionals at re-established vertical height. Upper anteriors have had full flap periodontal surgery with provisionals in place.

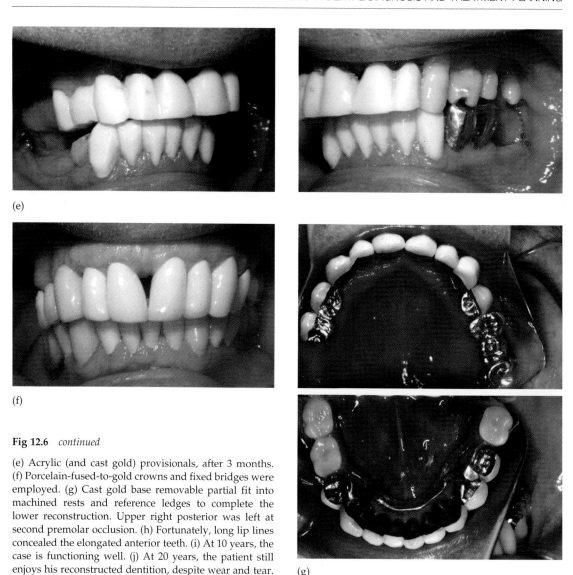

Fig 12.6 *continued*

(e) Acrylic (and cast gold) provisionals, after 3 months. (f) Porcelain-fused-to-gold crowns and fixed bridges were employed. (g) Cast gold base removable partial fit into machined rests and reference ledges to complete the lower reconstruction. Upper right posterior was left at second premolar occlusion. (h) Fortunately, long lip lines concealed the elongated anterior teeth. (i) At 10 years, the case is functioning well. (j) At 20 years, the patient still enjoys his reconstructed dentition, despite wear and tear.

planing. Endodontic treatment was carried out on no. 12, and a post and core placed. After 3 months preparatory treatment was complete, and the patient was comfortable and functional at the reestablished vertical dimension.

Crowns and fixed bridges were placed in the upper (upper right molars were left unreplaced, with fixed bridge fabricated from number 4 to 7–8) (Fig 12.6f). Crowns were placed on lower teeth, splinting 20–21, 27–28, with machined ledges and grooves in those units and in the crown no. 31, designed to accept a cast gold, lower partial denture (Fig 12.6f). Fortunately, the patient's long lip lines mask the elongated postperiodontal crown restorations (Fig 12.6h).

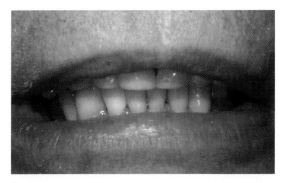

(h)

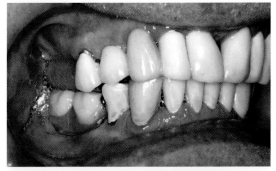

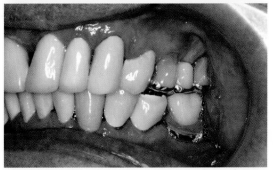

(i)

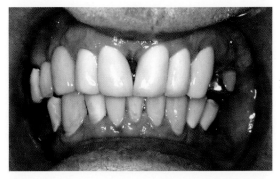

(j)

EPILOGUE CASE HISTORY 12.6

Regular maintenance visits and diligent home care kept this case going strong. At 10 years (Fig 12.6i) no further restorative or prosthetic treatment had been or was needed, and at 20 years (Fig 12.6j) the patient continues to do well. Of note is the fact that tooth no. 12, endodontically treated and restored with post/core and crown, failed at the 19-year mark. The patient was not bothered by loss of the crown, and the decision was made not to replace it. The patient has also discontinued wearing his lower removable partial denture. Now nearly 80 years of age, he functions adequately and comfortably without it, and has declined the offer of a new one.

Of note here is the fact that many bypass patients experience recurrence of cardiac-artery blockages, and often require further surgery or angioplasty within 7–10 years. This patient is now nearly 23 years post-surgery, and is aging gracefully. Achieving and maintaining good oral and dental health may well have played a part in his continuing general health.

As dentists, we may take pride in our role in cases such as these. At the same time, we should feel privileged that good people have placed their confidence in us, and allowed us to serve them for so many years.

TELESCOPE CASTINGS

Some clinical situations call for desperate measures. The case illustrated here began in crisis. The patient thought she had received good care, and was not in pain. Unfortunately, a great deal of grossly deficient dentistry put nearly every tooth at risk of loss.

Aside from the medical–legal issues (a lawsuit was brought and settled), it was impossible to predict the long-term outlook for many of the teeth. The use of post/copings on the upper teeth allowed maximum flexibility should one or more teeth be lost, and temporary cementation was employed to keep options open.

ILLUSTRATIVE CASE HISTORY 12.7

Endodontic retreatment: *Dr John Newman*

Concepts illustrated: *endodontic failure and retreatment, orthodontic eruption to gain physiologic width and clinical crown length, post/copings, telescope overcastings, temporary cementation.*

This 37-year-old businesswoman presented for routine check-up and cleaning, having recently moved to the area (Fig 12.7a). The dental hygienist who saw her first brought the bad news: that there were openings under the margins of her extensive bridgework. Examination confirmed this, and bite wing radio-graphs (Fig 12.7b) made it clear that there was more bad news to come. Subsequent full mouth radiographs revealed multiple silver point endodontic treatment, most of it showing serious and critical defects. Short fills, unfilled canals, and broken files in midcanal were the rule rather than the exception (Fig 12.7c).

The patient was advised of the problems, in as neutral a fashion as possible. She was urged to go back for consultation with her previous dentist, and was given copies of the radiographs and a brief written summary of the findings. The previous dentist was un-sympathetic, and disparaged the findings.

The patient, however, could clearly see the problems and returned for treatment. She also sought legal counsel, as mentioned above. The following problem list was developed:

Patient SN: 37-year-old businesswoman, in good general health
Chief complaint: initially, none. Subsequent to evaluation, concerned about significant problems with inadequate endodontic and restorative treatment
Dental goal: not to lose any teeth, if possible
Generally good periodontal health, with scrupulous home care. Local areas of gingival inflammation as a result of defective restorative margins
Grossly deficient endodontic treatment on many teeth, grossly deficient crowns and fixed bridgework

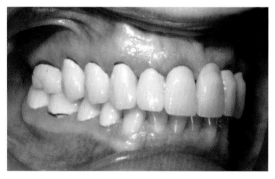 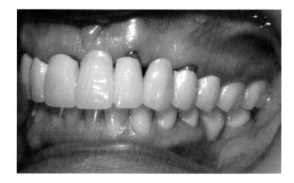

(a)

Fig 12.7

(a) New patient, presenting for routine check-up and cleaning.

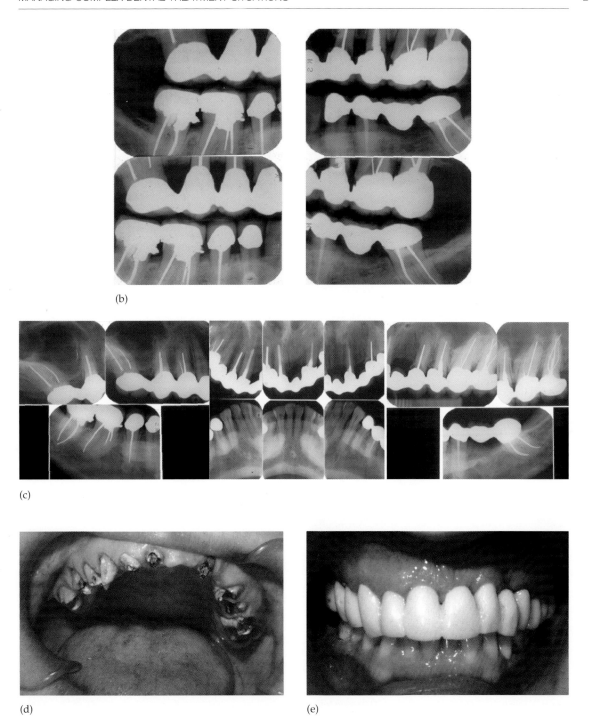

(b)

(c)

(d)   (e)

Fig 12.7 *continued*

(b) Bite wing radiographs revealed serious problems. (c) Full mouth periapicals brought even worse news. (d) Continuous upper arch splinted crowns and bridge were removed. (e) A full arch provisional was fabricated using pull-down shim.

Precise planning was not possible until the extent of the problems could be ascertained. The continuous upper fixed prosthesis was to be removed (Fig 12.7d), the task made easy as a result of the fact that the entire complex turned out to have been retained solely by the upper right canine no. 6. Once that unit was slit, the entire upper arch prosthesis fell out. As it did, several silver points also fell out and were sucked into the high-volume evacuator. After retrieving as many points as possible, a full arch temporary was fabricated, using a thin pull-down shim made on the original study cast (Fig 12.7e).

Endodontic retreatment was started, most canals filled with conventional gutta percha technique, some with apical surgery and reverse fills (Fig 12.7f). Only the mesial canals of no. 30, blocked by a broken file, were not amenable to either retreatment strategy. The distal canal was retreated, and

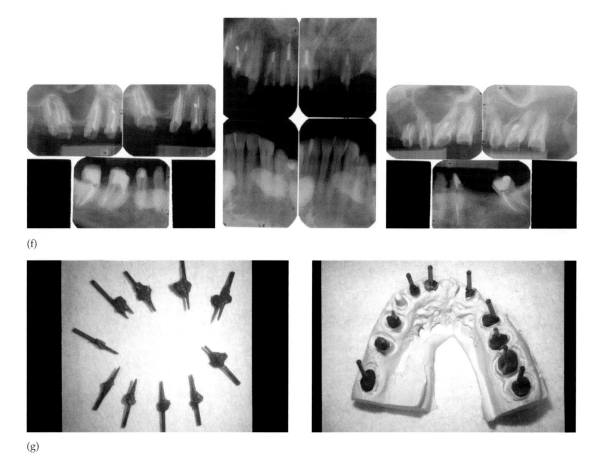

(f)

(g)

Fig 12.7 *continued*

(f) Endodontic retreatment was done, conventionally where possible, surgically where necessary. (g) Direct acrylic patterns were made in the mouth, using plastic sprues and Duralay. (h) Upper arch dies (before trimming) were used to fit direct patterns from the mouth onto/into each tooth (left). Copings were waxed over the acrylic to create post-coping patterns. Finish lines on anteriors are left short of the prepared beveled shoulder margins, to avoid showing the gold collars. Posteriors have collars, with finish lines entirely on the metal coping (right). (i) Castings of post-copings (left), were fitted back to the dies (center), and mounted in occlusion (right). The shim used for temporary fabrication also served to verify clearance for final restorations before insertion of post-copings in the mouth.

mesial canals sealed without retreating the apex. Once endodontic retreatment was completed, the task of rebuilding the dentition began.

The upper arch was stabilized first by the fabrication of post/copings on all teeth (coping only on vital no. 6). The post patterns, made directly in the mouth, would provide intracoronal retention, and were carried to stone dies to be waxed up into post/copings (Fig 12.7g).

Fitted to dies of the prepared 'stumps,' copings were waxed onto the post patterns providing some extracoronal retention, a ferrule effect to prevent longitudinal fracture, tight margins and gold gingival collars subgingivally, and cores on which to reconstruct the dentition (Fig 12.7h).

Ten post/copings and one coping were cast, finished, fitted to the dies, and the thin 'shim' again used to verify clearance for crown and bridge fabrication (Fig 12.7i).

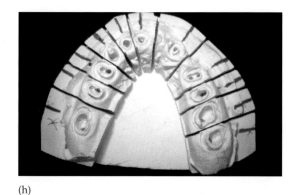
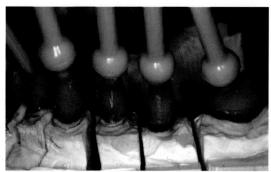

(h)

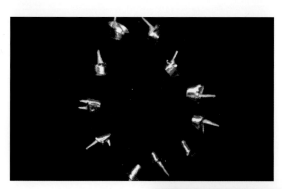
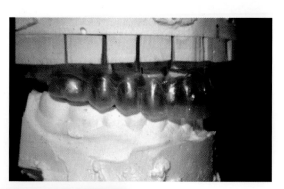

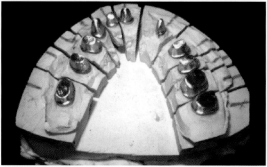

(i)

The coping on no. 10 was constructed with a lingual strut (Fig 12.7j) for reasons that will become clear. Another provisional was fabricated over the new post copings, and we paused to reassess.

The key to the upper arch was that delicate and fragile lateral incisor, no. 10. In the absence of teeth nos 9 and 11, it became critical to preserve no. 10, or else deal with an unacceptably long span from no. 8 to 12. Conceivably, double or triple abutments at each end of the span could support a fixed prosthesis, but having a center pier was the preferable option by far.

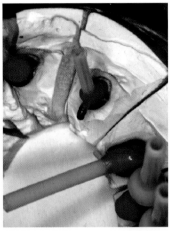

(j)

Fig 12.7 *continued*

(j) A lingual strut was cast on no. 10 post-coping. (k) The temporary was sectioned (left), to allow an orthodontic spring wire to be embedded into numbers 6, 7, 8–9. Provisional on no. 10 is slotted from the lingual to accommodate the strut (right). (l) The spring engaged the strut on no. 10, and was used to extrude the tooth (left), while the provisional remained in service.

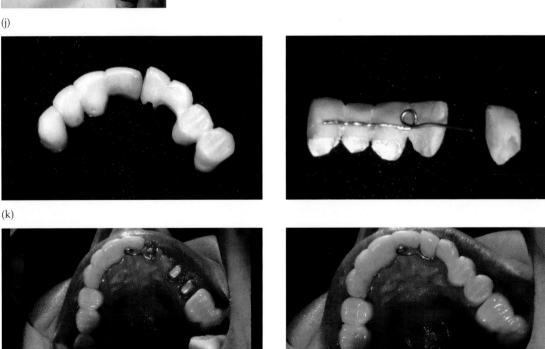

(k)

(l)

Unfortunately the defective bridgework, endodontics, and recurrent caries had left a thin root, barely extending above the alveolar bone. Orthodontic extrusion was necessary to gain enough sound tooth structure out of bone for adequate physiologic width and successful restoration. The temporary prosthesis was split (Fig 12.7k), an orthodontic spring wire embedded into the anterior segment, and no. 10 was extruded over a period of 3 months (Fig 12.7l).

Once no. 10 was in position (Fig 12.7m) reconstruction commenced, using gnathological techniques and principles.

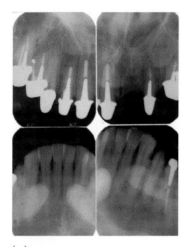

Fig 12.7 *continued*

(m) No. 10 now had adequate physiologic width (root out of bone). (n) Lower posterior quadrants were prepared, and mounted against a model of the upper provisional. (o) After dies were trimmed and prepared with blue spacer, the occlusal of the opposing model was reduced to permit occlusal development in a 'prospective' wax-up.

(m)

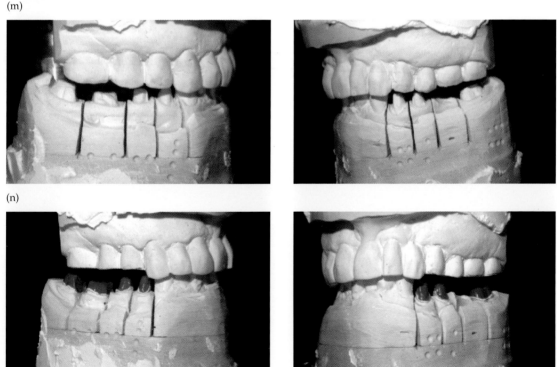

(n)

(o)

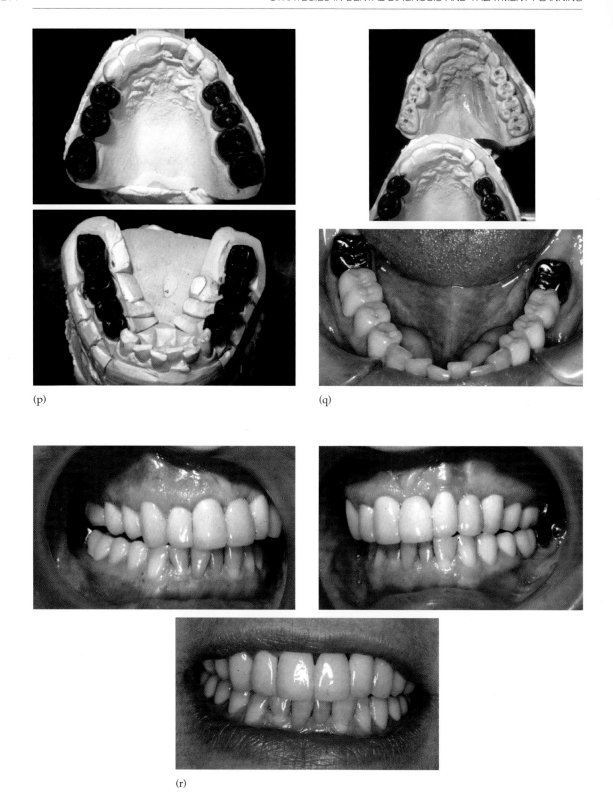

(p)

(q)

(r)

Lower posteriors were completed first, articulating against the upper provisional (Fig 12.7n). The occlusals of the upper were relieved (Fig 12.7o) to permit development of the posterior occlusion by wax-to-wax cone build-up (Fig 12.7p).

The upper wax-up was impressed, and replicated in die stone to provide an opposing model for the lower porcelain-to-gold posterior rehabilitation (Fig 12.7q). The lower crowns and bridge were cemented permanently because confidence was reasonably high, and recovery options, should one or more teeth fail, were fairly simple.

The upper arch was then restored with individual crowns and fixed bridge running from nos 7–8—10—12–13. To maintain flexibility, as there was no way to know which retreated teeth might and which might not survive, all upper units were cemented temporarily for approximately one year. At that time, with all the retreated teeth doing well, the patient swallowed one of the temporarily cemented units (which passed uneventfully), and the decision was made to cement permanently (Fig 12.7r).

EPILOGUE CASE HISTORY 12.7

At 5 years post-treatment, radiographs (Fig 12.7s) show no sign of periapical pathology, and the patient remains functional, comfortable, and esthetically content (Fig 12.7t).

The patient has maintained her reconstruction scrupulously, and regular maintenance

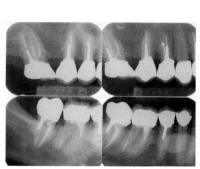
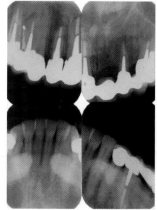
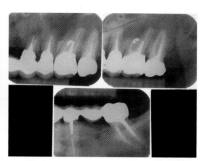

(s)

Fig 12.7 *continued*

(p) Upper prospective wax-up and lower definitive wax-up were done together using a cone build-up technique, as shown in previous cases. (q) Once the wax-up was complete, the upper model was duplicated and poured in die stone (top). The main centric stops are shown marked in red. The lower arch crowns and fixed bridge (bottom) were finished against the upper prospective model, and inserted in the mouth. (r) The completed reconstruction is shown face-on, and in left and right excursions. Anterior group function (with disclusion of posteriors and no balancing contacts) was established. (s) Full mouth radiographs at 5 years were most encouraging. (t) Clinical appearance at 5-year follow-up.

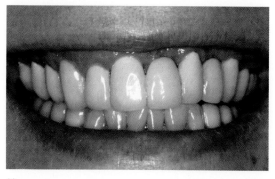

(t)

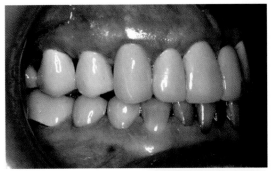
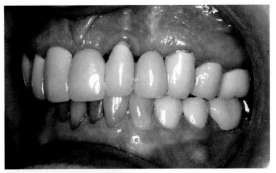

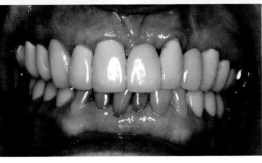

(u)

Fig 12.7 *continued*

(u) At 16 years, minor local recessions are evident, along with natural darkening of lower natural dentition.

follow-ups have been consistently positive. Now, 16 years later, the only findings of significance are local recessions, consistent with the passing of years (Fig 12.7u). At some future date recession in the anterior segments may necessitate replacement prostheses. Overall the prognosis remains good.

IMPLANTS, SIMPLE TO COMPLEX

The development and widespread application of osseo-integrated implants have provided dentists with solutions to many problems that were previously insoluble. It must be understood, however, that any implant application tends to make for 'complex' treatment, as a result of the necessary surgery, time, and cost associated with placing the fixtures, and the greater complexity of restorations or prostheses placed over them. The cases illustrated represent two extremes in the use of implants as a complex treatment strategy.

ILLUSTRATIVE CASE HISTORY 12.8

Implant surgeon: *Dr Brian Blocher*

Concepts illustrated: *use of implants in their most simple form to solve prosthetic problem, cast base upper full denture*

This 53-year-old businessman had worn upper and lower full dentures for at least 25 years. He had functioned reasonably well with them over that time, but had discussed getting into implants with several dentists. Although the proposal for multiple implant fixtures in both arches followed by fixed implant-supported prostheses was presented, the patient was discouraged by the cost, complexity, and time involved. He also questioned his own commitment and ability to perform the daily maintenance such cases demand. His problem list helped shape a more conservative approach:

Patient JN: 53-year-old businessman, in good general health
Chief complaint: long time denture wearer, would like more stable and retentive prostheses, especially the lower
Long-term ridge resorption, especially in the mandible. Conventional dentures not deficient, but not as stable and retentive as desired

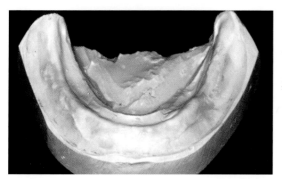

(a)

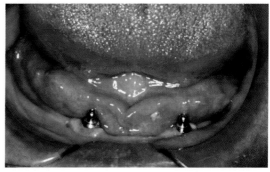

(b)

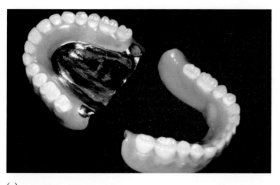

(c)

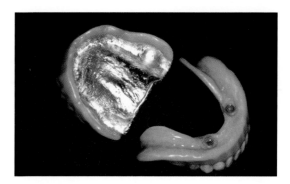

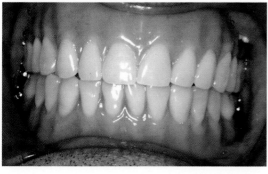

(d)

Fig 12.8

(a) After nearly three decades of full denture wear, the lower ridge was becoming atrophic. (b) Two osseo-integrated implant fixtures fitted with ball caps, to anchor lower full denture. (c) Upper cast chrome base, lower snap-on implant attachment. (d) Improved stability and fit of the upper, with excellent retention in the lower, provided patient with an excellent result.

The treatment option chosen and shown here is the simplest application of implant technology. Two lower anterior fixtures were placed into the atrophic lower ridge (Fig 12.8a) and allowed to 'sleep,' under his existing denture. Soft liner(s) were employed as necessary and new dentures made. Once integration could be assumed, implants were exposed, and simple ball-type fixtures attached (Fig 12.8b). Retentive caps with nylon bushings were then set into his lower denture.

To enhance the result, a new upper denture was made at the same time, using a cast chrome–cobalt base for better fit, stability, and cleanliness (Fig 12.8c). The patient readily accepted this plan which, although costly, was still done at a fraction of the cost proposed for full fixed implant-supported prostheses.

Treatment was carried out over a 6-month period, and the patient was extremely pleased with the result (Fig 12.8d).

ILLUSTRATIVE CASE HISTORY 12.9

Oral surgeon: Dr Phillip Hawkins (primary diagnosis, resection and implants)

Plastic surgeons: Dr Ben van Raalte (hemimandibulectomy), Dr David Larson (vascularized fibular graft)

Prosthodontist: Dr Kenneth J Waliszewski

Concepts illustrated: diagnosis and treatment of malignancy, use of implants in a complex and complicated surgical/prosthetic effort

Waliszewski Case 12.9

This 36-year-old electrician had presented to his physician and subsequently to an ear, nose and throat physician with a complaint of numbness in the lip and chin on the left side. No definitive diagnosis was made, and plane film studies were read as normal. His dentist likewise found nothing significant, but referred him to an oral surgeon concerning his complaint of paresthesia. Although a

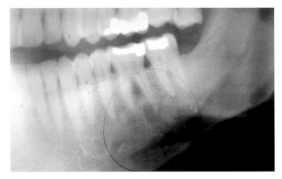

(a)

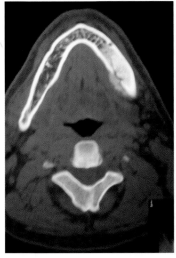

(b)

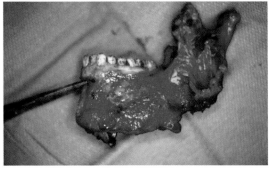

(c)

Fig 12.9

(a) Plane film suggests atypical anatomy inferior to the molars. (b) CT scan, clearly demonstrating osseous lesion. (c) Left hemimandible resected with negative margins.

panoramic film suggested some atypical findings (Fig 12.9a), no definitive diagnosis was made until a CT scan was obtained by the oral surgeon, revealing a radiodense lesion in the left mandibular body (Fig 12.9b). Biopsy, by way of a submandibular transcutaneous approach, confirmed an osteoblastic grade III osteosarcoma. Multiple consultations were obtained, and a combined chemotherapy and surgical approach was undertaken.

Three months after initiation of chemotherapy, a left hemimandibulectomy was performed (Fig 12.9c). Stabilization of the remaining hemimandible was obtained by the placement of a Luhr bone reconstruction plate, running from a prosthetic 'condyle,' serving as a 'provisional mandible,' and attaching to the unaffected side (Fig 12.9d).

After initial healing, and with reasonable confidence that the malignancy was eradicated, a vascular bone graft from the leg (fibula) was performed, retaining the metal prosthetic condyle and ramus (Fig 12.9e). Once healed, the grafted bone was exposed, and six implant fixtures were placed and left to 'sleep' (Fig 12.9f). Palatal autografts were performed to establish keratinized tissue over the implants (in place of mucosa), and a removable

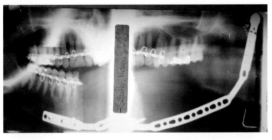

(d)

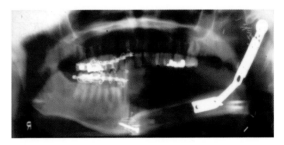

(e)

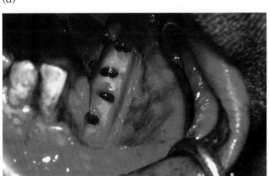

(f)

Fig 12.9 *continued*

(d) Mandibular bar 'analog' stabilizes right hemimandible, providing facial symmetry and mandibular 'continuity.' (e) Vascularized fibular graft serves as 'body' of reconstructed mandible. (f) About one year after the fibular graft, six implant fixtures were placed. (g) Left: Palatal autografts were placed over the sleeping implants to thin the soft tissue over grafted bone, and provide fixed tissue for later implant emergence. Right: Temporary unilateral removable partial denture used in the interim.

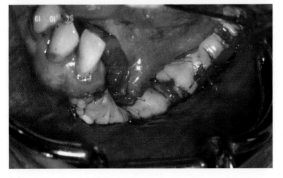

(g)

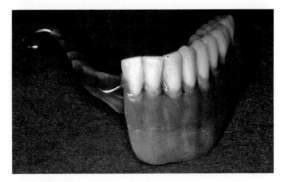

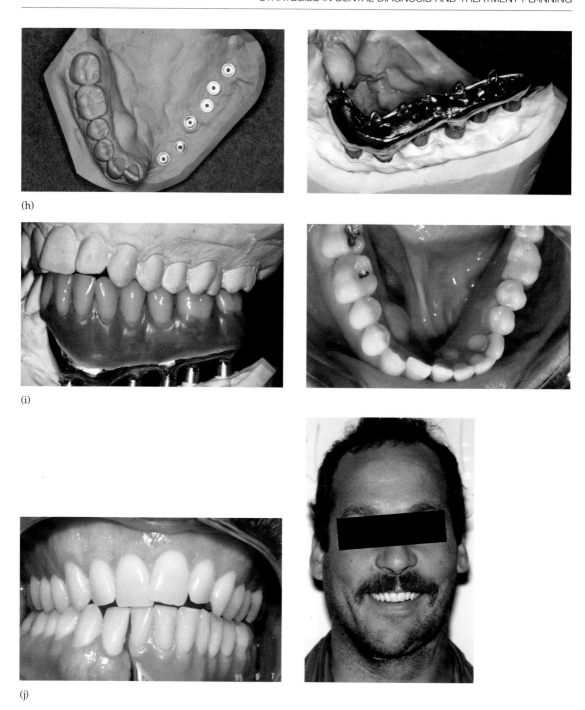

(h)

(i)

(j)

Fig 12.9 *continued*

(h) Implant fixtures (transfer analogs) were uncovered, and a cast gold precision overcasting made, which was retrievable. (i) Teeth and acrylic tissue were added to the overcasting, which was inserted and affixed (using the implant screws) to place. (j) Providing both functional and esthetic support and function, the prosthesis was well tolerated by the patient. The case is now 6 years after diagnosis without recurrence.

partial denture with soft base served as an interim dental prosthesis (Fig 12.9g).

After healing of the grafts, and presumptive osseo-integration, the implants were exposed, and a cast gold framework was fabricated over them (Fig 12.9h). Acrylic tissue and composite resin teeth were processed to the framework, and the fixed implant-supported prosthesis was inserted (Fig 12.9i). Access was preserved to the implant screws should retrieval of the appliance be necessary.

Now 6 years after surgery the patient remains healthy and functions comfortably with his prosthetic mandible and dentition (Fig 12.9j). This challenging and complex approach required careful planning and teamwork among the practitioners involved, and illustrates the far end of the implant spectrum in terms of complexity and risk. For this young patient, however, it provided the nearest thing to full rehabilitation after a life-threatening and, from a dental standpoint, potentially crippling disease.

Success in the treatment of complex cases depends greatly on a well thought-out plan and meticulous execution. There are few short cuts, and dentists who would take on the challenge of such treatment plans must be prepared to devote extra time and effort to them. The risks are greater, and the additional time required often makes for comparatively modest monetary rewards. The satisfaction to be gained from a successful 'save,' and the patients' gratitude and appreciation over the ensuing years are priceless, and make all the extra effort worth while.

PLANNING FOR FAILURE

It can be said that the prudent practitioner always hopes for success but plans for failure. By carefully assessing the factors that influence the prognosis, we can identify possible sources of failure. We may then attempt to build into the treatment plan some 'escape routes,' alternative approaches that can be followed without having to redo everything or start from scratch.

Indeed, there are many clinical situations in which the safest, most predictable treatment is not the most desirable option. It is often possible to opt for high-risk treatment plans, provided that an 'escape route' is established. Patients need to understand the risks of failure fully, and accept the potential time and costs should the 'fall back' plan become necessary.

On the other hand, treatment strategies that anticipate failure give the patient peace of mind knowing that, should a risky investment go bad, all is not lost; we can recover from small disasters if necessary. When successful, high-risk treatment approaches provide optimal comfort, function, and esthetics even if for a limited period of time. When and if some of the components fail, we should be able to implement the alternative approach with a minimum of time, money, and trauma to the patient. This is treatment planning at its most sophisticated. It requires great care and full patient involvement and, if applied judiciously, it is a powerful tool in dental treatment planning.

The examples shown represent a variety of such strategies. Obviously, the hope is that the 'parachutes' will not be needed, and in some cases this will be true. In other cases, however, we know that it is only a matter of time before the anticipation of failure becomes the reality, but many patients appreciate whatever time we can buy them and are understanding when the end comes, because we have shared the strategy with them.

DESIGN FLEXIBILITY IN PROSTHETIC APPLIANCES (ILLUSTRATED CASES)

ILLUSTRATIVE CASES 13.1 AND 13.2: BRIDGE CONVERTIBLE TO CANTILEVER

The most obvious example of anticipatory restoration and planning for failure is the use of a questionable distal abutment tooth for a fixed bridge, which is double abutted in the anterior and designed to convert to a cantilever bridge (Fig 13.1a). The schematic shows a lower second molar ('?') opposed by a questionable upper second molar, and a slightly supererupted upper first molar. If a lower fixed bridge is abutted on both canine and first premolar, and the pontic designed to be readily sectioned (this is critical), then should the distal abutment fail, a cantilever bridge may be created from the anterior portion, which retains the first molar occlusal stop (Fig 13.1b).

It is important when using this strategy to apply all the principles of cantilever bridge design (see Chapter 10) to enhance the prognosis should the conversion become necessary. Figure 13.2(a,b) shows such a case done in 1980. Both distal abutments were questionable, endodontically treated third molars. Figure 13.2(c,d) shows an 18-year follow-up (1998). Both bridges continue to serve, and both remain convertible if necessary.

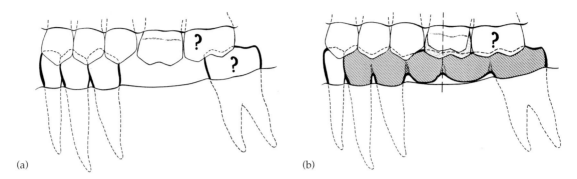

(a)   (b)

Fig 13.1

(a) Planning lower bridge – convertible to cantilever. Distal molar abutment is questionable, periodontally or otherwise. Upper first molar is slightly supererupted, second molar is also questionable. This is a fairly common clinical scenario. (b) Bridge design anticipates cantilever from mesial double abutment, with pontics designed to be sectioned at the appropriate place (vertical line). Note that the upper supererupted first molar has been crowned and shortened, correcting the curve of occlusion. Although this is always a good idea, it would be critical to the success of a cantilever, should the conversion be necessary.

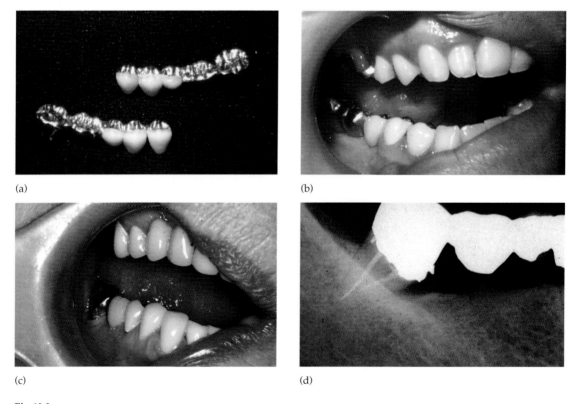

(a)   (b)

(c)   (d)

Fig 13.2

(a) Bilateral convertible to cantilever bridges using questionable distal molar abutments, placed in 1980. (b) Note the anterior prospective cantilever bridge is porcelain veneer, whereas the distal abutment and 'expendable' pontic are all gold. It is difficult to section through a porcelain-fused-to-gold pontic. (c) Eighteen-year follow-up, with bridge still intact. Contralateral side is also still stable and functioning well. (d) Radiograph at 18 years shows tipped and conical, endodontically treated, lower third molar abutment still in service.

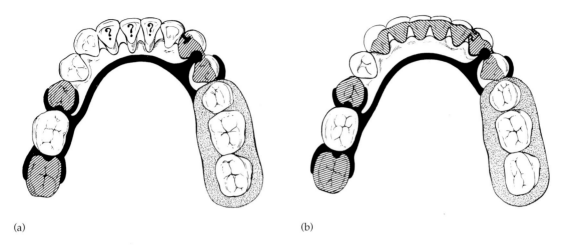

(a)   (b)

Fig 13.3

(a) Schematic of lower partial denture clasped to prepared crowns, including double abutment of nos 27–28. Questionable lower incisors might require an anterior fixed bridge at some future time, so a keyway is incorporated into the mesial of the canine crown, and filled with resin. (b) Questionable incisors have been removed, and lower anterior fixed bridge is placed from canine no. 22, to lateral incisor no. 26, and keying into the pre-planned attachment no. 27. Note: another option here would be to use a lingual plate instead of a bar on the partial, so that denture teeth could be added to replace missing incisors.

ILLUSTRATIVE CASES 13.3 AND 13.4: ANTICIPATORY RESTORATIONS AND ATTACHMENTS

The schematic in Fig 13.3a shows a lower partial denture using cast crown abutments lower left, and splinted canine–first premolar abutment lower right. Note that the canine crown has a mesial attachment set into it (which can be filled with acrylic), in anticipation of the possible need for additional stability should the questionable lower incisors ('?') be lost. That scenario is illustrated in Fig 13.3b, in which the questionable incisors have been removed and replaced with a fixed bridge abutting on nos 22 and 26, with a keyed non-rigid attachment locking into the pre-set cast female in no. 27.

The clinical case is a slight variation on this theme. Figure 13.4a shows a porcelain-to-gold veneer crown placed on no. 22 in 1978, with a distal cast attachment in anticipation of possible replacement of the very old fixed bridge from nos 18–20, cantilevering no. 21. As the patient was almost 70, this conservative approach seemed appropriate.

Within 3 years the old bridge did fail (Fig 13.4b), and was replaced with another, which again used nos 18 and 20 as abutments, but also keyed into the attachment previously placed in no. 22. At 9 years (Fig 13.4c), the quadrant remains sound, and continues so at 19 years (Fig 13.4d). The patient, nearing his 90th birthday, is a gracious and gentle man, pleased to have his own teeth at this point in his life.

ILLUSTRATIVE CASES 13.5 AND 13.6: BRIDGE CONVERTIBLE TO PARTIAL DENTURE ABUTMENT

The schematic diagrams in Fig 13.5 show a bridge using a questionable molar abutment, with the canine having been designed as a partial denture abutment. If the molar fails, the bridge can be sectioned distal to the canine with rests, guide planes, and undercuts already established. The clinical case is a slight variation on this theme. Figure 13.6(a,b) shows a long-time partial denture wearer who

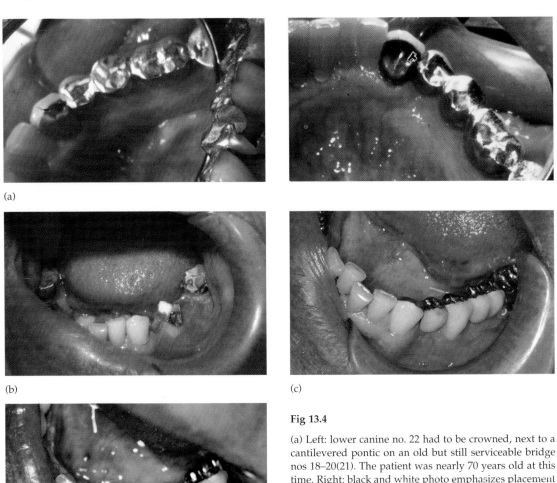

(a)

(b)

(c)

(d)

Fig 13.4

(a) Left: lower canine no. 22 had to be crowned, next to a cantilevered pontic on an old but still serviceable bridge nos 18–20(21). The patient was nearly 70 years old at this time. Right: black and white photo emphasizes placement of the attachment keyway. (b) As luck would have it, the old bridge came loose about 3 years later, and had to be remade. The patient was in good health at age 72. (c) Follow-up at 9 years, patient aged 78, still going strong. (d) Follow up at 19 years, patient aged 89, still going.

was about to lose an upper right first premolar as a result of root fracture, and whose upper right second molar abutment (no. 2) had been endodontically treated and was somewhat compromised periodontally. The patient was seeking a fixed prosthetic alternative, however, and so the sound canine was prepared as a partial denture abutment, with cast keyway, and a fixed bridge was fabricated that used the molar abutment but attached to the canine with a matching key and lingual bracing/retentive arm (Fig 13.6c,d).

The case was completed in 1986, and the patient was thrilled to be rid of her removable partial denture (Fig 13.6e).

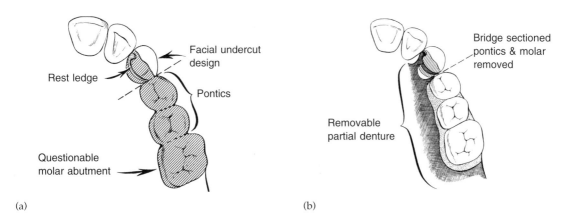

(a)   (b)

Fig 13.5

(a) Planning upper bridge – convertible to partial denture abutment. Distal abutment is questionable, anterior abutment is surveyed and predesigned as partial denture abutment. (b) If molar abutment fails, canine no. 11 is already designed with rest and lingual ledge, distal guide plane, distobuccal retentive undercut.

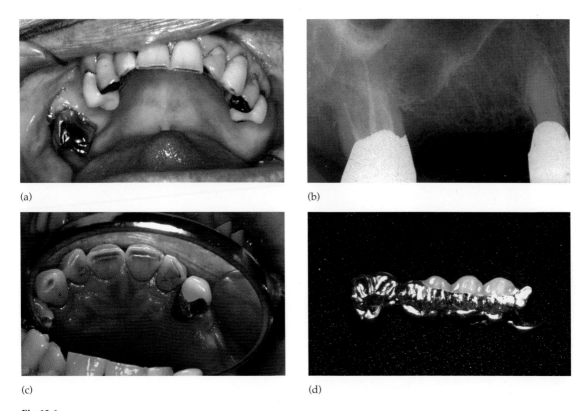

(a)   (b)

(c)   (d)

Fig 13.6

(a) Long-time partial denture wearer, aged 65, about to lose no. 5, interested in fixed option, employing cantilever upper left, fixed bridge from nos 2—6. (b) Questionable upper right second molar no. 2 (endodontically treated, furcation involved). (c) Canine no. 6 restored with distal keyway and lingual ledge. (d) Bridge made abutting questionable no. 2, attached to canine with matching key and lingual bracing/retentive arm.

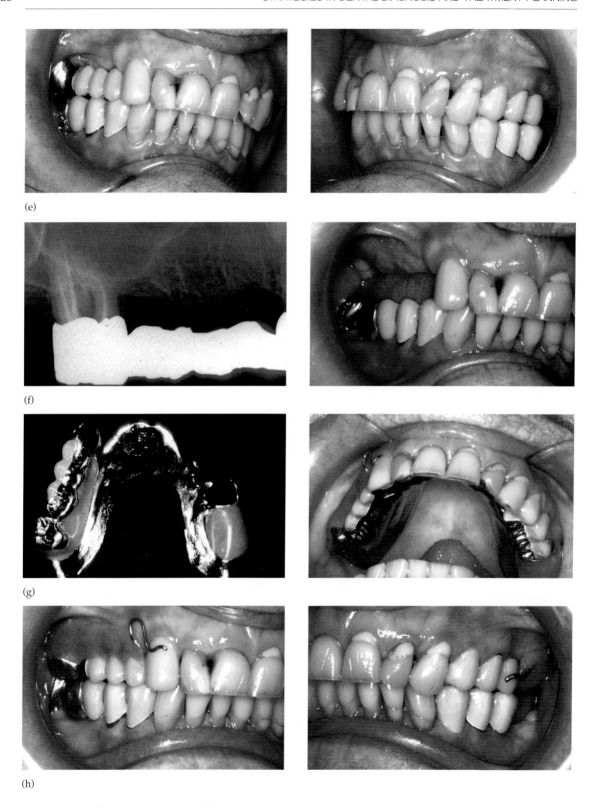

(e)

(f)

(g)

(h)

Fig 13.6 *continued*

(e) Completed case, 1986. (f) Left: 7 years later, 1993, periodontal breakdown threatens no. 2. Right: tooth no. 2 removed, with anterior canine abutment now ready for partial denture. (g) Left: the bridge was cleaned out and 'retrofit' onto the partial denture frame. Right: key and bracing arm fit into canine as before; a wrought wire projection clasp was employed on the buccal. Upper right cantilever bridge had been predesigned for partial denture as well. (h) Five years later, 1998, case is going strong. Patient is now in her late seventies.

Seven years later, in 1993, periodontal breakdown necessitated the removal of no. 2 (Fig 13.6f), and the bridge, with no. 2 removed from its casting, was incorporated into an upper removable partial denture (Fig 13.6g). The key and bracing arm which had fit in and on the canine continued to do so, only now as part of the removable appliance. The last follow-up (1998) shows the upper partial in place, with a wrought wire projection clasp lightly engaging the canine (Fig 13.6h). It should be noted that the upper left fixed cantilever bridge, when placed in 1986, was designed with rest, distal guide plane, and surveyed buccal undercut to accept a partial denture without further modifications.

ILLUSTRATIVE CASE 13.7: TOOTH-BORNE PARTIAL CONVERTIBLE TO DISTAL EXTENSION

Removable partial dentures can be comfortable and functional long-term solutions to tooth loss, but flexibility in design can be an effective strategy in their use. The case illustrated presents six lower anterior teeth, of which the central incisors are somewhat questionable, and two short-rooted lower third molars, tipped at nearly 90° to the anteriors (Fig 13.7a,b). Opposing is an upper full denture, which is comfortable and functional. To obtain an optimum result with flexibility, the 'key' anchor teeth, first premolar and canine on either side, were crowned and splinted. With difficulty, the third molars were prepared for full coverage crowns, designed with flat mesial guide planes, mesial rests, and 'normal' occlusal tables, at approximately 45° to the long axis (Fig 13.7c,d).

A cast gold base lower was fabricated with attachments engaging the anterior splinted abutments, and rests seating into the third molar crowns (Fig 13.7e,f). This strategy allowed maximum use of available teeth, but anticipated the possible future loss of distal abutments.

Now seventeen years into service, the partial denture is still stable and functioning comfortably (Fig 13.7g). Radiographs confirm the viability of all abutments, including the tipped third molars (Fig 13.7h).

Note that the lower central incisors continue to be of concern. As the partial denture base is gold, it will be feasible to add a small lingual plate and facings should either or both centrals be lost in the future. Again, design and fabrication choices have preserved flexibility.

A word of caution is in order. In planning for failure through design flexibility, there are two pitfalls. The first is attempting to preserve teeth or situations that are clearly already failing, and that have little or no chance for even short-term success. Much time and effort may be expended with nothing to show for it. The second pitfall is to be 'too clever by half,' employing overly complex restorative and/or prosthetic schemes which create more problems than they solve. Once again, the general rule of keeping it simple must be observed. We cannot always predict which teeth may fail, or how that failure may come about. I have designed an anterior bridge abutment to anticipate a future partial denture, when the posterior abutment was questionable, only to have the anterior anchor fail, not the posterior. We definitely cannot win them all.

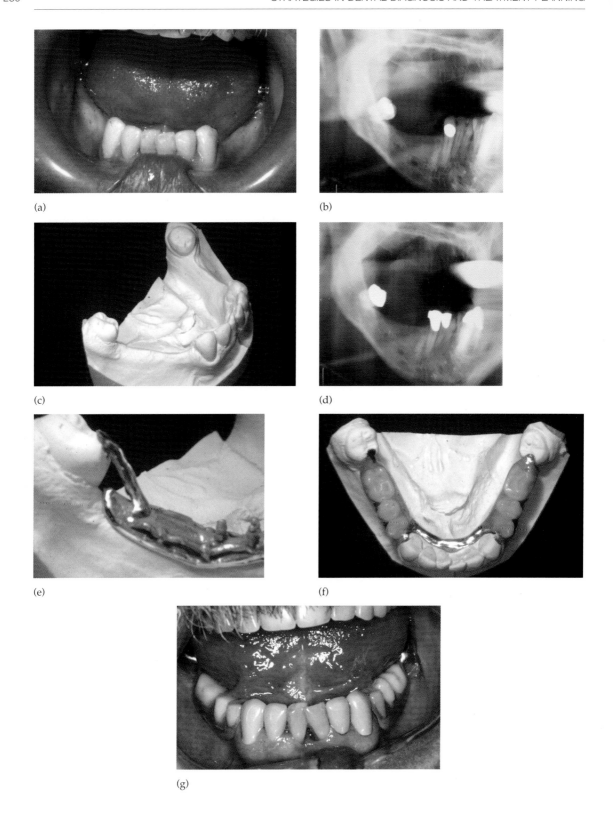

(a)

(b)

(c)

(d)

(e)

(f)

(g)

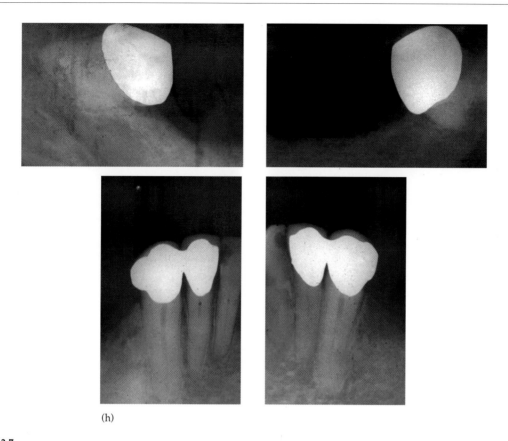

(h)

Fig 13.7

(a) Lower partial denture, with crowned splinted abutments (nos 22–23, 26–27) in the anterior. Semi-precision keyways set into canine crowns. (b) Severely tipped (both mesial and lingual) lower third molars present, but very questionable. Same situation on both sides. (c) Full cast crowns fabricated on lower third molars, correcting occlusal plane. (d) Radiograph shows severity of correction, and double-abutted crowns in anterior. (e) Cast gold base partial frame will have keyway-attached anterior. Posteriorly, cast struts engage mesial rests on third molar crowns. (f) Prosthesis nearly complete, with teeth set in wax. (g) Seventeen-year follow-up, with original partial denture still in service. (h) Radiographs at 17 years confirm viability of all abutments. Design would allow (even now) for loss of one or both distal abutments, followed by modification (not replacement) of partial.

OTHER STRATEGIES IN PLANNING FOR FAILURE

PROVISIONAL SPLINTING OF QUESTIONABLE TEETH

Throughout this book you have seen illustrated the use of acrylic or even cast provisional crowns or bridges for extended periods of time. After periodontal therapy teeth often exhibit marked mobility. Provisional splinting is useful to stabilize such teeth, and periodic removal of the splint allows evaluation of gingival health and mobility. Similar results can be obtained by extracoronal splinting using wire ligatures, or reinforcing fibers with composite resin, but these may create limitations in terms of effective hygiene and ease of removal for evaluation. Interim intracoronal provisional splinting can be done with the use of 'A' splints, cast or twisted-wire arches laid directly into grooves cut mesio-occlusal–distal through posterior biting surfaces. The splint wires are luted into the grooves with composite resin. Again, care must be taken to provide access for plaque removal interproximally.

ideal outcome, looking at the original bone involvement and severe pocketing in 1973, a quarter of a century of comfort and function is not a bad result. You will find many other examples of long-term splinting throughout this book.

LONG-TERM SPLINTING

Long-term splinting of mobile or periodontally compromised teeth has many advantages. Generally, splinting is not indicated for simple post-treatment mobility alone. It is appropriate, however, when periodontal bone loss leaves teeth vulnerable to secondary occlusal traumatism, that is, unable to withstand the normal occlusal forces likely to act upon them. The example shown in Fig 13.8a demonstrates splinting across the midline of two anterior bridges after periodontal surgery. At 5 years the prosthesis remained functional and stable. At 17 years (Fig 13.8b), the case was still holding, despite sporadic lapses in patient maintenance and recall. Now 25 years from the start of treatment, the periodontal disease has regained its hold, and we are in 'transitional' treatment, leading to a full upper denture. Although this is not the

PROVISIONAL CEMENTATION OF FIXED PROSTHESES

Fixed prostheses require a major investment of time, effort, and money and, once they are cemented permanently, they cannot be readily removed intact. When placing fixed bridges over teeth that have been compromised pulpally, periodontally, or mechanically, one assumes a measure of risk should any of the abutment teeth fail. This risk increases with the severity of the original problems, and with the complexity (length, number of units) of the bridge.

We may temper this risk through provisional cementation – that is, by placing the appliance on the teeth with a nonsetting or temporary cement to permit subsequent removal of the bridge. The advantages are obvious, in permitting assessment of abutment

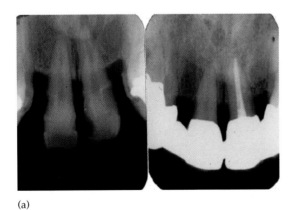

(a)

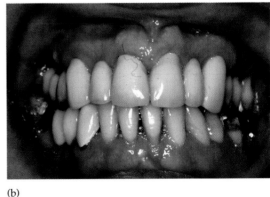

(b)

Fig 13.8

(a) Central incisors are badly involved periodontally (50% bone loss) and, after periodontal surgery and endodontic treatment, they are splinted into anterior bridge canine to canine. Radiograph is at 5 years. (b) At 17 years, anterior splint was still functioning. Now 25 years from initial treatment, many posterior teeth have been removed, and 'transitional' partial dentures are holding, with full dentures contemplated.

teeth over time (their pulpal and/or periodontal status) as well as assessing the form and function of the prosthesis itself. Defective solder joints, porcelain fractures, and unforeseen occlusal or esthetic problems can be rectified fairly easily if the fixed prosthesis can be removed.

Unfortunately, provisional cementation has a number of disadvantages that limit its use. Being removable, it is subject to accidental displacement through mastication of sticky foods, or failure of the cement seal. As cements must be selected carefully to ensure removal (the inability to remove a temporarily cemented prosthesis can be a major problem), loss of cement integrity must be anticipated. Accidental displacement raises the possibility of aspiration, ingestion, loss, or damage of the prosthesis. Cement leakage can lead to pulpal irritation and, over time, caries under the retainer.

Under the best of circumstances provisional cementation requires periodic inspections, removal, and recementation. Although it is a potentially valuable tool in planning for failure, the logistics and risks involved limit the length of time it should be employed. Generally, some target date should be set, whether 3, 6, or 9 months, at which time the prosthesis will be permanently cemented if all signs are positive.

Previous chapters (9 and 12) have included illustrations of complex crown and fixed prostheses which were cemented provisionally for varying lengths of time. The example in Chapter 12 included the use of telescope castings, which bears further comment in regard to provisional cementation.

In telescope castings, abutment teeth are over-prepared to allow a thin cast coping to be permanently cemented, over which the final crown or fixed bridge is then constructed, and often cemented temporarily. This allows longer periods of time between recementation, because there is no risk of pulpal irritation or recurrent caries should cement wash out. Indeed, in some cases the overcasting is not cemented at all, but retained with mechanical methods, or simply frictional fit. In one such case the patient, a dentist, preferred to remove his full arch overcasting bridge each day to clean the eight abutment copings, and access the gingival sulci with a brush.

Advantages of the telescope approach are flexibility, the potential for recovery should an abutment tooth fail, as well as the ability to use nonparallel abutment teeth by correcting the path of insertion with the coping (Fig 13.9).

Disadvantages of the telescope include the rather severe preparations necessary to avoid overcontour of the overcastings. If copings are placed on vital teeth, and the pulp is of normal size, it is often difficult to safely remove enough tooth structure to avoid a 'bulky' final product. Telescopes on endodontically treated teeth, or teeth with receded pulps, are more viable. Accidental or inadvertent loss of the overcasting is a risk if provisional cementation (or no cementation at all) is used. Finally, the significantly higher cost and complexity of telescope systems may render them impractical for many patients.

ENDODONTIC RECOVERY

Any tooth that has endured the rigors of dental disease and/or treatment may be compromised pulpally. Even virgin teeth may have sustained traumatic injury at some past time and, although they are asymptomatic, they may be pulpally compromised. In planning for failure, we must always consider the consequences of pulpal involvement of any given tooth. This is particularly critical when we involve teeth in multiple-abutment fixed prostheses or as removable partial denture abutments. We must consider the likelihood of pulpal problems, the feasibility of endodontic therapy should pulpal problems arise, and the significance of the tooth to the overall treatment plan.

Careful assessment of clinical and radiographic findings may reveal pulpal abnormalities in otherwise asymptomatic teeth. Pulp chambers that are larger or smaller than expected (compared with other teeth in the mouth) or that contain pulp stones should be considered suspect. Discolored teeth and teeth with questionable periapical appearance are also suspect. Electronic pulp testing might

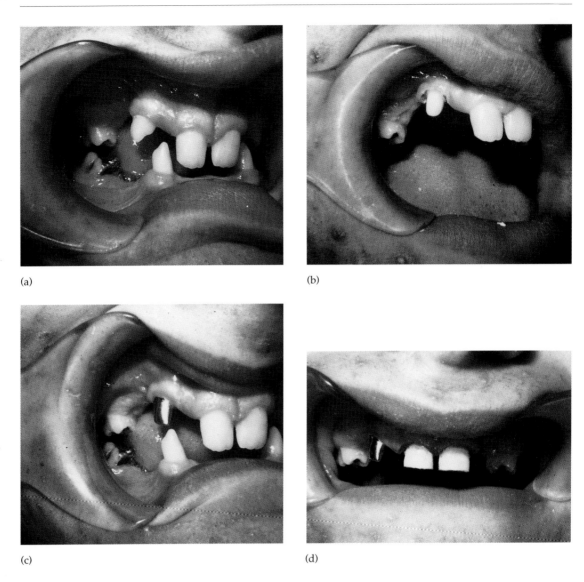

Fig 13.9

(a) Severe partial anodontia (see Chapter 9) had involved pre-prosthetic orthodontics, but no. 6 was left undisturbed, at 45° angle to the plane of occlusion. (b) Tooth is prepared for coping. Note 'shoulder prep,' which finished to collar subgingivally. (c) Coping is waxed to proper alignment, 90° to plane of occlusion, and parallel with other maxillary teeth. (d) Central incisors shortened, gingivoplasty performed; note relatively flat plane of occlusion and parallelism obtained with coping on no. 6.

reveal nonresponsive teeth that are otherwise asymptomatic. Indeed, it is likely that many asymptomatic and functional teeth are compromised pulpally and no one knows it. Even if we recognize a possible abnormality in pulpal appearance or reaction, we may choose simply to watch and reevaluate it periodically. If the tooth in question is not involved in an overall treatment scheme, does not require extensive restoration, and could

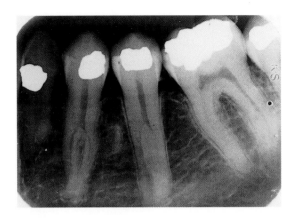

Fig 13.10

Lower first premolar, with deep amalgam restoration. Note the striking root and canal bifurcation of both lower premolars. Endodontic treatment would be a challenge.

the overall situation, a questionable tooth may simply be watched, receive preemptive endodontic treatment, or be extracted.

Finally, a word of caution about failure planning and endodontic recovery. Although root canals can often be performed successfully on teeth with cast restorations, it is not always easy. We must understand that the success rate may not be as high, and the chances of complications are greater. The use of metal rather than porcelain on occlusal and lingual surfaces may greatly facilitate later access to the pulp, as well as subsequent repair and restoration of the opening. Likewise, the prudent clinician will control the thickness of the casting over the occlusal so that, should endodontic access become necessary, one does not face the prospect of boring through 5 or 10 mm of cast alloy!

be treated or even removed and replaced without affecting other restorations and/or appliances, it is often better left alone.

If such teeth are involved directly (for example, abutments) or indirectly (adjacent to bridges or abutment crown) in the overall treatment plan, the feasibility of future endodontic therapy must be considered. A questionable upper incisor with normal pulp chamber and root morphology lends itself to successful conventional endodontic treatment, or to apical surgery if necessary. A questionable lower first premolar with atypical root morphology (Fig 13.10), whose proximity to mandibular and/or mental canals could complicate a surgical approach, is a poorer candidate for root canal therapy, and consideration must be given to preemptive endodontics or strategic extraction.

Pulpal failure of an anteroposterior bridge abutment which also retains a precision-attachment removable partial denture is more significant than if that same tooth were merely an abutment on a three-tooth posterior bridge. Likewise, the pulpal failure of that three-tooth bridge abutment is more significant than that of a single crowned tooth which, if lost, could be readily replaced without affecting other crowns or prostheses in the mouth. Depending on its relationship to

THE ROLE OF THE DENTAL LABORATORY

It is obvious that in any complex treatment plan – especially one attempting to 'plan for failure' – the laboratory procedures involved take on tremendous importance. The best approach is for the restorative dentist to carry out some or all of the key procedures 'in house,' or to employ a technician. When this is not practical, close communication is necessary between the dentist and a commercial laboratory. Not all laboratories are prepared to carry out sophisticated procedures effectively, and care must be taken in choosing the laboratory. Once a laboratory or specific technician is selected, face-to-face discussions about techniques and goals are often helpful, along with detailed written directions, sketches, diagnostic wax-ups, and verbal follow-up.

The dentist cannot do many of these things effectively unless there is a working familiarity with the laboratory procedures involved. The dentist who understands and can do laboratory procedures is a better clinical dentist, for many laboratory procedures can be simplified, or complicated, by the approach, design, and preparation format used. The dentist who attempts to employ sophisticated restorative and prosthetic approaches without an understanding of the attendant laboratory procedures is tempting failure.

COMPROMISE TREATMENT

The most difficult and frustrating problem faced in diagnosis and treatment planning is the need to carry out compromise treatment in the face of inevitable failure. Often, the patient's financial resources will not allow necessary definitive treatment, or else the prognosis is so clouded by a variety of factors that costly and extensive treatment is contraindicated. Total edentulation and full removable prostheses may be an alternative, yet even that approach is not without cost. Furthermore, removal of all teeth may simply not be necessary or justified at the time. The patient may be better served with an incomplete and debilitated natural dentition than with full dentures. The dentist is then left with a dilemma: unable to justify removing the teeth, and unable to replace or restore them properly. The only course available in many cases is patchwork dentistry, the application of add-on and wrap-around silver amalgams, composite resins, and/or various types of shell crowns in an attempt to forestall the inevitable.

When the situation requires it, patchwork is the treatment of choice and needs no apology. Patchwork, however, does not justify sloppiness or negligence. We need not make a bad prognosis worse by failure to remove caries, by improper occlusion, contour, or contact, or by rough, noncleansible margins or surfaces. Good quality patchwork can prolong the useful life of a terminal dentition and postpone total edentulation (Fig 13.11).

Techniques and strategies in this type of treatment are numerous. Their application requires that two criteria be met. First, the cost–benefit ratio must be considered – that is, is the time and money to be invested justified in light of the prognosis? For example, you would not place a massive multi-surface silver amalgam on a periodontally condemned molar that has already had acute periodontal flare-ups. On the other hand, a similarly involved

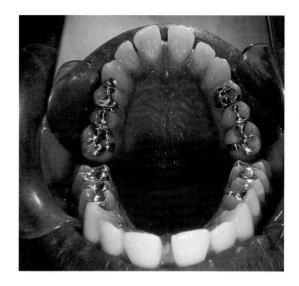

Fig 13.11

Financial limitations did not permit the crowns, onlays, etc, which are clearly indicated on some of these teeth. The silver amalgam 'patchwork' dentistry is a compromise, but quality is maintained.

molar with advanced periodontitis but no history of acute symptoms might provide a number of years of useful service, and the amalgam restoration might be justified. Second, the patient must know, understand, and accept this treatment approach for what it is – a temporary holding action, that is, patchwork.

If these criteria are met, a number of compromise treatment strategies are possible. The following are examples of a few such strategies.

RECOVERY FROM GROSS OVERHANG

Large overhanging margins on silver amalgams often require complete replacement of the restoration. In some cases, a fine needle-shape diamond point can be used to recontour interproximally (a tissue curettage is performed simultaneously) and smoothing can be done with a similarly shaped multiflute finishing bur and/or abrasive strips (Fig 13.12a).

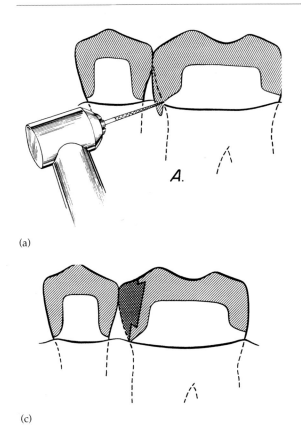

(a)

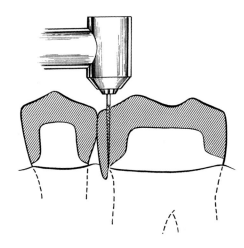

(b)

(c)

Fig 13.12

(a) Schematic of overhang removal, using fine diamond or finishing bur. Infiltration anesthesia is used, because a 'curettage' is unavoidable. (b) Often there is not good access simply to trim the overhang, and a slice approach, removing the entire mesial of the overhanging filling, is a better option. (c) The mesial aspect is restored, locking into the existing filling, eliminating the overhang, and maintaining/restoring good contact.

Difficulty of access sometimes makes this approach impossible, however, and another strategy is to cut away the entire mesial aspect of the overhanging restoration with a slice approach, and then replace just the proximal with silver amalgam, cutting a retentive box into the remaining alloy (Fig 13.12b).

If the existing restoration is large, but otherwise well condensed and contoured, the modification can be done quickly and without anesthetic in most cases (as cutting is primarily done on and in the restorative material). One such recovery is illustrated in Fig 13.13. Chronic gingival inflammation and hypertrophy have been cleared with electrosurgery (Fig 13.13a). The bite wing radiograph reveals the cause (Fig. 13.13b). Using the 'slice' approach illustrated, the overhang was removed, a retentive box cut, and a mesio-occlusal add-on amalgam was condensed,

with matrix band wedged at the gingival surface and burnished at the contact (Fig 13.13c). Five-year follow-up illustrates the continued service of the original amalgam with proper contour and contact established with the 'patch' (Fig 13.13d).

RECOVERY FROM OPEN CONTACT

The same strategy can apply when an existing restoration lacks proximal contact. By slicing to gain access, cutting a proximal box into the existing restoration (amalgam, resin, or even crown), and placing a well-wedged band tightly adapted to the proximal contact area, contact may be restored without removing and replacing the entire restoration, usually without anesthesia (Fig 13.12c).

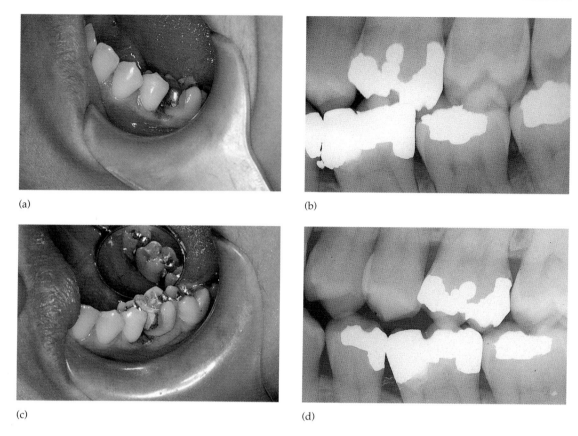

Fig 13.13

(a) After infiltration anesthesia, electrosurgery removes edematous and inflamed tissue mesial to number 19. (b) A large, otherwise acceptable filling has a gross mesial overhang. (c) After mesial 'slice,' retention is cut, for the most part in the old filling, and new filling material restores the mesial aspect of no. 19. (d) Radiograph illustrates the improved contour. Note also that the distal marginal ridge has been reduced to improve that contour as well.

PIN-RETAINED CROWN BUILD-UPS

When there is insufficient tooth structure to hold a restoration, retentive pins may be employed. Since the development of viable bonding agents and the recognition that such pins have some drawbacks, they have become less commonly used. In some cases, however, they remain an effective tool. The cases illustrated show two different approaches. In the first (Fig 13.14a) a vital lower incisor (no. 25) has fractured. The patient was stretched financially to have two abutment crowns and lower removable partial, and was not able to sustain the additional cost for endodontics, post and core, and crown. The decision was made to place pins and a direct composite resin build-up crown, with the 'fall back' option being to remove the tooth and add it to the partial denture.

Note: planning for failure in this case meant using a lingual plate on the partial denture rather than a bar, so that a tooth/facing could be added if necessary.

The case was followed for 5 years, at which time the pin-retained crown build-up was performing satisfactorily (Fig 13.14b).

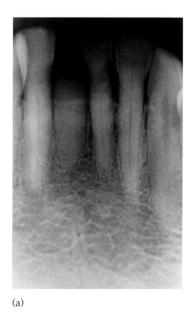

(a)

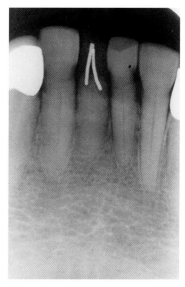

(b)

Fig 13.14

(a) Fragile lower incisor has fractured, without pulp exposure. Self-threading TMS mini-pins were used, along with bonding agent, to retain composite resin crown build-up. (b) Radiograph at 5 years demonstrates both successful pin placement, and reasonably good viability of this compromise treatment.

A related compromise approach is shown in Fig 13.15. In this case, a poorly condensed root canal was failing, as was the short post/composite resin restoring it. The patient had very limited financial resources, yet we did not want to extract the tooth. Instead, the endodontic treatment was redone, and a bonded resin was condensed into the 'post space' and used to form a new and esthetic composite crown (Fig 13.15b). Follow-up at 6 years shows resolution of the apical lesion, and continued integrity of the 'patchwork' restoration (Fig 13.15c).

TRANSITIONAL PROSTHESES

When used appropriately, a wrought wire and acrylic temporary partial denture can provide an esthetic solution, if not a highly functional one, for a terminal dentition. These 'transitional' appliances can permit patients to keep some of their weakened or debilitated natural teeth for many years, and can often be modified upon the loss of one or more teeth, into temporary full dentures.

When moving toward a full removable denture, it is sometimes feasible to retain two or more roots temporarily, amputating at the gumline, performing vital pulpotomy, and placing amalgam seals over the openings. These teeth act as overdenture abutments for an immediate denture, providing improved stability and proprioception to the patient losing his or her teeth. These teeth may be removed after a few months when the denture is to be relined, or if they are reasonably stable, endodontic therapy may be carried out for longer-term use. At worst, they can help make the transition to full dentures easier. Naturally, the patient must appreciate the transitory nature of such treatment.

Compromise treatment can be difficult, frustrating, and less rewarding personally or financially. It is, nevertheless, a service some patients desperately need and deeply appreciate. Applied indiscriminately, sloppily, and without careful communication and patient understanding, it is poor dentistry. Applied selectively and skillfully for an informed patient, it can be a legitimate strategy and a source of pride for the dentist who does it well (Fig 13.16).

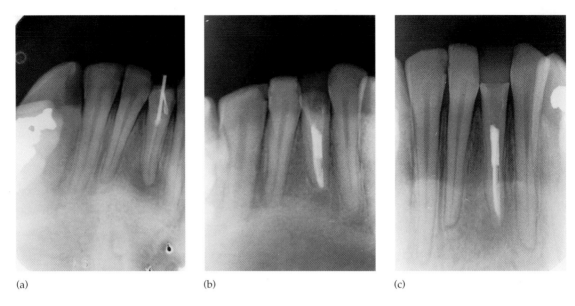

(a)   (b)   (c)

Fig 13.15

(a) Failed endodontic fill and post-retained resin. Finances were limited, but extraction was not a good choice. (b) Endodontic retreatment, followed by solid composite resin core and crown. Patient could not afford definitive restoration at the time. (c) 6-year follow-up demonstrates reasonable viability of compromise treatment.

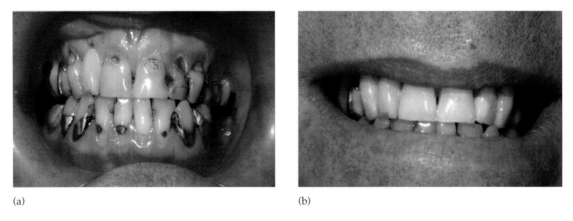

(a)   (b)

Fig 13.16

(a) A lifetime of recurrent caries and failed dental restorations made this patient hesitant to accept definitive (crown and fixed bridge) restoration. (b) Although clearly a compromise from the 'ideal,' in one appointment, bonded composite resins dramatically changed the appearance of this 35-year-old man. Years later, he accepted a more definitive treatment approach.

ESTABLISHING THE PROGNOSIS

The prognosis, our prediction of the likely outcome of dental treatment, is at best an educated guess. There are so many variables, so many factors beyond our ken and control, that we must take great care in giving patients their 'prognosis.' Nevertheless, we are ethically and practically required to give it our best effort, so that patients can make informed decisions, based on as much good information as we can provide.

When presented with treatment options, most patients would like to know the expected useful life of a given course of treatment. We must avoid answers such as 'it will last as long as you take proper care of your teeth,' which, although not a bad answer, may not be true. Dentists may fear that costly and extensive treatment may not be accepted if 'permanence' cannot be assured. Patients deserve (and sometimes demand) a more realistic assessment of their oral and dental future and often accept extensive treatment even if that future is bleak. They do so, however, knowing what the score is, having a reasonable idea of the odds in favor, or against, long-term success.

What kind of information can we provide in predicting the future? We often express the projected life of a restoration or prosthesis in years – a risky business unless we have a crystal ball. It is more prudent to discuss, in general terms, the patient's future dental situation based on factors that we can observe and discuss with the patient.

We must define what we see as the end-point. Taking a silver amalgam restoration on a molar tooth as an example, we can say that such a restoration will provide good function, comfort, and cleansibility, for as long as it lasts. If we have to put a time factor to the treatment, we must ask whether we are predicting the useful life of that restoration, or of the tooth itself. Dental treatment is, after all, a means to an end. The patient must understand that keeping teeth for a lifetime doesn't imply lifetime retention of any given restoration, but that dental treatment, restoration, and prostheses will enhance the overall outlook for the dentition over a lifetime.

If we must predict the useful life of a specific component of treatment, say the silver amalgam just mentioned, we can discuss with the patient the various ways in which the end-point might be reached.

Technical failure, including insufficient retention to cause the filling to fall out in short order, gross open or overhanging margins, or hyperocclusion requiring removal or gross reduction for relief of pain, is the dentist's responsibility, and the end-point is immediate. We would like to assume that a dentist will act with competence and integrity in this regard. Competence implies that treatment meets minimum standards of clinical acceptability; integrity demands that, should the treatment fall short of such standards for any reason, it would be corrected or redone before the treatment is considered complete.

Assuming that minimum standards have been met in placement, early mechanical failure can be an end-point. Breakage of filling material, or of surrounding tooth structure, can happen to anyone. Even healthy un-restored teeth suffer fractures. The patient should be made aware of this possibility, especially if the restoration is large or extensive, putting greater functional strain on the material, and usually implying relatively thin (hence weak) surrounding tooth walls. Indeed, the dentist must apprise the patient when a casting would better restore such a tooth, so that an informed choice based on relative cost and prognosis can be made.

Uncontrolled dental disease will often determine an end-point. Recurrent caries may require another restoration, or severe periodontal disease may result in the loss of the entire tooth. These things are primarily the patient's responsibility, but the dentist must have clearly apprised the patient of the situation, and provided the counseling and mechanical training necessary to control dental disease.

Wearing out after years of comfortable function and service is clearly the most desirable end-point we can envision. We must accept, and the patient must understand, that the delicate, miniature mechanical devices we place in the mouth must withstand tremendous forces and a hostile environment in which continual changes in humidity, huge temperature gradients, bacterial action, and physical stresses never stop. Consider that, in a one-year period, our hypothetical amalgam restoration must withstand well over 1000 mastication sessions (assuming three meals/snacks per day), and around half a million bracing occlusal contacts during swallowing (assuming 1200–2000 swallows per day). Temperature gradients from 0°F (hard ice cream from the freezer) to 180°F (hot coffee) may cycle as our patient has dessert, whereupon any organized plaques will immediately begin producing acids around our margins, measurable within seconds of the ice cream entering the mouth.

When a 10-year-old amalgam restoration breaks, or is to be replaced as a result of a marginal breakdown, surface roughness, corrosion, or wear, we must consider the 11 000 meals and 5 million swallowing contacts it has survived and marvel with that patient at this minor miracle of dental science, rather than explain why their 'permanent' filling must now be replaced. Just when, under ideal conditions, a given restoration or prosthesis is likely to wear out depends on many factors that are discussed here.

Finally, a dental end-point can be reached when a restored deciduous tooth exfoliates, or when the patient dies. Without being macabre, lifetime dentistry is most easily achieved with terminally ill patients. Conversely, young healthy patients must appreciate that they are likely to outlive a succession of dental restorations no matter how well they were done or cared for.

With this background, we can return to the problem of prediction. If, in our discussion with the patient, we hypothetically rule out the end-points caused by incompetence, accident, disease, or death, we can attempt to estimate the time it will take a restoration to wear out, to reach its 'natural' end-point. We may express this as a time, in years, at which we would declare a 'success.' Physicians treating cancer consider 5 years without recurrence to be a 'cure.' It is reasonable, then, to make conservative estimates of the minimum useful life of a restoration with the expectation that its actual tenure may be considerably longer. If, for example, a course of dental treatment is succeeding at 5 years, with

healthy tissues supporting sound dentistry, the prognosis for continued health and function is excellent.

Finally, in establishing a prognosis, it may be neither necessary nor desirable to attach a specific lifespan to the treatment and/or restorations; rather, we should attempt to relate the probable impact of the proposed or completed treatment on the long-term goals established before treatment planning and to rate the likelihood of the treatment serving to achieve those goals. For example, if the long-term goal is retention of all the teeth, a given course of treatment may result in a poor, fair, good, or excellent prognosis for achieving that goal, independent of the useful life of any given component of the treatment. The prognosis must be continually reassessed and updated. Observation over time is the most useful predictive tool, and a dismal prognosis may brighten, or a good prognosis become dismal, as time passes and conditions change.

FACTORS IN THE PROGNOSIS

In establishing a prognosis, many factors must be considered that will enhance or detract from the final outcome. Those pluses and minuses must be considered for each patient, because no two people are alike, and seemingly identical treatment done for seemingly identical problems may present very different prognoses based on individual factors. The following factors are highly significant in establishing the prognosis.

PATIENT BEHAVIOR

This is at once the most significant and least controllable factor in the dental prognosis. The ability and willingness to control plaque and carry out other daily preventive measures determines whether oral health will be maintained, or whether caries and/or periodontal disease will continue unabated. The choice of a healthy and relatively noncariogenic diet is also the patient's responsibility. Home-use fluoride regimens, the proper use and maintenance of dental appliances (for example, night guards, removable partial dentures), and the curtailment of potentially harmful, conscious oral habits are some of the areas that are under sole control of the patient.

The periodic recall visit to the dentist, an essential element in any comprehensive long-term oral health strategy, is also dependent on patient commitment and cooperation. The most sophisticated computer-generated recall system, using both phone and mail reminders, will not ensure every patient's return to the dental office.

It is essential that the dentist engage the patient intellectually from the first day of the relationship and emphasize the patient's vital role in establishing and maintaining oral health. Assuming that the dentist has discharged that responsibility, we may attempt to predict patient behavior based on a number or criteria, including past experience, present behavior, and future commitment.

Past experience

What level of oral health maintenance was being achieved when the patient was first seen? Was the patient brushing regularly and using floss? Did the patient admit high frequency of dietary sugars? Had the patient sought regular preventive care, at least annually, or merely when symptoms arose?

Although we must not prejudge behavior on the basis of past experience, we must realize that some habit patterns are difficult to change, and relapse into old habits is always a possibility. Especially significant is the regularity of preventive maintenance visits. We can reinforce plaque control and good dietary habits only if the patient returns on a regular, periodic basis. Likewise, small problems can be dealt with simply if they are diagnosed in early stages. Simple mechanical maintenance – smoothing a chipped tooth or restoration or adjusting an appliance – is possible on a regular recall regimen and can greatly enhance the prognosis.

A track record of poor oral health maintenance and/or sporadic dental care detracts from the prognosis, whereas a history of daily home care and regular recall visits enhances it.

Present behavior

Behavioral change, although difficult, is not impossible. Often the most satisfying moments in dentistry arise from the realization that, with our assistance, a patient has exchanged oral disease for oral health, making those adjustments in lifestyle that will ensure freedom from major dental problems and greatly enhance the prognosis of any treatment or restoration. If our course of dental treatment is unhurried, we have the opportunity to observe and encourage such new behavior as novelty develops into habit. Such gradual and apparently sustained changes in behavior bode well for the overall prognosis. On the other hand, if the patient is unwilling or unable to achieve effective health maintenance while undergoing dental treatment, the prognosis may be very poor. If the dentist must wipe the plaque away to place a restoration, it is unlikely that the restoration will succeed, and the overall prognosis is very poor.

Future commitment

Assuming that present behavior is at least reasonably effective in maintaining oral health, we must assess the strength of the patient's future commitment. If, for example, a patent has grudgingly accepted plaque control as a prerequisite to the desired dental treatment, the strength of the future commitment might be questionable, and the prognosis guarded. A frank discussion with the patient about the need for periodic recalls may reveal enthusiasm and commitment or apathy and resistance, and the effect on the prognosis can be assessed accordingly.

In our own dedication to oral health for ourselves and our patient we may, in effect, coerce the patient into commitments that he or she cannot or will not keep. Indeed, if we create standards of plaque control, dietary discipline, or frequency of recalls that the patient is not prepared to accept, we may invite failure. Feeling incapable of achieving unrealistic goals, the patient may give up, quit trying, and not return to the dental office.

The commitment must be based on the patient's honest assessment of what he or she feels capable of achieving, even if it is less than ideal. It might be better for a patient to commit to every-other-day flossing and succeed, than to commit to daily flossing, fail, and become discouraged. Annual recall visits, if they are kept by the patient, are preferable to 6-month check-ups if the latter are rejected by the patient and several years elapse before he returns. A sincere commitment to a reasonable recall schedule enhances the prognosis.

Host resistance

Host resistance is the innate resistance to injury or disease, regardless of behavior, that is unique to each individual. Why, in the presence of bacterial plaque, some individuals remain caries free, with little or no gingival inflammation or loss of attachment, we do not fully understand. Why, even with relatively good maintenance, some individuals succumb rapidly to oral disease, deteriorating almost before our very eyes, we are only beginning to fathom. We must, in rationally establishing a prognosis, accept the fact that some patients will survive dentally with or without us, and others will be continually on the brink, despite our best efforts on their behalf. Until research sheds more light on this issue, we can use two clinical indicators of host resistance, each requiring a good history, and each related to the other.

Apparent progress rate of existing disease

If we have the opportunity to observe a patient over a period of years, we can assess the progress rate of oral disease fairly well. For example, the patient who, in 6 months to a year, develops multiple new carious lesions has a much greater rate of disease than someone developing a similar number of lesions, but over a period of 3–5 years. If we follow two periodontally involved patients over time, we might see one whose pocket depths increase, and bone levels decrease, measurably from year to year and another who, although initially presenting with a similar clinical situation, might progress very little in the same time.

Often, however, we do not have the luxury of such continual surveillance and must employ a history to assess the progress rate of existing disease. A patient presenting with numerous caries who reports having had regular dental care (check-ups and treatment) on at least an annual basis shows a greater disease progress rate than someone with similar numbers of lesions, but who has not had dental care for 5 or 10 years. Obviously, the size and extent of lesions as a function of time are also significant.

The net effect of the progress rate is that the prognosis is good for patients whose disease rate is apparently slow, and not as good for those whose disease rate has been rapid. Keep in mind that, although striking changes in oral health and disease are possible with treatment and behavior modification, high rates of disease in the past must be taken into account in establishing the prognosis.

Age vs level of disease

This criterion is similar to the last, but differs in that it dwells less on the rate of existing disease states than on the general progress of oral disease over the patient's lifetime. This criterion has long been employed in assessing periodontal outlook, and used to be called 'bone factor,' the amount of bone loss relative to the patient age. Given a typical case of periodontal disease with 5-7 mm pockets and 10–15% bone loss, the prognosis may be dismal if the patient is 20, poor if the patient is 30, fair if 40, good if 50, excellent if 60, and may not call for treatment at all if the patient is 70 or older! This is because periodontal disease often begins early in adulthood and progresses slowly over long periods of time. Take a patient with 20% horizontal bone loss around first permanent molars at the age of 55. We must, in assessing prognosis, realize that the loss may have occurred over nearly half a century. In general, then, the prognosis is better when a given disease level is seen at older ages (assuming a reasonably healthy patient) and is worse when that same level is reached earlier in life.

This criterion is more applicable to periodontal disease than to caries, but it could be applied to either in some cases. A history is essential, but can be misleading, because periodontal disease may be present for some time and go unnoticed by the patient and undiagnosed by the dentist.

PHYSIOLOGIC ENVIRONMENT

Just as significant to the prognosis as patient behavior and host resistance is the oral environment in which we perform our treatment and place our dentistry. We must consider local biologic factors, mechanical factors, and general systemic factors.

Local biologic factors

These include the patient's musculature, oral habits, and periodontal status.

Heavy, well-developed muscles of mastication and perioral muscles may create a worse prognosis, because they may put greater stresses on the periodontium, and any restoration or prostheses that we may have placed. A normal or delicate musculature may improve the prognosis.

Clenching, grinding (bruxism), or uncontrolled tongue or lip habits worsen the prognosis, whereas the absence of such habits improves it. Indeed, the size and tonus of the oral and perioral musculature are often related to parafunctional muscle activity, such as bruxism. The prognosis may be improved through muscle retraining, protective appliances, and extra strength designed into restorations and prostheses.

After definitive therapy, the resulting periodontal status bears heavily on the overall prognosis. Post-treatment bone level, cleansibility of all sulcular areas, and integrity of the gingival attachment must be considered. A periodontal result that produces reasonably good bone levels, readily cleansible gingival architecture, and intact, keratinized gingivae improves the prognosis, which deteriorates if any or all of these factors are lacking.

Even in the absence of periodontal disease, the nature of the periodontium affects the prognosis. The patient with copious bone support and broad bands of keratinized gingiva will have a more favorable prognosis than one with thin, friable tissues, narrow keratinized gingiva, and prominent roots suggesting delicate alveolar bone.

Mechanical factors

In terms of pure mechanical advantage or disadvantage, we can relate prognosis to the number and position of key teeth in the dental arches (see Chapter 7). Mechanically, an intact dental arch with many key teeth will have a better prognosis than a restored arch with few or no real key teeth. A three-unit fixed bridge with two sound abutments and one pontic is mechanically more stable than a five- or six-unit bridge given the same two abutments.

Occlusal relationships also affect the mechanical factors. A normal healthy class I occlusion may produce fewer mechanical stresses on and restorations than a class II malocclusion with deep anterior overbite.

Obviously, this factor is closely related to the biologic factors just discussed in terms of potential stresses encountered. In addition to the musculature, oral habits, and periodontal status of the patient, we must also consider the great difference in mechanical stress when one arch is edentulous. This is an advantage for the arch with teeth (whether restored or replaced) because less force is generated; at the same time, it is a disadvantage to the edentulous arch as greater forces may be generated on the ridge beneath a full prostheses when it is opposed by natural dentition. The net effect on the prognosis often depends on which arch is edentulous. An upper full denture may do quite well against lower restored dentition, especially if forces are evenly distributed. Lower natural anterior teeth lacking good posterior support and opposing upper full denture can destroy the anterior segment of an upper edentulous ridge. A lower fully edentulous ridge is nearly always at risk when opposed by upper natural dentition.

Whatever the scenario, greater mechanical stresses on teeth, soft tissues, restorations, and protheses generally cloud the prognosis, whereas a mechanical environment that is harmonious and non-stressful enhances it.

Systemic factors

The general systemic health and well-being of the patient influence the oral environment and, thereby, the prognosis of dental treatment.

A healthy, well-adjusted individual has a better dental outlook than a debilitated, neurotic one. Systemic diseases and disorders are often reflected in the oral cavity by decreased resistance to disease, impaired healing, and lessened ability to maintain a plaque-free mouth. Problems such as diabetes, thyroid disorders, rheumatoid arthritis, Parkinson's disease, and various malignancies are but a few of the systemic problems that cloud the prognosis. Tobacco use clearly worsens it. Any disease state that impairs or decreases salivary flow is detrimental to long-term outlook, and nearly all oral medications can produce, or contribute to, a dry mouth.

On the other hand, a patient who has a history of general good health, or of rapid and full recovery from past diseases, presents a better dental prognosis.

QUALITY OF TREATMENT

Obviously, the quality of treatment rendered bears heavily on the prognosis and should be considered in two categories: the type and level of treatment selected, and the care, skill, and judgment brought to its execution.

Selected treatment approach

The prognosis is often directly related to the quality of the selected treatment approach. The prognosis for a course of operative dentistry is better if cast gold or other durable restorations are employed, and is less favorable if large silver amalgams are placed instead. Quality and durability of materials play an important role in prognosis. High-temperature glazed dental porcelains will generally outlast acrylic or composite, cast onlays will generally outperform amalgams or resins, and cast gold crowns will generally outlast stainless steel shell crowns.

However, there may be some situation in which the 'quality' treatment has a poorer prognosis than a less costly alternative. A continuous, full arch fixed bridge connecting 5 or 6 periodontally weakened teeth is a risky procedure, and the prognosis would probably be better (in terms of long-term viability) with a full denture or overdenture.

The patient and dentist select a treatment approach that satisfies certain criteria (cost, esthetics, comfort, function, longevity) but may sacrifice others. The selection of a course of treatment based on the patient's goals, felt needs, finances, and lifestyle will influence the prognosis both in terms of the useful life of the restorations and prostheses employed, and in the overall long-term retention of teeth.

Level of execution

The care, skill, and judgment applied in rendering dental treatment will vary greatly among different dentists and, at any given time and situation, will vary for the same dentist. Many factors influence the dentist's level of execution. Obviously no two dentists possess the same native ability or the same standards of excellence, quality of judgment, or concern for the patient's well-being. Training varies greatly among schools of dentistry, and commitment to and participation in advanced and continuing education vary even more.

Clinical results will vary among dentists, and the prognosis will depend on the quality of those results. Day-to-day variations must be expected for every dentist. Assuming that every dentist has his or her peak performance level, that performance can be compromised by fatigue (last patient in a long day), emotional distress (marital or family crises), physical discomfort (prodromal symptoms of the 'flu, incipient diarrhea), or any number of other impairments that, although not enough to prevent us from treating patients, may degrade the quality of that treatment, however slightly, and the prognosis as well.

Working conditions also greatly affect execution, especially those inherent to a given patient. A willing and cooperative patient with a 'wide' mouth presents an easier task than a resistant (consciously or not) patient with small mouth, large tongue, and quick gag reflex. The finest dentist may struggle to perform at a minimal level of quality in such an environment.

The net effect of all these variables is an execution level that may range from barely acceptable to undeniably excellent, and the prognosis will reflect that level. The dentist's critical self-assessment is essential in establishing a prognosis, as is an objective and non-judgmental evaluation of the patient's treatability.

IN CONCLUSION

The prognostic factors discussed here are not necessarily the only ones bearing on the outcome of dental treatment, nor should each factor be given equal or consistent weight when assessing its long-term effects. A single negative factor might result in failure of an entire treatment effort, and long-term success is often achievable even in the face of multiple negative factors. Assessing the factors is still critical, both in establishing the prognosis for and with the patient, and in identifying potential threats to the treatment plan. Anticipation of future problems allows us to plan for them, thereby enhancing the overall prognosis.

APPENDIX
RECORD KEEPING

The dental record is the primary tool for the documentation, organization, and delivery of dental care. It is also a legal document, protecting both dentist and patient relative to the process and outcome of care. Finally, it is an effective tool for quality assessment. This brief appendix addresses key elements of dental record keeping, and presents some examples of dental record systems.

The process of examination, diagnosis, and treatment planning as described in this text is useless without the development of an accurate and complete written record. This written record enables the dentist to review the collected data at leisure, so all findings are readily recalled. Certainly all frank pathologic findings must be considered in the diagnosis and treatment plan. Seemingly isolated pathologies may often be related, and that relationship is often not obvious until the record is compiled and reviewed. Even seemingly innocuous and unrelated findings may, when viewed as part of the overall picture, fit into an overall pattern of disease or dysfunction.

The diagnosis or diagnoses made from the findings must be documented to facilitate the development of an appropriate plan of treatment. That treatment plan must then be put in writing, in sequence, with appropriate codes and/or fees to facilitate presentation to the patient, and the orderly execution of the plan over time.

Lastly, all treatment rendered must be documented, along with any complications, changes in treatment plan, or further diagnostic discoveries. This continuing chronicle of patient care serves to inform future diagnosis and treatment. Memory will not serve these purposes; documentation is essential.

The dental record is also a legal document. The dentist/patient relationship is a contract, whether written or not, and the dental record is of prime importance should any questions arise as to the nature of that contract. When a third party looks at dental records that are complete, comprehensive, and well organized, a presumption of competence is hard to avoid. Conversely, sloppy or incomplete records suggest similar levels of care, whether true or not. It is important to note here that the standard for dental record keeping does not derive from statutes or courtrooms, but from our own profession. Records that meet the standard as tools for the organization and delivery of dental care generally meet, by definition, any 'legal' standard. Creating voluminous and sometimes irrelevant documents as a defense against potential lawsuits is silly, and may even be counterproductive.

Although we often think of the legal aspects of dental records primarily in terms of defense against malpractice litigation, records are also of legal significance in other types of situations, including the collection of fees, tax issues (for both patient and dentist), and, forensically, in the positive identification of deceased persons.

Finally, quality assessment schemes often rely on dental record reviews as an efficient and non-intrusive mechanism to evaluate care. An audit of a representative sample of active patient files can provide a good picture of what level of care is being performed, how it is organized and delivered, and, of course, how well it is being documented.

CRITERIA FOR ALL DENTAL RECORDS

There are three general criteria for all dental records.

ACCURACY

The need for accuracy in any medical or dental record is self-evident. For example, if the wrong tooth is marked for extraction, the results can be disastrous. Such details as the spelling of a patient's name or having a correct current address can prevent gross errors and/or embarrassment. Inaccuracies or omissions in the record tend to cast doubt on the entire record and on the integrity of the treatment.

LEGIBILITY

To be of use, the record must be readable, not only by the dentist, but by anyone who might need the information in the record – an auxiliary, another dentist, or even an attorney. To that end, record entries should be made neatly in ink (unless visual charting entails colored pencil, etc.) and the record protected against soil, water spots, and the like.

COMPREHENSIVENESS

The question of how much information needs be recorded and at what depth of detail is of prime importance. We see extremes in dental records from the grossly inadequate (the old 'recipe card'), to the overblown (voluminous charts with so much information that they become too cumbersome to use). Although better to err on the side of completeness, a reasonable minimum is a good compromise.

Figure A.1 shows an example of an inadequate dental record.

ESSENTIAL COMPONENTS OF A RECORD SYSTEM

Any record system devised or adopted must strike a happy medium. It should facilitate clear and concise recording of all essential information and allow for greater depth and detail where necessary. It should be geared to the practitioner using it, the type of practice, and the routine systematic approach being employed. Any record system must have

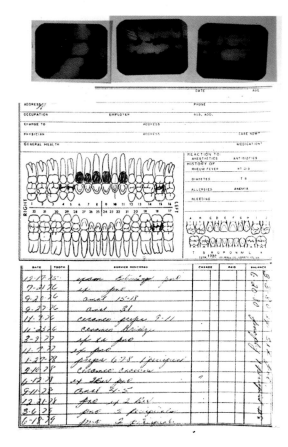

Fig A.1

Example of an inadequate dental record. This note card, along with the radiographs shown, represents the total clinical record documenting nearly 5 years of general dentistry. It was produced in the course of a lawsuit alleging failure to diagnose and/or treat periodontal disease. It is, of course, a grossly inadequate record, although it may accurately reflect the level of care rendered, which was also grossly inadequate. Although such records are becoming rare, many dental records still fail to reach a minimum standard of care. The guidelines and recommendations in this Appendix are aimed at meeting or exceeding that standard as it stands today, at the 'turn of the century'.

certain essential elements, however, and they include the following:

• Business information, including patient's name, address, and phone number; party responsible for the account, and so on. It is obvious that the dentist must know who he is treating and record that information.

- Patient histories, both medical and dental, including chief complaint.
- Record of soft tissue examination, findings of the head/neck and intraoral soft tissue examination.
- Record of periodontal examination, including a provision for the charting of periodontal pockets, and a written periodontal diagnosis. The patient's oral hygiene status, both at the outset of care and ongoing, must be part of the record as well.
- Dental chart, whether pictorial or numerical, including charting of existing conditions, restorations, missing teeth, clinical and radiographic pathologic findings, and restorations placed or treatment rendered.
- Record of functional evaluation, including occlusion, temporomandibular joint, and myofunctional findings.
- Diagnostic summary, either drawn as a formal 'problem list', or evidenced within the various component parts of the diagnostic data chart.
- A written treatment plan, including approximate fees, date presented to patient, patient's acceptance or rejection, modifications, or changes made during the course of treatment.
- Dental radiographs, mounted with patient's name and date the radiograph was taken.
- Treatment record (progress notes), including an accurate summary of all treatment rendered, procedures performed, prescriptions written, fees charged, and communication with the patient regarding same, dated and signed or initialed by the responsible party – dentist, hygienist, chairside assistant, etc. Progress notes should, of course, be legible and consistent in format.
- Other material obtained or generated at the discretion of the dentist which may be pertinent to a given patient. A wide variety of 'special records' addressing everything from daily diet to nocturnal bruxing may be employed. Study casts may become part of the patient's record (although generally not stored in the same location), if they are better evidence of critical findings than the written record. In many cases such models are reasonably discarded, along with impressions, bite records, and the like, once treatment is done.
- Correspondence to, from, and about the patient (specialty referral letters, etc.) should be maintained in the dental record system.

It is obvious that there is no limit to the depth of detail possible in compiling such a record. The three progress notes shown here all describe the same procedure, and range from a paucity to a wealth of information, yet even the most detailed is still concise. Figure A.2 shows three versions of the same progress note.

9-21	L6 O/A	$45
9-21-95	#3 O/A, BASE, ANES. BUR NICKED RT. BUCCAL	
	MUCOSA – PT. INFORMED AND ADVISED. RBM	$45
9-21-95	#3 OCCLUSAL CARIES, CaOH BASE, AMALGAM	
	RESTORATION. GAVE XYLOCAINE c̄ 1:100,000	
	EPINEPHRINE VIA INFILTRATION. BUR NICKED	
	RT. BUCCAL MUCOSA WHEN PT. MOVED	
	SUDDENLY. INFORMED PT. OF SAME AND	
	RECOMMENDED SALINE RINSES IF	
	UNCOMFORTABLE. RB MORRIS DDS	$45
	NEXT APPT: ANTERIOR OPERATIVE	

Fig A.2

Three versions of the same progress note. The first entry is inadequate: the date fails to include the year, and no mention is made of base material or anesthetic. One cannot deduce that there was a complication during the procedure (noted in the other two entries). The record does not provide sufficient detail to be an effective tool. The third entry is clearly sufficient for effective management and care. It gives a diagnosis of the problem being treated, describes the treatment performed and the complication that arose, and even includes a reminder of treatment planned for the next appointment. The second entry, although considerably briefer, is adequate if certain conditions are met. Specifically, it may be assumed that the occlusal restoration implies a diagnosis of occlusal caries. 'Base' may be sufficient information if the same base material is used in all or nearly all of that dentist's procedures. Likewise 'Anes' may be sufficient if the same local anesthetic agent is used exclusively. If two agents are used, one without vasoconstrictor, then 'Anes' or 'Anes w/o epi' could be used. The complication is described adequately, provided that the dentist routinely informs patients of such complications and offers consistent advice on how the patient may deal with them. Should medicolegal questions arise, however, it may be necessary to obtain testimony from a third partly (chairside or other auxiliary) that such information and instruction were indeed routine practice. An office manual outlining instructions to be given to patients might also be helpful in supporting a sketchy dental record.

At the time the record is being made, economy of time and space may seem of prime importance; indeed, a brief and concise record has much to recommend it. Should later developments of a dental (pain or sensitivity in the restored tooth) or legal nature (parotid swelling thought to be precipitated by the bur nick incident) require thorough recall of the procedure, it is better to have a more detailed record. Years after a routine procedure is performed, memory alone will not serve. A complete and comprehensive dental record is an essential tool not only in diagnosis and treatment planning, but in the practice of dentistry in general.

SELECTING A RECORD SYSTEM

Many commercially available record systems are used in dentistry, and the practitioner may select a system, modify it according to individual needs, or even develop a totally customized record in this age of ubiquitous desktop publishing. Issues to address in selecting or creating a system include the following:

- Does the record system provide for all the essential components of a complete dental record? If there is no specific place on the chart to record certain findings, they may be overlooked.
- Do all the component areas provide sufficient depth and detail? A medical history that simply asks 'are you in good health?' will be inadequate unless accompanied by a more exhaustive oral history, which must then be written into the record.
- Is the system logical in its layout and sequence? Whatever routine sequence is used by the dentist ought to be reflected in the chart system, so information can be recorded easily in the order in which it is obtained.
- Is the system appropriate to the practice? A pedodontist does not need questionnaires about past denture experience,

nor is a prosthodontist likely to require much in the way of thumbsucking history.
- Is there a significant amount of irrelevant or extraneous material in the chart? If large sections of a chart system seem unnecessary, then time will be wasted in gathering and recording trivial information, or patients will be unhappy to find that, after completing lengthy forms, their responses are ignored. Furthermore, some sections of a complicated and overly detailed chart system may be left blank, giving the impression of an incomplete job.

Records are tools. It is important to select the correct tool for the task at hand. Good systems can be assembled from commercial sources, or modified to individual taste. Many dentists prefer to develop and produce their own personal system, which in this age of computer-assisted 'desktop' publishing is easy, and quite affordable. There are many sources of expert help in this area, particularly if you have computer-literate children. The sample chart systems shown here represent two ends of the spectrum.

The first example (Fig A.3) is a complete system, marketed by the Wisconsin Dental Association, and reproduced here with their permission. Used in its totality, it is quite detailed, but it may be modified simply by deleting or changing any of its components. It is a good example of an 'off the shelf' record system, ready to go.

The second example (Fig A.4) is a completely customized system, the components of which were designed to follow the routine systematic approach described in this text, and to keep pages and forms to a minimum. All the diagnostic data can be documented on one page, and additional 'special' records can be added and inserted.

This system, or any system, can be augmented with 'special' records pertinent to certain patients or conditions (Fig A.5). Such forms can be 'off the shelf', or custom made. Custom charts and forms have the advantage of flexibility: they are easily modified or updated.

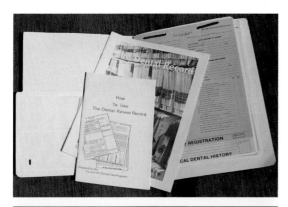

Fig A.3.1

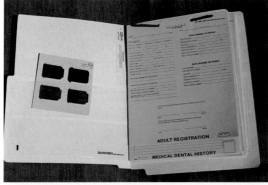

Fig A.3.2

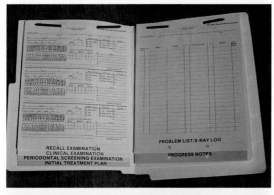

Fig A.3.3

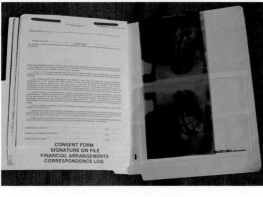

Fig A.3.4

Fig A.3

Example of a commercially available record system. This record system (Fig A.3.1) was developed by and for dentists and is marketed commercially by the Wisconsin Dental Association. It is in a divided folder format, with each section containing elements which are clipped into place. The first section (Fig A.3.2) has demographic and business information, medical and dental histories, and a pocket for current radiographs. The second section (Fig A.3.3) has clinical examination records, problem list, and progress notes. The third section (Fig A.3.4) has consent and signature forms, financial arrangements, and another pocket for 'old' radiographs, correspondence, prescription copies, laboratory forms, etc. The record is complete and nicely organized, but somewhat lengthy. It is flexible, in that the component pieces can be mixed and matched, and custom forms substituted or incorporated as needed. For illustration, some of the system's components include:

PATIENT NUMBER

© 1985 Wisconsin Dental Association

PATIENT'S NAME _____
Last   First   Initial

Date _____ Date of Birth _____

PARENT'S NAME _____

DENTAL INSURANCE 1ST COVERAGE

RESIDENCE - STREET _____

EMPLOYEE NAME _____

CITY _____ STATE _____ ZIP _____

EMPLOYEE DATE OF BIRTH _____

BUSINESS ADDRESS _____

EMPLOYER _____ #YRS. _____

TELEPHONE: RESIDENCE _____ BUSINESS _____

NAME OF INSURANCE CO. _____

PARENT EMPLOYED BY _____

PROGRAM OR POLICY # _____

PRESENT POSITION _____ HOW LONG HELD _____

UNION LOCAL OR GROUP _____

SPOUSE EMPLOYED BY _____

SOCIAL SECURITY NUMBER _____

PRESENT POSITION _____ HOW LONG HELD _____

DENTAL INSURANCE 2ND COVERAGE

WHO WILL PAY THIS ACCOUNT _____

EMPLOYEE NAME _____

PURPOSE OF CALL _____

EMPLOYEE DATE OF BIRTH _____

OTHER FAMILY MEMBERS IN THIS PRACTICE _____

EMPLOYER _____ #YRS. _____

_____

NAME OF INSURANCE CO. _____

PROGRAM OR POLICY # _____

WHOM MAY WE THANK FOR THIS REFERRAL _____

UNION LOCAL OR GROUP _____

_____

SOCIAL SECURITY NUMBER _____

SOMEONE TO NOTIFY IN CASE OF EMERGENCY
NOT LIVING WITH YOU _____

DENTAL HISTORY	YES	NO
Is this the child's first visit to a dentist _____	__	__
If not, how long since his last visit to the dentist _____	__	__
Does child eat between meals _____	__	__
Does child eat sweets, such as candy _____	__	__
soda pop, chewing gum _____	__	__
Does child eat a well balanced diet _____	__	__
Does child brush teeth upon arising _____	__	__
when going to bed _____	__	__
right after eating meals _____	__	__
after eating any food _____	__	__
Do you have fluoridated water in the home _____	__	__
Have teeth been treated with fluorides _____	__	__
Have any cavities been noted in the past _____	__	__
Were any teeth (baby or permanent) removed _____	__	__
by extraction _____	__	__
Was it suggested that the space be maintained _____	__	__
Was appliance placed _____	__	__
Have there been any injuries to teeth —		
falls, blows, chips, etc. _____	__	__
Has child had any unfavorable dental experience _____	__	__
How many children in your family _____		__
Has child been recommended for othodontics _____	__	__
Has child received a local anesthetic _____	__	__

MEDICAL HISTORY	YES	NO
Is child now in good health _____	__	__
Is child under care of physician _____	__	__
If yes, why _____		
_____		
Name of physician _____		
Has child had surgery _____	__	__
Is surgery contemplated _____	__	__
Is child subject to heavy bleeding _____	__	__
Is child subject to nervous disorders _____	__	__
fainting _____	__	__
dizziness _____	__	__
Is child allergic to penicillin _____	__	__
or other drugs, anesthetics _____	__	__
Is child receiving any medication _____	__	__
Has child had history of diabetes _____	__	__
*hemophilia _____	__	__
*heart trouble _____	__	__
asthma _____	__	__
kidney infection _____	__	__
*rheumatic fever _____	__	__
toothache _____	__	__

Parent's signature _____

CHILD REGISTRATION

MED. ALERT

Fig A.3.5

Child registration: includes a medical and dental history tailored to the pediatric patient.

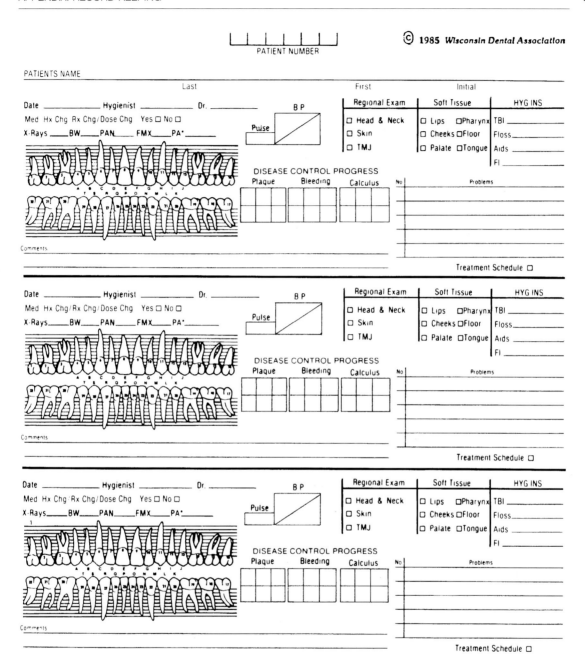

RECALL EXAMINATION

Fig A.3.6

Recall examination form: a brief charting is repeated and recorded at each recall visit. Another strategy is to 'update' previous charting, noting changes, and placing date and initials at each new recall.

PATIENT NUMBER

PATIENTS NAME
_____

Last   First   Initial

I hereby authorize _____
DOCTOR'S NAME

and whomever he/she may designate as his/her assistants, to perform upon me the following operation and/or procedures:

and if any unforeseen condition arises in the course of these designated operations and/or procedures calling, in their judgment, for procedures in addition to or different from those now contemplated, I further request and authorize him/her to do whatever he/she deems advisable.

I consent to the above treatment plan after having been advised of the alternate plans of treatment available, the known material risks of the treatment to be used and the consequences if this treatment were withheld.

I am informed and fully understand that inherent in any type of surgery are certain unavoidable complications. In oral surgery, the most common of these complications include post-operative bleeding, swelling or bruising, discomfort, stiff jaws, loss or loosening of dental restorations. Less common complications can include infection, loss or injury to adjacent teeth and soft tissues, nerve disturbances (e.g., numbness in mouth and lip tissues), jaw fractures, sinus exposure and swallowing or aspiration of teeth and restorations, and small root fragments remaining in the jaw which might require extensive surgery for removal.

I further consent to the administration of local or general anesthesia, antibiotics, analgesics or any other drugs that may be deemed necessary in my case, and understand that there is a slight element of risk inherent in the administration of any drug or anesthesia. This risk includes adverse drug response (e.g., allergic reactions), cardiac arrest, and aspiration; and thrombophlebitis (e.g., irritation and swelling of a vein), pain, discoloration and injury to blood vessels and nerves which may be caused by injections of any medications or drugs.

A more complete explanation of all complications of surgery and anesthesia is available to me upon my request from the Doctor.

I realize that in spite of the possible complications, my contemplated surgery/treatment is necessary and desired by me. I am aware that the practice of dentistry and surgery is not an exact science and I acknowledge that no guarantees have been made to me concerning the results of the operation or procedure.

I realize that it is mandatory that I give as accurate and complete medical and personal history as possible, follow any and all instructions as directed and permit prescribed diagnostic procedures.

_____   _____
SIGNATURE OF PATIENT   DATE

_____   _____
SIGNATURE OF PARENT OR GUARDIAN   DATE

_____   _____
SIGNATURE OF WITNESS   DATE

CONSENT FORM

Fig A.3.7

Consent form: a good attempt at a 'blanket' consent; a simpler statement may be preferable.

⌐ ⌐ ⌐ ⌐ ⌐

PATIENT NUMBER

© **1985 Wisconsin Dental Association**

PATIENTS NAME _____

Last   First   Initial

I _____ have had my treatment plan and options explained to me and hereby

authorize this treatment to be performed by Dr. _____

Patient's Signature _____ Date _____

(Parent or Guardian MUST sign if patient is a minor)

I also understand that the cost of this treatment is as follows and that the method of paying for the same will be:

Total (Partial) estimate of treatment $_____
          Less:
              Initial Payment   − _____
              Insurance Estimate If Applicable − _____
              Other _____   − _____

          Balance of Estimate Due $_____

              Terms: Monthly Payment $_____ over a _____ mo. period.

PLEASE CONTACT THE BUSINESS OFFICE IF YOU ARE UNABLE TO MEET YOUR FINANCIAL OBLIGATION.

The Truth In Lending Law enacted in 1969 serves to inform the borrowers and installment purchasers of the true Annual Interest charged on the amounts financed. This law applies to this office whenever the office extends the courtesy of Installment Payments to our patients, even when no finance charge is made.

The signatures below indicate a mutual understanding of the ESTIMATE for treatment and the acceptable schedule of payment as noted.

Today's Date _____
                    Signature of Responsible Party

_____   _____
         Financial Advisor   Phone #

NOTE: THIS IS AN ESTIMATE ONLY, if treatment plan should change please request an amended estimate should it not be offered by our staff. This estimate is valid for 90 days from the date above IF treatment has not begun within that period. A patient's voluntary termination of treatment makes this agreement invalid.

FINANCIAL ARRANGEMENTS

Fig A.3.8

Financial arrangements: in a fee for service relationship, a clear statement of estimated fees and how they will be paid is in the best interest of dentist and patient alike.

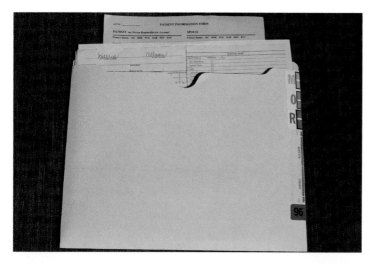

Fig A.4.1

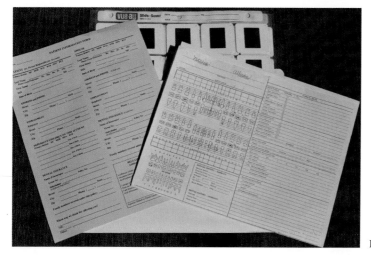

Fig A.4.2

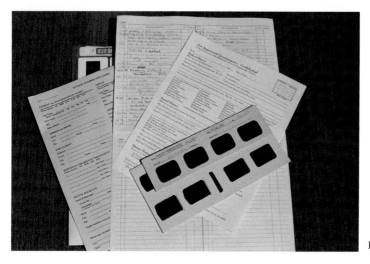

Fig A.4.3

Fig A.4

Example of a custom-designed record system. This record system fits in a 'pocket' type of envelope (Fig A.4.1). All records are kept in the pocket, including the yellow diagnostic data chart, treatment planning form, and progress notes which were custom designed and taken to a printer to set up the 11 × 17 inch format, which folds to standard stationery size (Fig A.4.2). Kept in the 'fold' are medical/dental histories, current radiographs, and other 'active' records, which are selectively retrieved when the yellow folded chart is taken out (Fig A.4.3). Business records, 'old' radiographs, correspondence, and other forms and documents are retained in the 'pocket', but need not come out every time the clinical chart is accessed. For illustration, some of the system's components include:

ACCT # _____

PATIENT INFORMATION FORM

PATIENT *(or, Person Responsible for Account)*

Primary Dentist: MC MOR WAL KAR HOV RYP

Last Name _____
  Please Circle Preference: Mr. Mrs. Ms. Dr. Atty. _____

First Name _____ MI _____

SSN _____ - _____ - _____

Date of Birth _____

ADDRESS and PHONE

Street _____

City _____ State _____

Zip _____ Phone (_____) _____

EMPLOYMENT

Employer _____

Street _____

City _____ State _____

Zip _____ Phone (_____) _____

DEPENDENT CHILDREN ON THIS ACCOUNT
Primary Dentist: MC MOR HOV RYP

_____ Date of Birth _____

_____ Date of Birth _____

_____ Date of Birth _____

_____ Date of Birth _____

_____ Date of Birth _____

DENTAL INSURANCE

Name of Insurance _____

  Group No: _____ **Policy No:** _____

  Policyholder _____
  (if different than above)

Street _____

City _____ State _____

Zip _____ Phone (_____) _____

Family members covered under this policy: _____

_____

Whom may we thank for referring you?

_____
Name
_____
Address

SPOUSE

Primary Dentist: MC MOR WAL KAR HOV RYP

Last Name _____
  Please Circle Preference: Mr. Mrs. Ms. Dr. Atty. _____

First Name _____ MI _____

SSN _____ - _____ - _____

Date of Birth _____

ADDRESS and PHONE *(if different)*

Street _____

City _____ State _____

Zip _____ Phone (_____) _____

EMPLOYMENT

Employer _____

Street _____

City _____ State _____

Zip _____ Phone (_____) _____

DENTAL INSURANCE *(if different)*

Name of Insurance _____

  Group No: _____ **Policy No:** _____

  Policyholder _____
  (if different than above)

Street _____

City _____ State _____

Zip _____ Phone (_____) _____

Family members covered under this policy: _____

_____

RELEASE OF INFORMATION
ASSIGNMENT OF BENEFITS

I authorize release of all information required to process dental insurance claims and permit a copy of this authorization to be used in place of the original assignment.

I assign to Wm. Nequette & Associates any benefits I am entitled from my insurance company for services provided and understand I am financially responsible for all charges regardless of type or level of insurance coverage.

_____   _____
Signature (Patient or Parent/Guardian)   Date

Fig A.4.4

Patient information (registration) form: organized according to our current computer scheme, that is, information is laid out in the order the computer asks for it, for ease of entry.

Get Acquainted Questionnaire: Confidential
So that we may treat you safely and effectively, please answer all questions fully. Thank you.

UPDATES:	W/INITIALS
/ /	____
/ /	____
/ /	____
/ /	____
/ /	____
(office use only)	

Name _____ Age____ Date of Birth___/___/____

Medical History
When was your last physical exam? _____ Reason for exam? _____

Are you seeing a physician at this time? Yes / No   If so, for what?_____

Physician's name_____   Party to notify in case of emergency_____

Please list any medications (prescription or non-prescription) you are taking, and what they are for:

_____

_____

Are you allergic, or do you react to anything (drugs, food, etc.)   Yes / No   If so, what? _____

❑ Are you allergic to latex?

Do you now, or have you ever had: (check if yes)
❑ Arthritis	❑ Pacemaker	❑ Jaundice
❑ Diabetes	❑ High Blood Pressure	❑ Hepatitis
❑ Thyroid Problem	❑ Pain in Chest on exertion	❑ Liver Disease
❑ Asthma	❑ Swollen Ankles	❑ Contact with AIDS virus
❑ Tuberculosis	❑ Abnormal Bleeding	❑ Venereal Disease
❑ Heart Problems/murmur	❑ Anemia	❑ Epilepsy
❑ Rheumatic Fever	❑ Blood transfusion	❑ Fainting Spells
❑ Heart Valve Problems	❑ Fatigue Easily	❑ Nervous disorder/
		Psychiatric Care

❑ Malignancy or Tumor
❑ Radiation Therapy
❑ Artificial Joint
❑ Do you smoke? How much? ____ /day
❑ History of alcohol/drug use or abuse
❑ (female) Is there any chance you could be pregnant?

Dental History
What is your main problem/reason for coming?_____

Who referred you to us?_____   Any concerns about dental treatment   Yes / No

How do you feel about the condition of your teeth?_____

How do you feel about your past dental experiences?_____

_____

Do you now, or have you ever had, (check if yes)
❑ Clicking or popping in jaw joint	❑ Regular dental check-ups	❑ Bridgework or partial dentures
❑ Clenching or Grinding, day or night	❑ Any missing teeth	❑ Bleeding Gums
❑ Pains in or near the ear	❑ Toothaches	❑ Gum Surgery, or non-surgical
❑ "TMJ" splint, or other types of treatment	❑ Bad Breath	treatment—root planing
❑ Other sore or painful areas in mouth	❑ Pain in Chewing	❑ Orthodontic treatment (braces)
	❑ Canker Sores	❑ Root Canal Work

When was your last dental visit?_____   Did you have x-rays at that time?   Yes No

Have you been instructed on how to brush and floss? Yes No   How often do you brush? ____Times per day / week

If so, When and By Whom?_____   When, usually?_____Type of brush: hard / soft

What kind of toothpaste?_____   Do you use dental floss?   Yes / No / Occasionally

Dietary History
Do you eat or drink between meals during the day? Yes No   In the Evening? Yes No   Does your diet include:

❑ Chewing gum	❑ Candy bars	❑ Hard candy	❑ Soft drinks, soda, fruit juice
❑ Cookies/pastry	❑ Sugar in coffee/tea	❑ Lifesavers	❑ breath mints or cough drops?

Thanks again for taking time   ___/___/___   _____
to complete this form!   today's date   signature

Greenbrook DENTISTRY, S.C. 13780 West Greenfield Ave. Suite 780 Brookfield, WI 53005 (414) 782-4860

Fig A.4.5

Medical, dental, and dietary history (see Figs 2.7 and 2.8): printed with the Oral Health Progress Record (see Fig 4.18A–C) on the back, and can be updated, or modified easily.

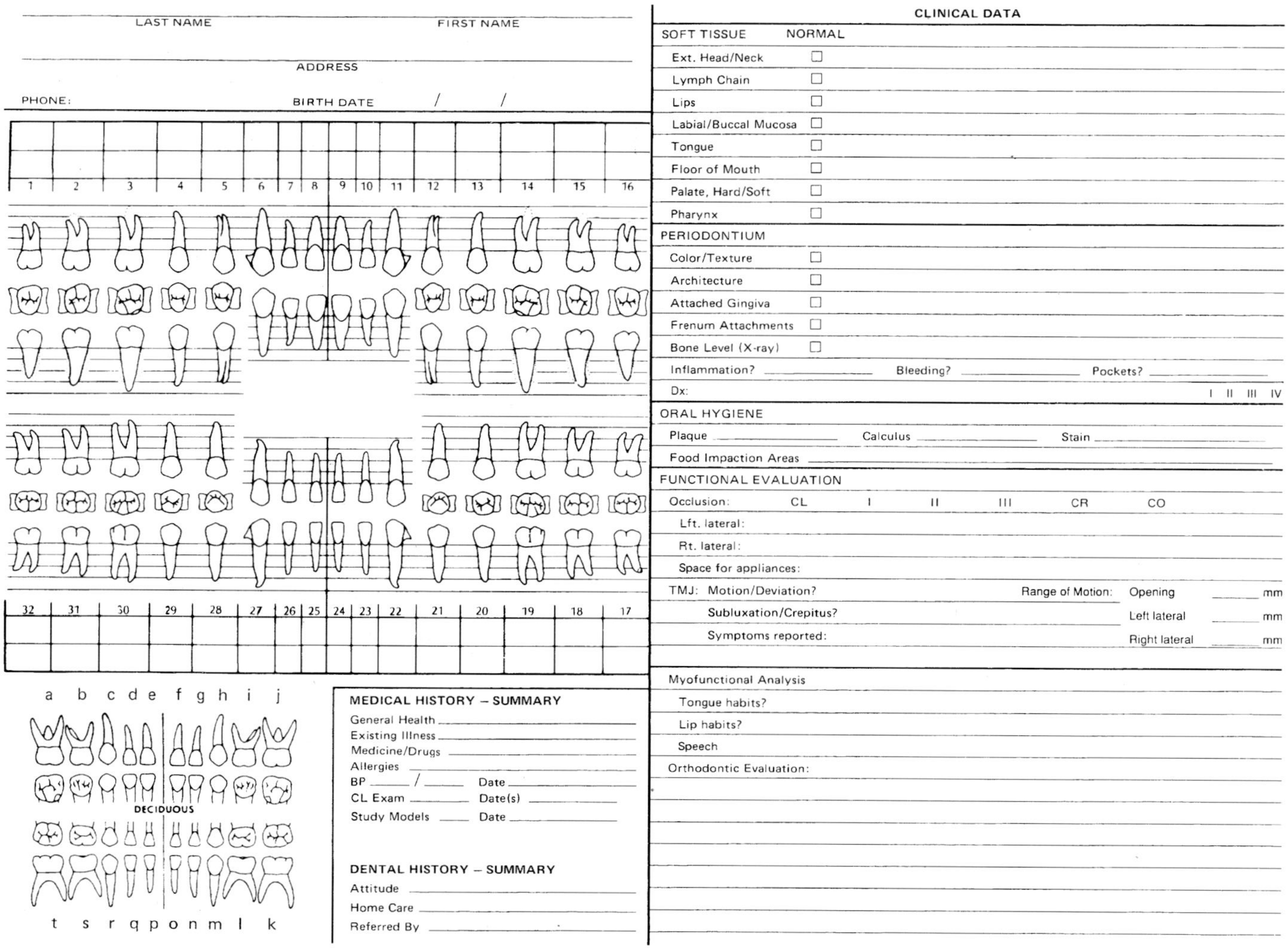

CLINICAL DATA

SOFT TISSUE — NORMAL
- Ext. Head/Neck ☐
- Lymph Chain ☐
- Lips ☐
- Labial/Buccal Mucosa ☐
- Tongue ☐
- Floor of Mouth ☐
- Palate, Hard/Soft ☐
- Pharynx ☐

PERIODONTIUM
- Color/Texture ☐
- Architecture ☐
- Attached Gingiva ☐
- Frenum Attachments ☐
- Bone Level (X-ray) ☐
- Inflammation? _____ Bleeding? _____ Pockets? _____
- Dx: _____ I II III IV

ORAL HYGIENE
- Plaque _____ Calculus _____ Stain _____
- Food Impaction Areas _____

FUNCTIONAL EVALUATION
- Occlusion: CL _____ I II III CR CO
- Lft. lateral:
- Rt. lateral:
- Space for appliances:
- TMJ: Motion/Deviation? _____ Range of Motion: Opening _____ mm
- Subluxation/Crepitus? _____ Left lateral _____ mm
- Symptoms reported: _____ Right lateral _____ mm

Myofunctional Analysis
- Tongue habits?
- Lip habits?
- Speech
- Orthodontic Evaluation:

LAST NAME _____ FIRST NAME _____
ADDRESS _____
BIRTH DATE ___ / ___ / ___
PHONE:

1 2 3 4 5 6 7 8 9 10 11 12 13 14 15 16

32 31 30 29 28 27 26 25 24 23 22 21 20 19 18 17

a b c d e f g h i j
DECIDUOUS
t s r q p o n m l k

MEDICAL HISTORY – SUMMARY
- General Health
- Existing Illness
- Medicine/Drugs
- Allergies
- BP ___ / ___ Date _____
- CL Exam _____ Date(s) _____
- Study Models _____ Date _____

DENTAL HISTORY – SUMMARY
- Attitude
- Home Care
- Referred By

Fig A.4.6

Diagnostic data chart: allows for all examination and radiographic data to be recorded on a single page, including pictorial permanent and deciduous tooth charts.

SERVICES NECESSARY	FEES
1	
2	
3	
4	
5	
6	
7	
8	
9	
10	
11	
12	
13	
14	
15	
16	
17	
18	
19	
20	
21	
22	
23	
24	
25	
26	
27	
28	
29	
30	
31	
32	

Fig A.4.7

Treatment planning form: flexible, and can be used in a number of ways. 'Services necessary' is numerical, tooth no. 1 through no. 32.

History for TMJoint Dysfunction
So that we may treat you safely and effectively, please answer all questions fully. Thank you.

Name _____   Age_____   Date ____/____/____

I. Chief Complaint: _

_ _

_ When did the problem start? (Date) _ _ _ _ _ _ _

II. Do you experience pain in the face, head or neck?   *Yes / No*   If yes, please complete the following:

A. Where is the pain located:

R	L		R	L		
_____	_____	joint	_____	_____	back of head	Other (describe): _ _ _ _ _ _ _ _ _ _ _ _ _ _ _
_____	_____	ear	_____	_____	eyes	_ _
_____	_____	lower jaw	_____	_____	sinuses	_ _
_____	_____	forehead	_____	_____	neck	_ _
_____	_____	temples	_____	_____	shoulders	_ _

B. What kind of pain do you have?

			How long does the pain last?	
_____ sharp	_____ burning	_____ mild	_____ minutes	_____ all day
_____ dull	_____ pulsating	_____ moderate	_____ hours	_____ days
_____ aching	_____ severe			

C. When is the pain more severe?

_____ morning   _____ at meal time

_____ evening   _____ no particular time

D. What do you do to relieve the pain?

_____ medication {what kind (s) } _

_____ hot applications   _

_____ cold applications   _

_____ massage

_____ rest

_____ other {describe } _

III. Have you ever had trauma to your face, jaws or neck?   _____Yes   _____ No

A. Do you have grating, clicking or popping in your jaw joint?   _____Yes   _____ No
    If yes: _____ left joint   _____ right joint   _____ both joints

B. Have you had an episode where your jaw was stuck and could not open?   _____Yes   _____ No

C. Do you feel limited in your ability to open wide?   _____Yes   _____ No

D. Has your mouth ever locked open so you unable to close it?   _____Yes   _____ No

E. Do you have ringing, noise, or fullness in your ears?   _____Yes   _____ No

F. Do you have difficulty swallowing?   _____Yes   _____ No

Fig A.5

Examples of 'special' records. Fig A.5.1: history for temporomandibular joint dysfunction (two pages, front and back). This form is employed when the initial comprehensive examination reveals temporomandibular or facial pain problems, or when the presenting chief complaint is of this nature.

III. Habits

A. Are you aware of ever bracing or resting your jaw by holding your front
       teeth in contact?   _____ Yes   _____ No

B. Are you aware of clenching your teeth during the day?   _____ Yes   _____ No

C. Have you been told you grind your teeth in your sleep?   _____ Yes   _____ No

D. Do you ever awaken with an awareness in your jaw as if you had your teeth
       clamped together in your sleep?   _____ Yes   _____ No

E. Have your teeth or muscles ever been sore from biting your teeth? _____ Yes   _____ No

F. Do you bite your nails, cheek, or tongue?   _____ Yes   _____ No

IV. Dental History

A. Have you had your teeth straightened (braces) ?   _____ Yes   _____ No

B. Have you had your bite adjusted?   _____ Yes   _____ No

C. Have you had previous treatment for bite problems?   _____ Yes   _____ No

D. Have you had impacted wisdom teeth removed?   _____ Yes   _____ No

V. Medical History

A. Are you currently being treated by a physician?   _____ Yes   _____ No

B. Are you taking any medication at this time?   _____ Yes   _____ No

C. Do you feel you are under stress, tension or anxiety?   _____ Yes   _____ No

D. Do you have other current non-dental physical problems or diseases? _____ Yes   _____ No

E. Do you have any of the following:

_____ arthritis   _____ sinus infection   _____ blood vessel disease

_____ osteoarthritis   _____ ear infection

_____ rheumatoid arthritis   _____ swollen glands

V. Please write any other pertinent information not covered above: _ _ _ _ _ _ _ _ _ _

- -

- -

- -

- -

- -

- -

- -

- -

Greenbrook Dentistry   July, 1998

Fig A.5.1: continued

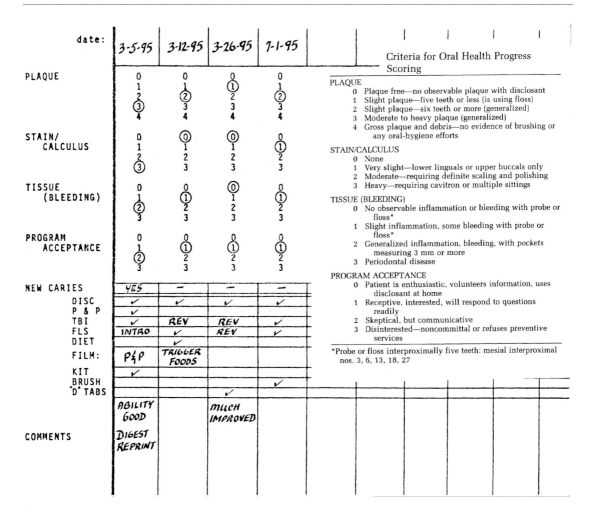

Fig A.5.2

Oral health progress record: this tool has been discussed and illustrated (see Fig 4.18A–C), and is an efficient way to monitor and document a number of aspects together, and over time.

PERIODONTAL EVALUATION

LAST NAME _____ FIRST NAME _____ DATE _____

WILLIAM L NEQUETTE, D.D.S.
CHARLES W. McCAULEY, D.D.S.
ROBERT B. MORRIS, D.D.S.

THOMAS S. RYPEL, D.D.S.
KENNETH J. WALISZEWSKI, D.D.S., M.S.
JAMES C. HOVE, D.D.S.

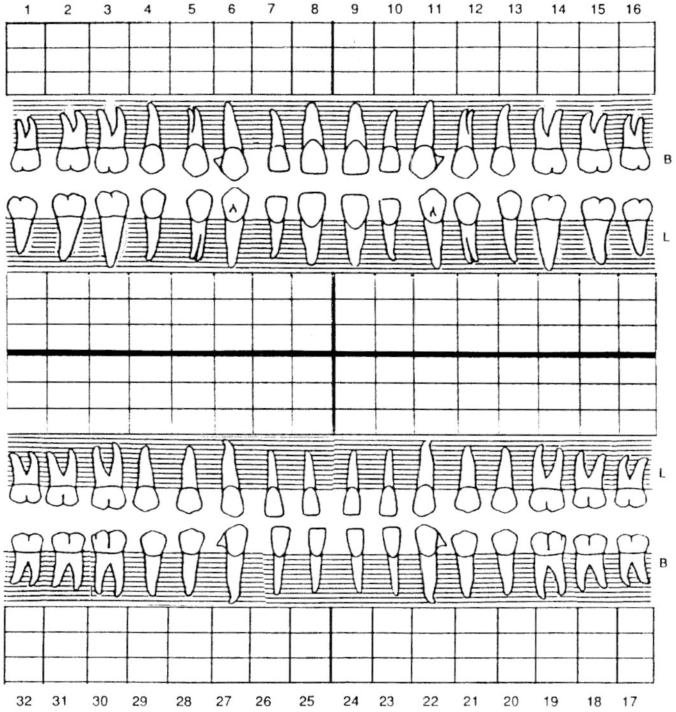

HOME CARE REGIMEN

___ Brush/Floss

___ Home Use Fluoride

___ Therapeutic Rinse
      Peridex/_____

Other Aids:
___ Proxabrush
___ Superfloss
___ Rubber Tip
___ Irrigator
___ Perio Aid

TREATMENT PLAN

INITIAL TREATMENT: fee

(4341 A) Scale/Root Plan--w/anesthetic
(4341 B)
(4341 C)
(4341 D)

DEFINITIVE SURGERY/REPAIR:

MAINTENANCE-- Q _____ Mo.:

(4910)

DATE

16 15 14 13 12 11 10 9 8 7 6 5 4 3 2 1

B

L

L

B

32 31 30 29 28 27 26 25 24 23 22 21 20 19 18 17

Periodontal Diagnosis: _____

CL   I   II   III   IV

Type I
Most pockets 1-3 mm but with an occasional 4 mm pocket.
Slight bleeding upon probing.
Mobilities of less than 0.5 mm.
No furcation involvement.

Type II
Most pockets 1-3 mm but with some 4-5 mm's in depth.
Moderate bleeding upon probing, and more generalized than Type I.
Most mobilities normal, but with some Class I's recorded.
No furcation involvements or only Grade I furcations noted.

Type III
Pocket depths are generally 3-5 mm, with possibility of some 6-10 mm's.
Generalized bleeding upon probing.
Mobilities of 1 to 2 are recorded.
Grade I with possibility of Grade II furcata present.

Type IV
Pocket depths are generally 3-6 mm, with possibility of some 7-12 mm pockets.
Generalized bleeding upon probing.
Mobilities of 1, 2 and 3 are present.
Grade I, II furcation involvements or only Grade I furcation involvements recorded.
Grade I, II and possibly III furcation involvements recorded.

Fig A.5.3

Periodontal evaluation/re-evaluation. A variety of forms is available to emphasize periodontal findings, and changes over time. Ease of use is critical. This form has boxes for three successive probings, a written periodontal diagnosis, and check-off treatment plan section.

3 DAY FOOD INVENTORY

Before starting to fill out this form, please read and then follow the instructions given on the reverse, carefully.

Name __________ Date __________ Phone __________

1st Day	PROT.	Ca++	A.A.	GOOD	BAD	2nd Day	PROT.	Ca++	A.A.	GOOD	BAD	3rd Day	PROT.	Ca++	A.A.	GOOD	BAD
Breakfast						Breakfast						Breakfast					
Midmorning Snack						Midmorning Snack						Midmorning Snack					
Noon						Noon						Noon					
Between Meals Snack						Between Meals Snack						Between Meals Snack					
Evening						Evening						Evening					
Bedtime Snack						Bedtime Snack						Bedtime Snack					

CER: 152 – Dental Printing, P. O. Box 730, Paradise, Calif. 95969

From: Dr. A. Chari

Fig A.5.4

Food inventory (2 pages, front and back). Another example of specialized information which may be gathered and documented on a 'customized' form, this one used by permission of Dr Carl Rieder.

The foods you eat have much to do with your general and oral health. To help in evaluation of your diet, please record in detail the food and drink you have consumed for a period of at least _____ day___. Recommendations and suggestions, if any, will constitute part of your treatment.

INSTRUCTIONS FOR THE USE OF THE FOOD DIARY

1. In the proper squares on the reverse side, immediately after each meal, record the time and all the food and drink you have consumed.

2. It is important that you continue your normal eating habits during the recording period.

3. Please list all the items in detail. Do not leave even the smallest item out (gum, colas, cakes, etc.)

4. Please use the following abbreviations:

T — tablespoonful	cn — canned	sm — small	gl — glass
t — teaspoonful	s — sugar	md — medium	bl — black
c — cup	sl — slice	lg — large	

5. Be sure to state the amount of each food eaten, such as:

INCORRECT	CORRECT
Juice	4 oz. Fresh Orance Juice
American Cheese Sandwich	American Cheese 2 sl., white bread 2 sl 1 leaf lettuce, ½ tomato, butter
Coffee	1 c coffee, 2 ts, with 2 T milk
Dessert	1 c peaches, cn
Vegetables	½ c peas, cn
Potato	1 md baked potato

6. **Please write clearly:**

Medications _____ Vitamins _____ Prescribed/Self _____ Height _____ Weight _____

Most recent weight gain or loss. Gain _____ Loss _____ lbs. Period of time _____

Meals: Regular _____ Irregular _____ Family _____ Alone _____

Appetite: Good _____ Bad _____ Cigarettes per day _____

Liquid intake glasses per day: Water _____ Coffee _____ Tea _____ Juice _____

Approximate meat consumption in lbs. per day: _____

Urinating frequency during the day _____ at night _____

Food dislikes: _____

Food allergies: _____

Food preferred: _____

General well being: Excellent _____ Good _____ Tired _____

Or use your own words in describing how you feel: _____

_____

D   Is your diet medically controlled? _____

D, 3-day food inventory (back side).

Fig A.5.4: continued

LEGAL ASPECTS OF DENTAL RECORDS

This is not intended to be a detailed treatise on forensics, but will touch briefly on a few key issues.

The first is the advent of electronic data management, or the so-called 'paperless record'. Many software applications are, and will be, available that assist in gathering data using touch-screen or even voice recognition to make a dental record. Although offering advantages in efficiency, speed, and access to data, such systems are subject to all the vagaries of our computer age. We turn our computers off during electrical storms, and occasionally the system is 'down', preventing both entry and retrieval of information. The paper chart may occasionally be 'misplaced', but it cannot be degraded by a refrigerator magnet! Storage capacity is another issue which is currently in question, especially if your paperless record includes graphic images, radiographs, and clinical photos, which can use up tremendous amounts of computer memory.

As yet unsolved is the question of authenticity of digital records, given the ease with which such files can be changed or manipulated. For legal documents, ink on paper will continue to serve us well, and it is not unusual to see a computer-aided record system used to produce 'hard copy' documents for day-to-day use.

Another key issue is the use of dental records in the identification of human remains. Although the advent of DNA identification has enabled forensic specialists to make identification from mere fragments of tissue, the technology is expensive and time-consuming. An accurate set of dental records and radiographs will continue to be a standard method of positive identification which can be rapidly employed with considerable confidence.

Litigation, and professional and peer review raise the third key issue, wherein records are called upon to protect both dentist and patient relative to the process and outcome of care. Records will not necessarily prevent litigation, but are critical to successful resolution of such issues. With this in mind, here are some key points for the dentist to consider.

MAKE AND KEEP RECORDS

As obvious as it may seem, there have been cases of litigation in which the dentist had no written records pertaining to the patient in question. Whether records were lost, misplaced, or never made in the first place, failure to keep records can put your word (and memory) against that of a complainant. As record keeping is an accepted standard of practice, the lack of records alone may be legally damning. In financial matters, lack of record may allow a taxing agency to make its own estimate of your income and tax you accordingly.

Granted, if one is doing something clearly illegal or unethical, documenting those acts may not be a good idea, but if errors of judgment or execution are made in the course of good-faith treatment, the patient should be informed and the event documented. In informing the patient it is not necessary to admit negligence or apologize: the disclosure should be made in neutral terms. Such candor with the patient may even prevent the initiation of litigation and, if not, the fact that disclosure was made is likely to help mitigate the circumstances. Failure to disclose can easily trigger a complaint when another practitioner discovers a problem and tells the patient. To err is human, to cover up the error often creates more trouble than the error itself!

MAKE AND KEEP *GOOD* RECORDS

Redundant, perhaps, but clear and detailed records have stopped a good many adversarial actions in their tracks. As an example, in an actual case attempts to collect an unpaid fee resulted in threats of a suit claiming that fees charged were twice the original estimate. The dental records included a written plan with estimated fees corresponding to actual fees charged, notes documenting case presentation in which the fee was presented, insurance coverage discussed, and payments agreed upon, and a follow-up letter sent to the patient reviewing and reiterating the agreement. Upon receipt of copies of these documents, the plaintiff's attorney dropped the action, and collection attempts resumed without complication.

You can do your own quality assurance survey, pulling several patient charts at random each week, and pretending that they have been subpoenaed for an impending legal action. Would they measure up? Would you care to testify about the patient's care using them as your only memory aid? Would you be tempted to add to or alter them? Don't do it! Altering records could result in criminal charges. Better to resolve that all future records will be up to standards and hope you won't need those that aren't. If your record sample has deficiencies, resolve to upgrade them as patients return on recall visits. Fill in the blanks and put the charts in order as patient care continues.

RETENTION AND CONTROL

Records are the property of the practitioner, not the patient. Patients pay for interpretation and diagnosis, not the physical records themselves. The dentist may be required to produce originals or copies of records upon court order, subpoena, or search warrant. When possible, make copies, and keep originals.

Many states have laws mandating that records be made available to patients, on the premise that individuals have rights to information therein. Indeed, it is good practice to release copies of records to other practitioners whom the patient may be seeing for more informed diagnoses and possibly less radiation exposure (in the case of dental radiographs).

Guidelines for the release of dental records include the following:

1. Release records only on written request of patient or parent/guardian. This may be a letter, a form kept on file (authorizing release to insurance carriers, etc.), or even a simple handwritten note.

2. Release only copies of records and radiographs, never the originals themselves. Double film packs provide duplicate radiographs of equal quality. Radiograph duplicating film and simple duplicating devices are also acceptable, but care must be taken to produce as good a quality copy as possible. Too many duplicate radiographs are unreadable, and useless. Charts can obviously be copied by machine.

   An exception to the copy-only rule might be the submission of preoperative radiographs for predetermination of benefit, or consultation with a specialist or another dentist for second opinion. In these cases diagnostic quality may be critical, and the radiograph would be returned before treatment. If original records are released for any reason, when and where they were sent should be noted in the patient chart and logged again when they are returned.

3. Never release more than is authorized or requested, but when 'all' records are demanded, be sure to copy and include everything, no matter how insignificant it may seem.

   The question of how long to retain dental records has no good answer. The safe policy is to retain them forever, but this is not a practical option for most dentists. Common sense suggests that, once applicable statutes of limitation have run out on potential litigation, the records may be safely destroyed. This time will vary from state to state, and keeping records well beyond the statute is not a bad idea. Be careful with records belonging to minor children, because the legal statute may not start to run until they reach adulthood! Likewise, certain individuals (including prisoners, the mentally incompetent, and other groups) are considered legally 'disabled', and the statute may never run out!

   Retirement or even death of the dentist does not mean that records can be destroyed, because legal actions can be brought against the estate of the deceased. Provision for retention and control of original dental records must be made in any event.

The 'magical signature'

Many people believe that a signature on some document gives it greater significance than may be the case. For example, if questions arise about information gathered in a health history, having the patient's signature affixed to the history may be beneficial. However, the existence of an unsigned written history, whether completed by the patient or taken orally and completed by the dentist, is probably just as useful as one signed by the patient. Most laypeople underestimate the weight of simple testimony by the professional. The dentist who can testify that he or she did take a health history for a patient in question, that it is his or her regular practice to do so, and that the written (albeit unsigned) history in the patient's dental chart reflects the information gathered, need not worry that the patient signature is not affixed. Conversely, a signed, dated, and witnessed history that does not ask about drug allergies will be of little value should a patient have an anaphylactic reaction to your prescription.

Consent

It is very difficult to do dentistry without consent. Our patients have to 'hold still and open wide' before we can do much to or for them. For us, informed consent simply means that the patient understands what you are proposing to do for them, and agrees to let you do it. The patient who calls our office and makes an appointment for cleaning, examination, and necessary radiographs has, in effect, consented to those procedures. This does not mean that a routine explanation of what is going to be done is not a good idea; it simply means that obtaining a written consent to perform those services may be superfluous. The obvious exception is a case in which the patient is not a legally responsible adult. If you are dealing with a minor child, or any legally disabled individual, the consent of parent or guardian is essential. Again, the act of bringing the child to your office for an examination/cleaning is sufficient. An unaccompanied child, even a teenager, cannot be treated without parental consent.

Beyond the diagnostic phase, a course of treatment is outlined and proposed to the patient. A written record of that proposal is essential, along with a record of the patient's acceptance of the plan. If the treatment and its possible complications (those most likely to occur) have been explained, and the patient elects to proceed, informed consent has been obtained. It is also important to discuss the consequences of nontreatment, so that the patient can consider risks and benefits fully.

Beyond this minimum requirement, the patient-oriented dentist will explain at the outset of every appointment what is to be done and why, and whether there are likely complications. This is the best way to ensure informed consent, because people often forget what they are told at the outset. With this brief background on consent, we return to the 'magical signature' and what it can and cannot do for us. If a treatment plan has been presented to the patient, is accepted, and the discussion documented in the record, the patient's signature on a consent 'form' is nice, but not necessary. Conversely, a lengthy and legalistic pre-printed consent form, which can be fairly described as 'difficult to understand', may be of little use, even with a patient signature! It is more important what is said between patient and dentist, than what is on the written consent. If, in fact, that patient has been informed, and has agreed to proceed, it is unlikely that a complaint will arise later of 'failure to inform'. Dentists should not attempt to blanket themselves with lengthy and legalistic-sounding consent forms, without taking the effort actually to talk with the patient about their problems, treatment options, risks, and benefits. Figure A.6 gives an example of an informed consent.

SERVICES NECESSARY		FEES		PLAN:
1 EXT ANES	65	20	80	SCALE/POL/OHI — DONE
2				RCT #14
3				CLOSE DIASTEMA 8-9
4				PVC #14
5				BRIDGE #18-20
6				EXT #1 — TIMING ELECTIVE
7				
8 MI COMPOSITE	95		190	8/3/98 DISCUSSED PLAN AT
9 MI ''	95			LENGTH W/PATIENT. PT.
10				ACCEPTED PLAN (BENEFITS
11				AND RISKS). WILL PAY 1/3
12				TO START ($1050), 1/3 AT
13				COMPLETION OF BRIDGE ($1050)
14 RCT, PVC	450	600	1050	BALANCE @ $350/MO - 3 MOS.
15				
16				
17				RB MORRIS DDS
18 FCC	600			
X PV PONTIC	600		1820	
20 PVC ANES	600	20		
21				
22			3140	
23				
24				
25				
26				
27				
28				
29				
30				
31				
32				

Fig A.6.1

Example of informed consents. This chart entry documents presentation and acceptance of a plan of treatment.

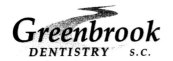

Charles W. McCauley, D.D.S.
Robert B. Morris, D.D.S.
Thomas S. Rypel, D.D.S.
James C. Hove, D.D.S.
Kenneth J. Waliszewski, D.D.S., M.S.
Michael B. Karczewski, D.D.S.,M.S.

August, 1998

Jane Doe
123 Elm St.
Brookfield, WI

Dear Jane,

This letter is to follow up and confirm our discussion of last week regarding your dental treatment. The problems we need to address include the following:

Abscess on upper left first molar—not painful now, but clearly visible on the x-rays.
Space between upper front teeth, which you don't like, and want to close.
Missing lower left first molar, with some tipping/drifting of the second molar.
Upper right wisdom tooth supererupted.

We discussed some options for treatment, and the risks and benefits of various choices. The treatment plan you accepted, and estimated costs are as follows:

Root canal therapy upper left molar, 2 to 3 visits	$ 450
Bonded composites on upper front teeth to close gap	190
Porcelain veneer crown on root canal tooth	600
Three tooth bridge lower left replacing missing molar	1820
Removal of upper right wisdom tooth—timing is up to you	80
Estimated total	$3140

You indicated you would like to spread the payments out, and will pay one third ($1050) when we start, one third ($1050) when we complete the lower bridge, and the balance over the following three months, at $350 per month.

Good dental health and successful treatment is dependent on your good maintenance. We recommend regular six month recall check-ups, and will send you a reminder, but you are the most important person in keeping your teeth healthy. Thank you for letting us help you do that.

If you have any questions regarding this treatment please feel free to call.

Sincerely,   Accepted by:

Dr. Morris

Robert B. Morris, DDS   _____/_____
                                       Jane Doe   Date

Please sign and date one copy and send or bring it to the office next time. Thanks.

13780 W. Greenfield Avenue, Suite 780 • Brookfield, WI 53005 • *Phone* (414) 782-4860 *Fax* (414) 782-7720

Fig A.6.2

It is supplemented nicely with a follow-up letter which further documents the consent, or may even be signed and returned by the patient.

PATIENT NUMBER

© **1985** *Wisconsin Dental Association*

PATIENTS NAME   *DOE, JANE*
       Last   First   Initial

I hereby authorize   *DR. ROBERT MORRIS*
                                 DOCTOR'S NAME

and whomever he/she may designate as his/her assistants, to perform upon me the following operation and/or procedures:

Root canal therapy upper left molar, 2 to 3 visits	$ 450
Bonded composites on upper front teeth to close gap	190
Porcelain veneer crown on root canal tooth	600
Three tooth bridge lower left replacing missing molar	1820
Removal of upper right wisdom tooth—timing is up to you	80
Estimated total	$3140

and if any unforeseen condition arises in the course of these designated operations and/or procedures calling, in their judgment, for procedures in addition to or different from those now contemplated, I further request and authorize him/her to do whatever he/she deems advisable.

I consent to the above treatment plan after having been advised of the alternate plans of treatment available, the known material risks of the treatment to be used and the consequences if this treatment were withheld.

I am informed and fully understand that inherent in any type of surgery are certain unavoidable complications. In oral surgery, the most common of these complications include post-operative bleeding, swelling or bruising, discomfort, stiff jaws, loss or loosening of dental restorations. Less common complications can include infection, loss or injury to adjacent teeth and soft tissues, nerve disturbances (e.g., numbness in mouth and lip tissues), jaw fractures, sinus exposure and swallowing or aspiration of teeth and restorations, and small root fragments remaining in the jaw which might require extensive surgery for removal.

I further consent to the administration of local or general anesthesia, antibiotics, analgesics or any other drugs that may be deemed necessary in my case, and understand that there is a slight element of risk inherent in the administration of any drug or anesthesia. This risk includes adverse drug response (e.g., allergic reactions), cardiac arrest, and aspiration; and thrombophlebitis (e.g., irritation and swelling of a vein), pain, discoloration and injury to blood vessels and nerves which may be caused by injections of any medications or drugs.

A more complete explanation of all complications of surgery and anesthesia is available to me upon my request from the Doctor.

I realize that in spite of the possible complications, my contemplated surgery/treatment is necessary and desired by me. I am aware that the practice of dentistry and surgery is not an exact science and I acknowledge that no guarantees have been made to me concerning the results of the operation or procedure.

I realize that it is mandatory that I give as accurate and complete medical and personal history as possible, follow any and all instructions as directed and permit prescribed diagnostic procedures.

X

SIGNATURE OF PATIENT   DATE

SIGNATURE OF PARENT OR GUARDIAN   DATE

SIGNATURE OF WITNESS   DATE

CONSENT FORM

Fig A.6.3

This broad 'blanket' consent is certainly detailed and complete, but could be considered a bit difficult for the average layman to read and understand.

Greenbrook Dentistry, S.C.

NAME _JANE DOE_ DATE _8/98_
ADDRESS _123 ELM ST._ PHONE _ _

At this time, the following services are to be performed:

☒ PREVENTIVE TREATMENT _DONE – MAINTAIN 6 MO RECALLS_

☐ PERIODONTAL TREATMENT _____

☒ ORAL SURGERY _REMOVE UPPER (R) 3RD MOLAR_

☒ OPERATIVE DENTISTRY _2 COMPOSITE RESINS – TO_
(fillings) _CLOSE SPACE IN FRONT_

☒ CROWNS/BRIDGES _1 CROWN UPPER (L)_

☐ ORTHODONTICS _3 UNIT BRIDGE LOWER (L)_

☒ OTHER _ROOT CANAL THERAPY UPPER (L)_
FIRST MOLAR

At a total estimated fee of _3140_

INSURANCE: — _NONE_
Pre-estimate of coverage: _____
Patient's portion (approximate) _____

The treatment summarized above and its possible complications have been discussed with me, and I have consented to proceed with it. I also agree to pay the fee (or my portion) on the following basis:

☐ FULL AMOUNT (CASH OR CHECK) AS TREATMENT PROCEEDS WITH 5% DISCOUNT.
☐ MASTERCHARGE/VISA, CHARGED AS TREATMENT PROCEEDS.
☐ FULL AMOUNT ON MONTHLY STATEMENT WITHIN 10 DAYS OF RECEIPT.
☒ IN THE FOLLOWING INSTALLMENTS: _____
⅓ ($1050) AT START,
⅓ ($1050) AT INSERTION OF BRIDGE,
$350/MO UNTIL PAID (~3 MOS)

There is no finance or interest charge to be paid provided the payment arrangement is adhered to. This arrangement is for the above treatment only and further treatment will be paid when rendered, or on the basis of future arrangements.

_____ X_____ _____
Signature of Dentist or Staff Signature of Patient Date
  (or Parent if Patient is minor)

Fig A.6.4

This summary plan and estimate includes a very simple consent statement (mid-page), which is clear and concise.

CONSENT FOR ORAL OR PERIODONTAL SURGERY

I request and authorize doctors and staff of *Greenbrook Dentistry , S.C.* to perform the following operations and/or procedures for me:

I understand that in any type of surgery there are possible unavoidable complications. In oral surgery the most common include post-operative bleeding, swelling or bruising, discomfort, and stiffness of the jaw. Less common complications can include infection, loss of or injury to adjacent teeth and soft tissues, nerve disturbances (such as persistent numbness), fractures, sinus exposure, and swallowing or aspiration of teeth and restorations.

I consent to the administration of local anesthetics or other drugs that may be necessary in my case and understand that there is an element of risk involved in the administration of any drug, including allergic reaction or other adverse effects.

I realize that it is essential that I give an accurate and complete medical history, take medications exactly as prescribed, and follow the instructions I am given.

I understand that despite the possible complications the surgery planned is necessary and it is my wish to have it performed. I know that the practice of dentistry and surgery is not an exact science and that no guarantees can be made as to the results of the operation or procedure. A full explanation of the operation and possible complications is available upon my request from the Doctor.

Date ____/ ____/ ____   Signed _____

==

FOR YOUR COMFORT AND PROTECTION FOLLOWING ORAL OR PERIODONTAL SURGERY

1. Following extraction, keep steady pressure on the site with dampened gauze for 20 minutes to and hour, as needed. Some prolonged bleeding is not unusual and you may repeat the gauze pressure if necessary.

2. Do not rinse, swish, or gargle for 24 hours. You should refrain from smoking, alcohol, and mouthwashes for a day or two. Avoid drinking through a straw or creating pressure in the mouth. A warm salt water rinse may be used after 48 hours (approximately 1/2 teaspoon salt in a tall glass of warm water).

3. No food or liquids for two (2) hours after surgery. After that, eat or drink whatever is comfortable; a soft bland diet is best for a few days.

4. Swelling sometimes occur and can be reduced by using an ice pack on the outside of the face. Apply ____ minutes on, ____ minutes off, for the first 4 to 6 hours after surgery.

5. If you have been given a prescription, follow directions exactly. Antibiotics such as penicillin, etc. must be taken for the full time prescribed; pain relievers may be taken only as needed.

6. If you have problems or unusual symptoms call your dentist. Office phone: (414) 782-4860

Special instructions: Home phone:

~~~ *Greenbrook Dentistry . S.C.*   13780 W. Greenfield Ave. Ste. 780 Brookfield. WI 53005 ~~~

Fig A.6.5

A combination pre-surgical consent form, with a detachable post-operative instruction sheet, can be very useful to document both informed consent, and that post-operative instructions were given.

BIBLIOGRAPHY

Chapter 1

Geboy MJ, *Communication and behavior in dentistry.* Williams & Wilkins: Baltimore, MD, 1985.

Morris RB, *Principles of dental treatment planning.* Lea & Febiger: Philadelphia, PA, 1983.

Roblee RD, *Interdisciplinary dentofacial therapy.* Quintessence Publishing Co: Chicago, IL, 1994.

Wright R, LeBloch DS, Lapin L, *Winning communications for the successful practice.* American Dental Association, Council on Dental Practice: Chicago, IL, 1986.

Chapter 2

Bernstein L, Bernstein RS, Dana RH, *Interviewing: A guide for health professionals.* Appleton-Century-Crofts: New York, 1974.

Bricker SL, Langlais RP, Miller CS, *Oral diagnosis, oral medicine, and treatment planning.* Lea & Febiger: Philadelphia, PA, 1994.

Coleman GC, Nelson JF, *Principles of oral diagnosis.* Mosby-Year Book: St Louis, MO, 1993.

Froelich RE, Bishop FM, *Clinical interviewing skills: A programmed manual for data gathering, evaluation, and patient management.* Mosby: St Louis, MO, 1977.

Geboy MJ, *Communication and behavior in dentistry.* Williams & Wilkins: Baltimore, MD, 1985.

Halsted CL, et al, *Physical evaluation of the dental patient.* Mosby: St Louis, MO, 1982.

Hardin JF, Hellman LF, *Clark's clinical dentistry.* Harper & Row: Hagerstown, NY, 1976–98.

Kerr DA, Ash MM, Millard HD, *Oral diagnosis.* Mosby: St Louis, MO, 1983.

Lindsay SJ, Millar K, Milgrom P, *Dental health psychology.* Harwood Academic: New York, 1993.

Mitchell DF, Standish SM, Fast TB, *Oral diagnosis, oral medicine.* Lea & Febiger: Philadelphia, PA, 1978.

Morris RB, *Principles of dental treatment planning.* Lea & Febiger: Philadelphia, PA, 1983.

Seidel HM, Ball JW, Dains JE, Benedict GW, *Mosby's guide to physical examination.* Mosby-Year Book: St Louis, MO, 1987.

Tullman MJ, *Systemic disease in dental treatment.* Appleton-Century-Crofts: New York, 1982.

Wright R, LeBloch DS, Lapin L, *Winning communications for the successful practice.* American Dental Association, Council on Dental Practice: Chicago, 1986.

Chapter 3

The Dental Radiographic Patient Selection Panel, *The selection of patients for x-ray examination: dental radiographic examinations.* Public Health Service, Food and Drug Administration Pub. No. 88-8273. US Government Printing Office: Washington, DC, 1987.

Goaz PW, White SC, *Oral radiology, principles and interpretation.* Mosby: St Louis, MO, 1987.

Hardin JF, Hellman LF, *Clark's clinical dentistry.* Harper & Row: Hagerstown, NY, 1976–98.

Langland OE, Langlais RP, *Principle of dental imaging.* Williams & Wilkins: Baltimore, MD, 1997.

Manson-Hing LR, Clark DE, *Fundamentals of dental radiography.* Lea & Febiger: Philadelphia, PA, 1990.

Morris RB, *Principles of dental treatment planning.* Lea & Febiger: Philadelphia, PA, 1983.

Razmus TF, Williamson GF, *Current oral and maxillofacial imaging.* WB Saunders: Philadelphia, PA, 1996.

Whaites E, *Essentials of dental radiography and radiology.* Churchill Livingstone: New York, 1996.

Chapter 4

Bricker SL, Langlais RP, Miller CS, *Oral diagnosis, oral medicine, and treatment planning.* Lea & Febiger: Philadelphia, PA, 1994.

Coleman GC, Nelson JF, *Principles of oral diagnosis.* Mosby-Year Book: St Louis, MO, 1993.

Dawson PE, *Evaluation, diagnosis, and treatment of occlusal problems.* Mosby-Year Book: St Louis, MO, 1989.

Hardin JF, Hellman LF, *Clark's clinical dentistry.* Harper & Row: Hagerstown, NY, 1976–98.

Kerr DA, Ash MM, Millard HD, *Oral diagnosis.* Mosby: St Louis, MO, 1983.

Mitchell DF, Standish SM, Fast TB, *Oral diagnosis, oral medicine.* Lea & Febiger: Philadelphia, PA, 1978.

Morris RB, *Principles of dental treatment planning.* Lea & Febiger: Philadelphia, PA, 1983.

Okeson JP, *Management of temporomandibular disorders and occlusion.* Mosby-Year Book: St Louis, MO, 1997.

Seidel HM, Ball JW, Dains JE, Benedict GW, *Mosby's guide to physical examination.* Mosby-Year Book: St Louis, MO, 1987.

Chapter 5

Barsh LI, *Dental treatment planning for the adult patient.* WB Saunders: Philadelphia, PA, 1981.

Blinkhorn AS, Mackie IC, *Practical treatment planning for the paedondontic patient.* Quintessence Publishing Co.: Chicago, IL, 1992.

Bricker SL, Langlais RP, Miller CS, *Oral diagnosis, oral medicine, and treatment planning.* Lea & Febiger: Philadelphia, PA, 1994.

Cameron AC, Widmer RP, *Handbook of Pediatric Dentistry.* Mosby-Year Book: St Louis, MO, 1997.

Cohen B, Thomson H, *Dental care for the elderly.* Year Book Medical Publishers: Chicago, IL, 1986.

Coleman GC, Nelson JF, *Principles of oral diagnosis.* Mosby-Year Book: St Louis, MO, 1993.

Gehrman RE, *Dental photography: today's camera and the growing practice.* PennWell Books: Tulsa, OK, 1982.

Hardin JF, Hellman LF, *Clark's clinical dentistry.* Harper & Row: Hagerstown, NY, 1976–98.

Holm-Pederson P, Loe H, *Geriatric dentistry: a textbook of oral gerontology.* Munksgaard: Copenhagen, 1986.

Kerr DA, Ash MM, Millard HD, *Oral diagnosis.* Mosby: St Louis, MO, 1983.

Mitchell DF, Standish SM, Fast TB, *Oral diagnosis, oral medicine.* Lea & Febiger: Philadelphia, PA, 1978.

Morris RB, *Principles of dental treatment planning.* Lea & Febiger: Philadelphia, PA, 1983.

Papas AS, Niessen LC, Chauncey HH, et al, *Geriatric dentistry: aging and oral health.* Mosby Year Book: St Louis, MO, 1991.

Rose LF, Kaye D, *Internal medicine for dentistry.* Mosby: St Louis, MO, 1990.

Tullman MJ, *Systemic disease in dental treatment.* Appleton-Century-Crofts: New York, 1982.

Wander PA, Gordon PD, *Dental photography.* British Dental Journal: London, 1987.

Chapter 6

Barsh LI, *Dental treatment planning for the adult patient.* WB Saunders: Philadelphia, PA, 1981.

Bell W, *Orofacial pains: differential diagnosis.* Mosby-Year Book Medical Publishers: St Louis, MO, 1989.

Bengel W, Veltman G, Loevy HT, Taschini P, *Differential diagnosis of diseases of the oral mucosa.* Quintessence Publishing Co: Chicago, IL, 1989.

Bricker SL, Langlais RP, Miller CS, *Oral diagnosis, oral medicine, and treatment planning.* Lea & Febiger: Philadelphia, PA, 1994.

Coleman GC, Nelson JF, *Principles of oral diagnosis.* Mosby-Year Book: St Louis, MO, 1993.

Elderton RJ (ed.) *Clinical dentistry in health and disease,* Vol 3. Heinemann Medical Books: Oxford, 1990.

Eversole LR, *Clinical outline of oral pathology, diagnosis and treatment.* Lea & Febiger: Philadelphia, PA, 1992.

Falace DA, *Emergency dental care: diagnosis and management of urgent dental problems.* Williams & Wilkins: Baltimore, MD, 1995.

Halsted CL, et al, *Physical evaluation of the dental patient.* Mosby: St Louis, MO, 1982.

Hardin JF, Hellman LF, *Clark's clinical dentistry.* Harper & Row: Hagerstown, NY, 1976–98.

Katzberg RW, Westesson, P-L, *Diagnosis of the temporomandibular joint.* WB Saunders: Philadelphia, PA, 1993.

Kerr DA, Ash MM, Millard HD, *Oral diagnosis.* Mosby: St Louis, MO, 1983.

Levine JF, Munroe CO, Desjardins RP, et al, *Current treatment in dental practice.* WB Saunders: Philadelphia, PA, 1986.

Mitchell DF, Standish SM, Fast TB, *Oral diagnosis, oral medicine.* Lea & Febiger: Philadelphia, PA, 1978.

Morris RB, *Principles of dental treatment planning.* Lea & Febiger: Philadelphia, PA, 1983.

Schafer WG, Hine MK, Levy BM, *A textbook of oral pathology.* WB Saunders, Philadelphia, PA, 1983.

Scully C (ed.) *Clinical dentistry in health and disease,* Vol 1. Heinemann Medical Books: Oxford, 1988.

Scully C (ed.) *Clinical dentistry in health and disease,* Vol 2. Heinemann Medical Books: Oxford, 1989.

Scully C, Flint SR, Porter SR, *Oral diseases: an illustrated guide to diagnosis and management of the oral mucosa, gingivae, teeth, salivary glands, bones and joints*. Martin Dunitz: London, 1996.

Wood NK, Goaz PW, *Differential Diagnosis of Oral Lesions*. Mosby-Year Book Inc: St Louis, MO, 1991.

Zegarelli EV, Kutscher AH, Hyman GA, *Diagnosis of diseases of the mouth and jaws*. Lea & Febiger: Philadelphia, PA, 1978.

Chapters 7–13

Barsh LI, *Dental treatment planning for the adult patient*. WB Saunders: Philadelphia, PA, 1981.

Elderton RJ (ed.) *Clinical dentistry in health and disease*, Vol 1. Heinemann Medical Books: Oxford, 1990.

Engelman MJ, *Clinical decision making and treatment planning in osseointegation*. Quintessence Publishing Co: Chicago, IL, 1996.

Grummons D, *Orthodontics for the TMJ–TMD patient*. Wright & Co. Publishers: Scottsdale, AZ, 1994.

Gutmann JL, Dumsha TC, Lovdahl PE, *Problem solving in endodontics: prevention, identification,* and *management*. Year-Book Medical Publishers: Chicago, IL, 1988.

Hall WB, *Decision making in periodontology*. Mosby: St Louis, MO, 1998.

Hall WB, Roberts WE, La Barre EE, *Decision making in dental treatment planning*. Mosby: St Louis, MO, 1994.

Hardin JF, Hellman LF, *Clark's clinical dentistry*. Harper & Row: Hagerstown, NY, 1976–98.

Laney WR, Gibilisco JA, *Diagnosis and treatment planning in prosthodontics*. Lea & Febiger: Philadelphia, PA, 1983. WB Saunders: Philadelphia, PA, 1986.

Levine JF, Munroe CO, Desjardins RP, et al, *Current treatment in dental practice*. WB Saunders: Philadelphia, PA, 1986.

Morris RB, *Principles of dental treatment planning*. Lea & Febiger: Philadelphia, PA, 1983.

Roblee RD, *Interdisciplinary dentofacial therapy*. Quintessence Publishing Co: Chicago, IL, 1994.

Scully C (ed.) *Clinical dentistry in health and disease*, Vol 1. Heinemann Medical Books: Oxford, 1988.

Scully C (ed.) *Clinical dentistry in health and disease*, Vol 2. Heinemann Medical Books: Oxford, 1989.

Sherman JA, *Oral radiosurgery*. Martin Dunitz Ltd: London, 1997.

Wood NK, *Treatment planning: a pragmatic approach*. Mosby: St Louis, MO, 1978.

INDEX

Note: page numbers in *italics* refer to figures